Case Based Echocardiography

Theodore P. Abraham
(Editor)

Allison Hays • Sourabh Verma • Erin Michos
(Associate Editors)

Case Based Echocardiography

Fundamentals and Clinical Practice

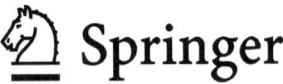 Springer

Editor
Theodore P. Abraham
Division of Cardiology
Johns Hopkins University
Baltimore, MD
USA

Associate Editors
Allison Hays
Division of Cardiology
Johns Hopkins University
Baltimore, MD
USA

Erin Michos
Division of Cardiology
Johns Hopkins University
Baltimore, MD
USA

Sourabh Verma
Division of Cardiology
Johns Hopkins University
Baltimore, MD
USA

ISBN 978-1-84996-150-9   e-ISBN 978-1-84996-151-6
DOI 10.1007/978-1-84996-151-6
Springer London Dordrecht Heidelberg New York

British Library Cataloguing in Publication Data
A catalogue record for this book is available from the British Library

Cover design: eStudioCalamar, Figueres/Berlin

Printed on acid-free paper

Springer is part of Springer Science+Business Media (www.springer.com)

Preface

Echocardiography remains the most commonly used cardiac imaging modality in clinical care despite the emergence of competing technologies such as magnetic resonance and computed tomography. Indeed, it is now considered an extension of the stethoscope and physicians without a primary interest in cardiac imaging, such as interventional cardiologists and internists, often view and interpret echocardiograms. Such an expansion of use has been further driven by the availability of smaller devices including some that are only slightly larger than a smartphone. Coincident with these developments there have been several technology advances in echocardiography such as tissue Doppler/strain and three-dimensional echocardiography. Furthermore, cardiac imaging is rapidly extending beyond the heart and laboratories are now incorporating various vascular imaging protocols as part of their clinical activity. Lastly, the emerging focus on continuing education and certification in echocardiography puts pressure on physicians to keep abreast of basic and new echocardiography.

There are several well-written echocardiography textbooks and atlases available. The intent of developing this particular handbook was: (1) to offer a succinct guide to echocardiography incorporating topics ranging from fundamental physical principles to important cardiac pathologies and novel technologies, (2) to provide this knowledge in a novel, condensed format enabling easy and quick reference to topics, (3) to enable a sonographer or echocardiographer to be able to use this handbook as a bedside guide to performance and interpretation of echocardiography and (4) to present content that would assist readers in preparing for competency tests in echocardiography, such as the echocardiography boards.

To give the reader the benefit of most meaningful and up-to-date content, this book sought to bring together a group of renowned experts in echocardiography with substantial experience in clinical echocardiography and particular expertise in various specific echocardiography technologies. The result is a compact yet highly informative handbook that provides as much if not more knowledge than most textbooks with a significantly less investment of time.

The concept and motivation to develop this book was born out of my years of interaction with cardiology trainees and sonographers in various echocardiography programs. Unbeknownst to them, I learnt as much from them about echocardiography as they did from me. More importantly, they all helped me develop into a better teacher. Although memory and space preclude me from mentioning all those who have helped in getting me here, there are several individuals who have been particularly helpful with developing this book. This list will unfairly exclude many others who have been equally instrumental in our success and I ask their pardon. My deepest gratitude goes out to Allison Hays, Sourabh Verma, and Erin Michos, our associate editors. The book would not materialize without their efforts. I am also highly appreciative of the kind and generous contributions of all the authors, despite their hectic schedules, that have resulted in the outstanding content in this book. Others who have played a major role in getting us here include Hsin-Yueh Liang, Lea Dimaano, Aurelio Pinheiro, Jacob Abraham, Sue Phillip, Heather Richardson, Ken Cresswell, Vickie Spearman, Joe Wassil, and Nancy Grap. Many thanks to Mary Corretti, Ed Kasper, and Gordon Tomaselli for allowing me the time to complete this book. I would also like to particularly thank Cate Rogers and Grant Weston from Springer who were a delight to work with despite all the delays in the production of this book. Lastly, I am deeply indebted to Roselle and Anya Marithea whose understanding and patience allowed me to do this work, and my parents Marjorie and John, my brothers Jason and Francisco, whose help and encouragement all my life and assistance in the last several months allowed me to bring this book to fruition.

Theodore P. Abraham

Contents

Contributors

Jacob Abraham, MD
Department of Medicine,
Johns Hopkins Hospital,
Baltimore, MD, USA

Theodore P. Abraham, MD
Division of Cardiology,
Johns Hopkins University,
Baltimore, MD, USA

Luis Afonso, MD
Department of Cardiology,
Detroit Medical Centre,
Wayne State University,
Detroit, MI, USA

Nausheen Akhter, MD
Division of Cardiology,
The Feinberg School of Medicine,
Chicago, IL, USA

Naser M. Ammash, MD
Department of Internal Medicine,
Mayo Clinic, Rochester, MN, USA

Khaled Bachour, MD
Internal Medicine, Division of Cardiology,
University of Pittsburgh,
Farrell, PA, USA

Jeroen J. Bax, MD, PhD
Department of Cardiology,
Leiden University Medical Center,
Leiden, The Netherlands

Gabe B. Bleeker, MD, PhD
Department of Cardiology,
Leiden University Medical Center,
Leiden, The Netherlands

Mary C. Corretti, MD, FACC, FAHA
Division of Cardiology,
Johns Hopkins University,
Baltimore, MD, USA

Veronica Lea J. Dimaano, MD
Division of Cardiology,
Johns Hopkins University School
of Medicine, Baltimore, MD, USA

Hisham Dokainish, MD
Department of Cardiology,
Baylor College of Medicine,
6620 Main Street-11A.08, 77030,
Houston, TX, USA

Allison G. Hays, MD
Division of Cardiology,
Johns Hopkins University,
Baltimore, MD, USA

Eduard R. Holman, MD, PhD
Department of Cardiology,
Leiden University Medical Center,
Leiden, The Netherlands

Kenneth D. Horton, RCS, RDCS, FASE
Echo/Vascular Laboratory,
Intermountain Medical Center,
Murray, UT, USA

Julie A. Humphries, MBBS, BHMS(Ed) (Hons)
Department of Cardiology,
Heart Care Partners,
Greenslopes, Queensland,
Australia

Sebastian Kelle, MD
Department of Cardiology,
German Heart Institute Berlin,
Berlin, Germany

Anupama Kottam, MD
Department of Cardiology,
Detroit Medical Centre,
Wayne State University,
Detroit, MI, USA

Bijoy K. Khandheria, MD
Division of Cardiovascular Diseases,
Mayo Clinic, Rochester, MN, USA

Christopher J. Kramer, BA, RDCS
Advanced Hemodynamic
and Cardiovascular Laboratory,
Aurora Medical Group,
Milwaukee, WI, USA

Roberto M. Lang, MD
Department of Medicine,
University of Chicago Medical Center,
Chicago, IL, USA

Hsin-Yueh Liang, MD
Division of Cardiology,
Department of Medicine,
China Medical University Hospital,
Taichung, Taiwan

Shizhen Liu, MD, PhD
Department of Cardiovascular
Medicine, The Ohio State University
Medical Center, Columbus, OH, USA

Anil Mathew, MD
Detroit Medical Centre,
Wayne State University,
Detroit, MI, USA

Issam A. Mikati, MD
Department of Medicine,
Northwestern University Feinberg School
of Medicine, Chicago, IL, USA

Farouk Mookadam, MBChB, FRCPC, FACC
Department of Cardiology,
Mayo College of Medicine,
Scottsdale, AZ, USA

Sherif E. Moustafa, MBBCh, MSc, FASE, MRCP
Department of Cardiovascular Diseases,
Mayo Clinic Arizona,
Scottsdale, AZ, USA

Christian D. Nagy, MD
Pediatric Cardiology/Adult Cardiology,
Johns Hopkins University Medical Center,
Baltimore, MD, USA

Alina Nicoara, MD
Department of Anesthesiology,
Yale University School of Medicine,
West Haven, CT, USA

Vuyisile T. Nkomo, MD, PhD
Division of Cardiovascular Diseases
and Internal Medicine,
Mayo Clinic, Rochester, MN, USA

Aurelio C. Pinheiro, MD, PhD
Department of Cardiology,
Johns Hopkins University,
Baltimore, MD, USA

Elizabeth V. Ratchford, MD
Department of Medicine, Division of
Cardiology, Johns Hopkins University
School of Medicine,
Baltimore, MD, USA

Richard E. Ringel, MD
Pediatric Cardiology,
Johns Hopkins University,
Baltimore, MD, USA

Partho P. Sengupta, MD
Cardiovascular Division,
University of California,
Irvine, USA

Mengistu Simegn, MD
Detroit Medical Centre,
Wayne State University,
Detroit, MI, USA

Lissa Sugeng, MD, MPH
Section of Cardiology, Department of
Medicine, Non-Invasive
Cardiovascular Imaging Laboratory,
University of Chicago Medical Center,
Chicago, IL, USA

**Madhav Swaminathan,
MD, FASE, FAHA**
Division of Cardiothoracic
Anesthesiology and Critical Care
Medicine, Duke University,
Durham, CA, USA

Yasuhiko Takemoto, MD, PhD
Department of Internal Medicine
and Cardiology, Osaka City University
School of Medicine, Osaka, Japan

W. Reid Thompson, MD
Pediatric Cardiology,
Johns Hopkins University School
of Medicine, Baltimore, MD, USA

Nico R. Van de Veire, MD, PhD
Department of Cardiology,
Leiden University Medical Center,
Leiden, The Netherlands

Mani A. Vannan, MBBS, FACC
Department of Cardiovascular Medicine,
The Ohio State University Medical Center,
Columbus, OH, USA

Tahlil A. Warsame, BS, RDCS, FASE
Cardiovascular Ultrasound Imaging
and Hemodynamic Laboratory,
Mayo Clinic Arizona, Phoenix, AZ, USA

Lynn Weinert, BS
University of Chicago Medical Center,
Chicago, IL, USA

Ilan S. Wittstein, MD
Department of Medicine,
Johns Hopkins University School
of Medicine, Baltimore, MD, USA

Minoru Yoshiyama, MD, PhD
Department of Internal Medicine
and Cardiology, Osaka City University
School of Medicine, Osaka, Japan

Physics and Artifacts

Kenneth D. Horton

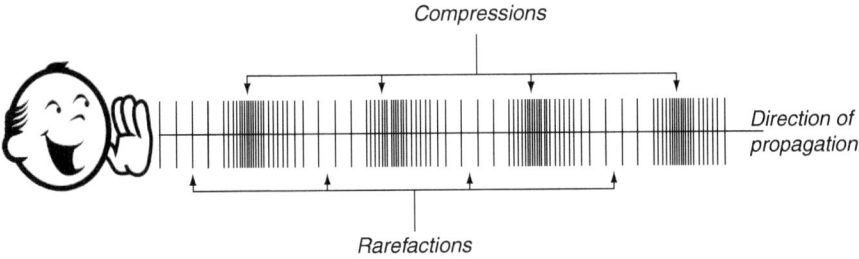

Fig. 1.1 Definition of sound and ultrasound. Sound is a mechanical vibration that consists of *compressions* and *rarefactions*. Sound waves *propagate* (travel) through various mediums by interactions between the particles that comprise the medium. Therefore, sound cannot travel through a vacuum. The range of hearing in the human ear is 20–20,000 Hz. Sound above 20,000 Hz is called *ultrasound*

K.D. Horton
Echo/Vascular Laboratory, Intermountain Medical Center,
Murray, UT, USA
e-mail: kd.horton@comcast.net

T.P. Abraham (ed.), *Case Based Echocardiography*,
DOI: 10.1007/978-1-84996-151-6_1, © Springer-Verlag London Limited 2011

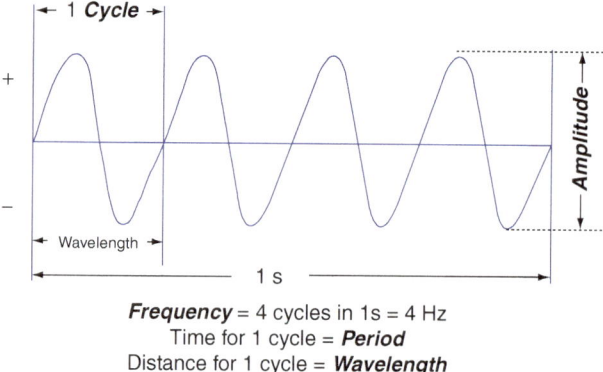

Frequency = 4 cycles in 1s = 4 Hz
Time for 1 cycle = Period
Distance for 1 cycle = Wavelength

Fig. 1.2 Wave terminology. The combination of one compression and one rarefaction is called one *cycle*. The number of cycles completed in 1 s is called the *frequency*. The frequency is measured in units of Hertz or, for ultrasound, megahertz (one million cycles/s). The distance occupied by one cycle is called the *wavelength* and the amount of time occupied by one cycle is the *period*. The strength of the ultrasound signal is the intensity. The higher the *amplitude*, the greater the intensity of the ultrasound signal

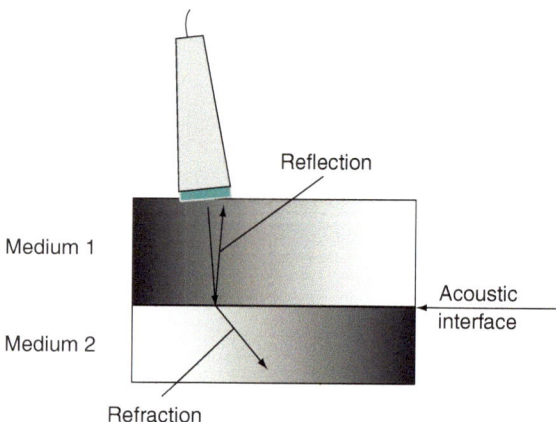

Fig. 1.3 Interactions with tissue. As a sound wave strikes, a difference in the medium (*acoustic interface*) it is traveling through, some of the sound is reflected back to the transducer (*reflection*) and some continues to travel through the next medium (*refraction*). As the sound wave travels through a medium, it loses its strength or intensity. This is called attenuation

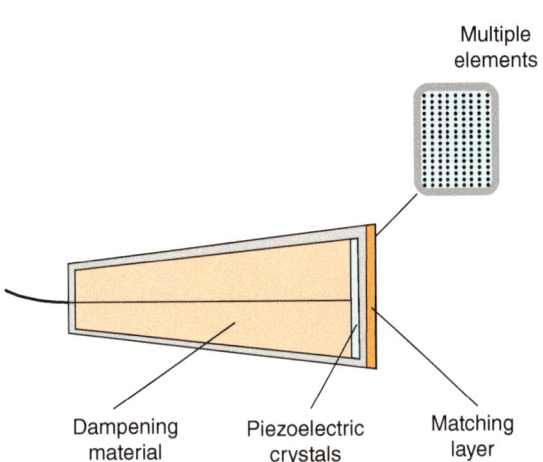

Fig. 1.4 Transducers. A transducer is a device that changes types of energy. An ultrasound transducer has multiple *piezioelectric crystals* (elements) that can change electrical energy to mechanical energy – or vice versa. The crystal is surrounded by a *dampening material* that prevents "ringing" when the crystal is activated. The *matching layer* has an acoustic impendence between that of the transducer and skin and facilitates the transmission of sound into the body

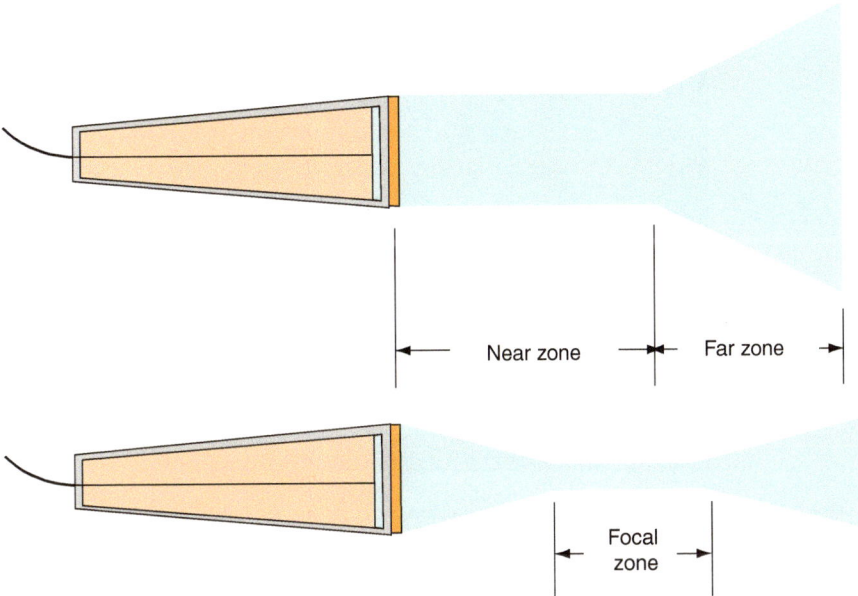

Fig. 1.5 Beam characteristics. In an *unfocused* transducer, sound leaves the transducer, travels parallel for a period of time and then begins to diverge. The area prior to the divergence is called the *near zone* and the area after the divergence is called the *far zone*. Using electronic timing or an acoustic lens, the beam can be *focused*. The resolution is highest in the area of the *focal zone*. Ultrasound systems have the ability to move the focal zone along the beam to improve the resolution in areas of interest

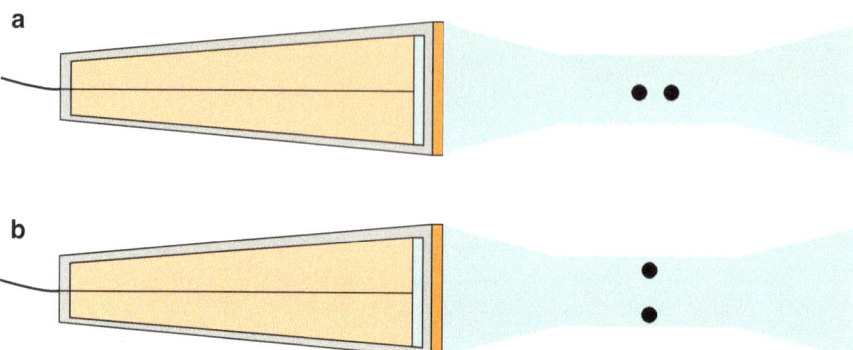

Fig. 1.6 Resolution. Resolution is the ability to see two different objects in the imaging field as two different objects and is measured in unit of distance (millimeters). There are multiple types of resolution in ultrasound. The two most common are (**a**) *longitudinal resolution* – resolution along the axis parallel to the direction of the sound propagation and (**b**) *axial resolution* – resolution on the axis perpendicular to the direction of the sound propagation

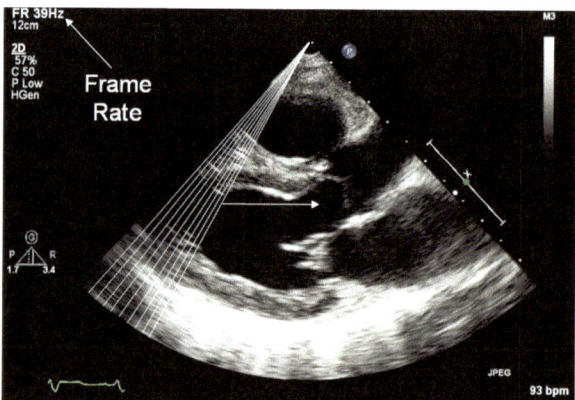

Fig. 1.7 Frame rate. An ultrasound image is created one scan line at a time. When the scan lines are processed across the field of view (sector) one frame is created. The number of frame that is created in 1 s is called the frame rate and is measured in Hertz. The temporal resolution of a system is determined by the frame rate. The higher the frame rate, the better the temporal resolution. In 2D echocardiography, you should attempt to image at the highest frame rate possible

Fig. 1.8 M-mode echocardiography. M-mode (motion-mode) echocardiography is a graphical depiction of the ultrasound signal along a single scan line. The temporal resolution of an M-mode tracing is superior to all other echocardiographic modes because the image is only processing the signal from a single scan line and can be updated thousands of times per second

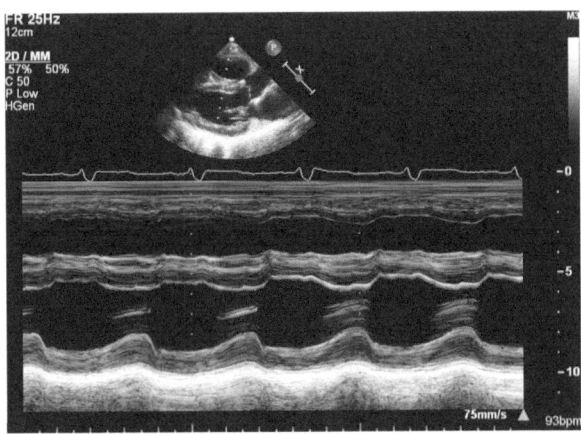

Fig. 1.9 2D Echocardiography. 2D echocardiography is a 2D depiction of the heart. It is usually acquired as a moving picture allowing for assessment of the heart throughout systole and diastole. 2D images are either captured on video tape or as digital loops

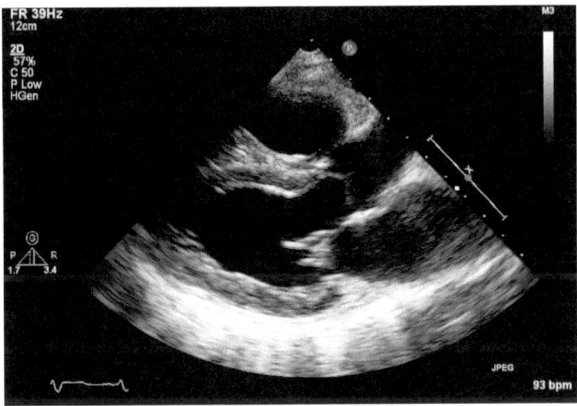

Fig. 1.10 Doppler echocardiography. As its name implies, Doppler images are created using the Doppler effect. Spectral Doppler tracings can be created using either continuous wave (CW) Doppler or pulsed wave (PW) Doppler. CW and PW Doppler each have distinct advantages and disadvantages that determine when each is used. (**a**) PW Doppler has the advantage of range resolution, or being able to measure flow of a specific point. Its main disadvantage is there is a limit to how high of a velocity it can measure (Nyquist limit). (**b**) CW Doppler has an unlimited Nyquist limit and therefore can measure very high velocities. Its disadvantage, however, is it does not have range resolution and measures all flows along the cursor

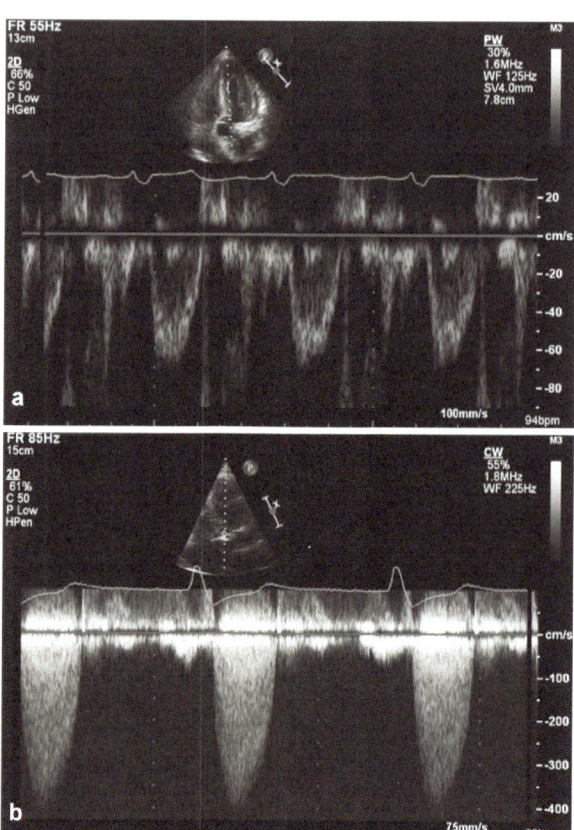

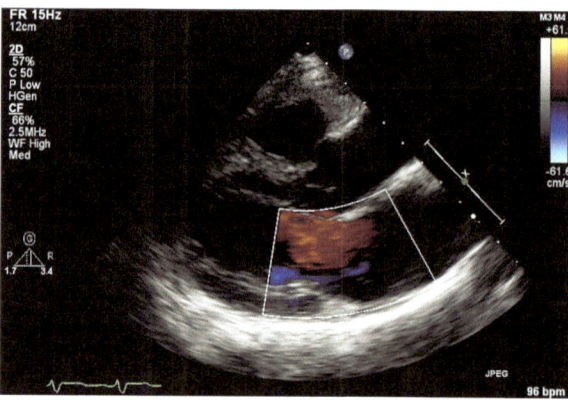

Fig. 1.11 Color flow imaging. Color flow imaging is used to detect the direction and velocity of blood flow. Flow is measured at thousands of points within the color flow sector. By convention, flow toward the transducer is colored *red-yellow* and flow away from the transducer is colored *blue-white*. Low flow velocities begin with darker shades and the shade increases as flow velocity increases

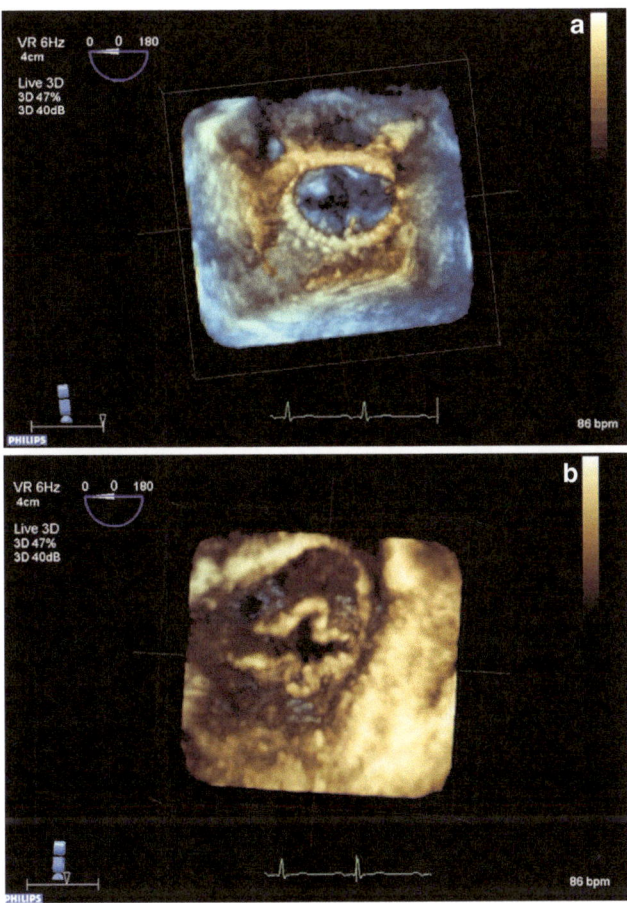

Fig. 1.12 3D echocardiography. 3D images are obtained using a pyramidal volume of pixels (voxels). Once the image is obtained, it can be rotated and cropped to better visualize any structure within the image. In this example, a mitral annular ring was placed. (**a**) Assessment of the annular ring from the LA perspective (looking down into the LV) and (**b**) assessment from the LV perspective (looking up into the atrium). Both images were obtained in the same acquisition

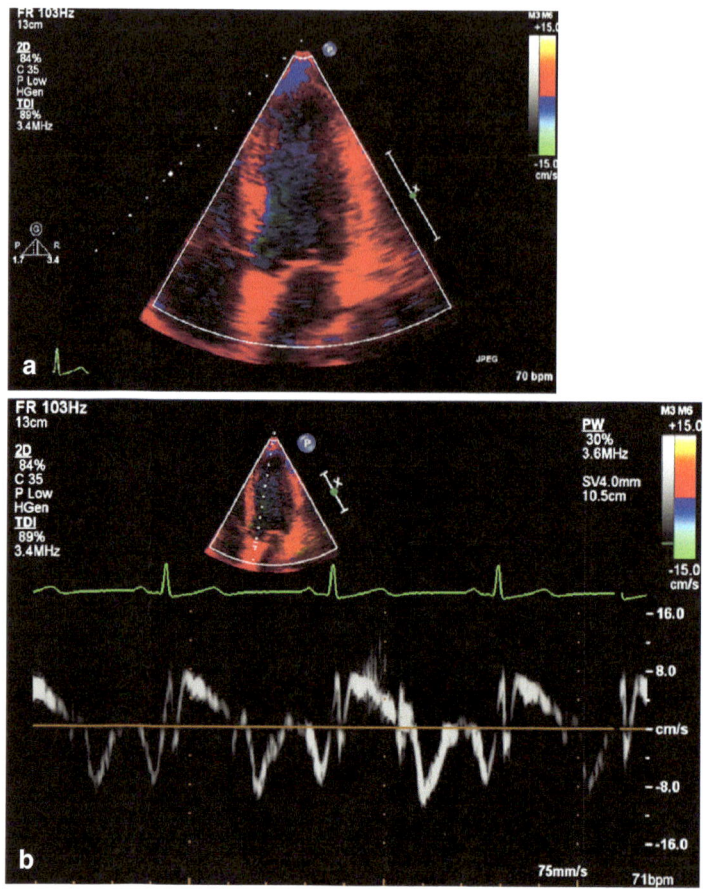

Fig. 1.13 Tissue Doppler Imaging (TDI). Tissue Doppler imaging is a technology that is used to assess the diastolic and systolic velocities of the heart. (**a**) TDI measures the direction and velocity of the myocardium (instead of blood flow) and color encodes the signal from the myocardium as red or blue depending on the direction of motion. (**b**) Using special filters, pulsed wave Doppler is used to measure the velocities during (1) systole, (2) early diastole, and (3) late diastole

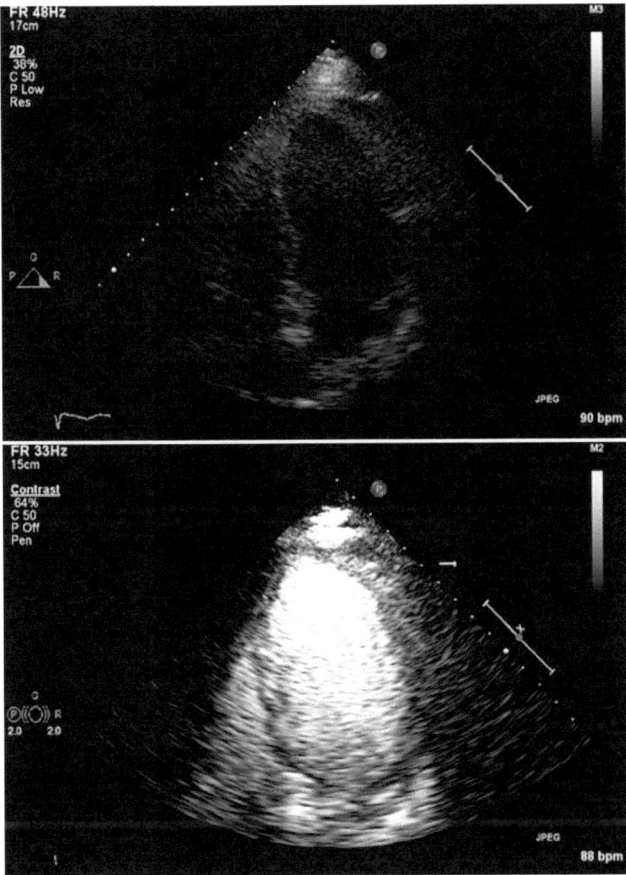

Fig. 1.14 Imaging artifacts – suboptimal images. The quality of the ultrasound image varies greatly from person to person. Even with today's excellent ultrasound systems, there are patients in whom diagnostic imaging is not possible. Assessment of the heart from multiple windows and image optimization using the ultrasound system controls do not always help. In most cases, the use of commercial contrast media (Definity or Optison) can make an undiagnostic ultrasound study diagnostic

Fig. 1.15 Imaging artifacts – shadowing. The amount of ultrasound that is returned to the transducer for processing is proportional to the difference in the media forming an acoustic interface. The stronger the acoustic interface, the more of the signal that returns to the transducer leaving little or none to continue to travel forward. It is the areas beyond that acoustic interface where shadowing occurs. Shadowing is overcome by imaging all areas in multiple windows and views

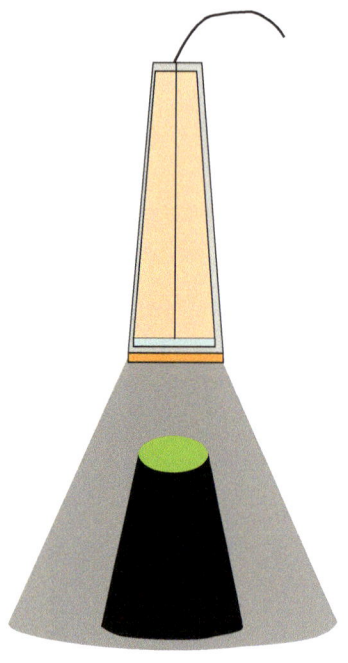

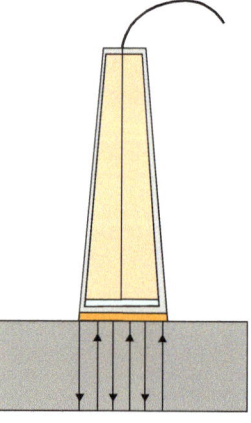

Fig. 1.16 Imaging artifacts – reverberation. Reverberation artifact occurs when an ultrasound signal is bounced back and forth between two acoustic interfaces before returning to the transducer. This results erroneously displayed objects in the imaging sector

——————————— Real object
···························· Reverberation artifact
···························· Reverberation artifact

Fig. 1.17 Imaging artifacts – side lobes. Although the majority of the ultrasound signal is processed from the center of the ultrasound beam, there are small lobes on each side of the signal that also processes returning signals. These are called side lobes. The ultrasound system may receive signals from structures within the side lobes and erroneously display them in the center of the imaging sector

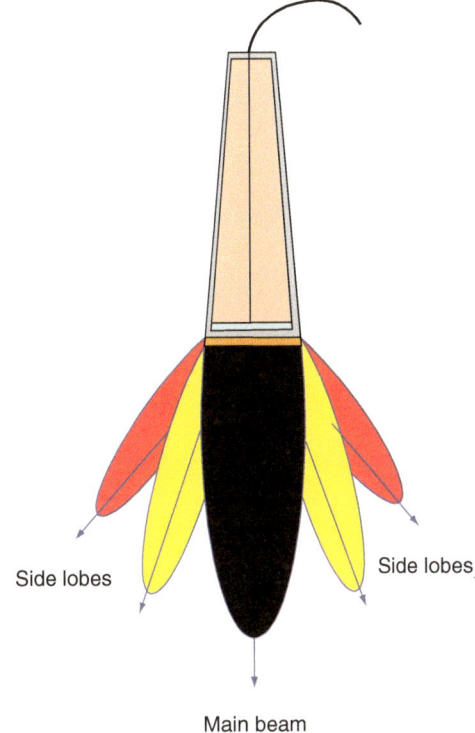

Side lobes   Side lobes

Main beam

Fig. 1.18 Imaging artifacts – range ambiguity. Ultrasound images are processed under the assumption that the sound wave is traveling directly to a structure and then being reflected directly back to the transducer. It is also assumed that sound travels at a constant 1,540 m/s. If either of these assumptions is violated, structures will be displayed at the incorrect depth within the imaging sector. In the pictured example, the depth of the reflected interface would be too deep because the signal was delayed in returning to the transducer

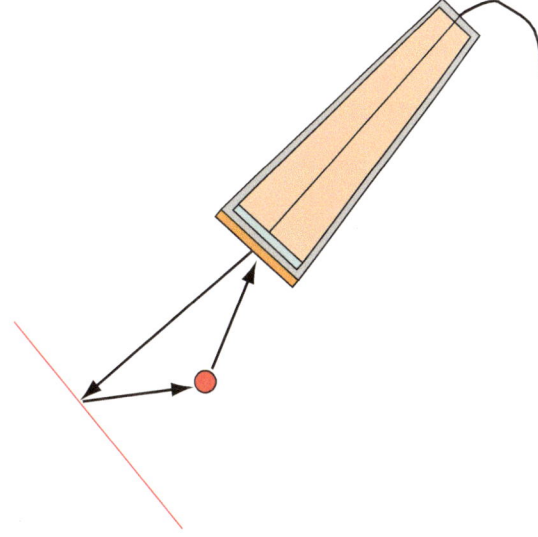

Basic Ultrasound Views

Kenneth D. Horton

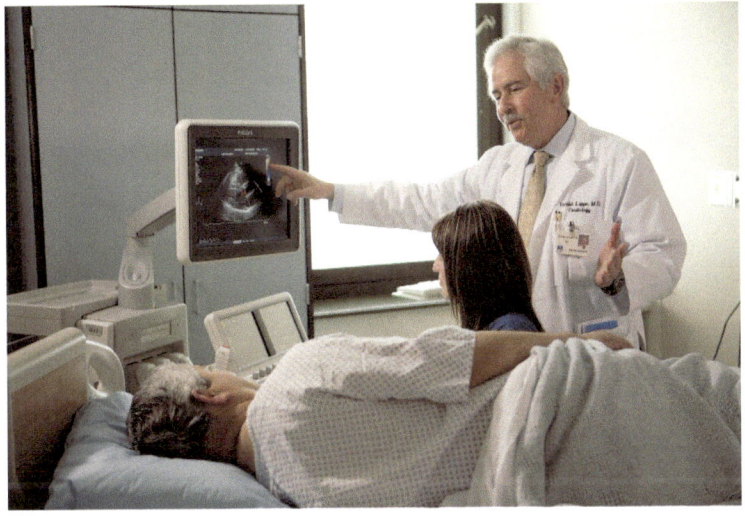

K.D. Horton
Echo/Vascular Laboratory, Intermountain Medical Center,
Murray, UT, USA
e-mail: kd.horton@comcast.net

T.P. Abraham (ed.), *Case Based Echocardiography*,
DOI: 10.1007/978-1-84996-151-6_2, © Springer-Verlag London Limited 2011

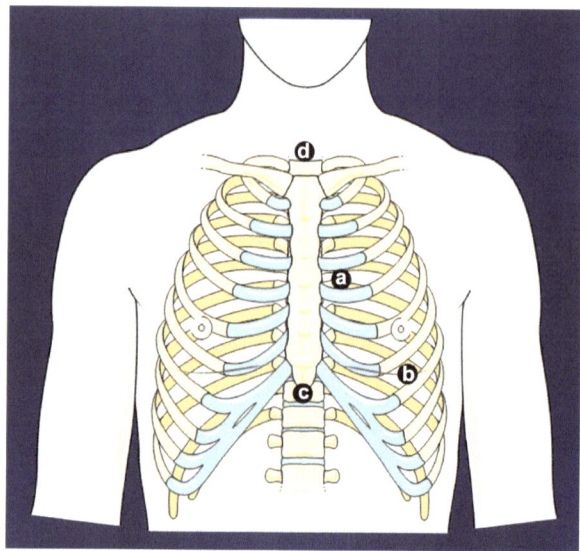

Fig. 2.1 Echocardiographic windows. When performing an echocardiogram, the transducer is placed in multiple areas of the chest. These areas are commonly referred to as "windows." The most common echo windows are: (**a**) the left parasternal window, (**b**) the apical window, (**c**) the subcostal window, and (**d**) the suprasternal notch. In certain circumstances, imaging from nonstandard windows is required. Some of the nonstandard windows include the right parasternal window and the mid-clavicular window. In some cases, imaging may need to be performed from any area of the chest from where an image can be obtained (Adapted from Servier Medical Art, www. servier.com, with permission)

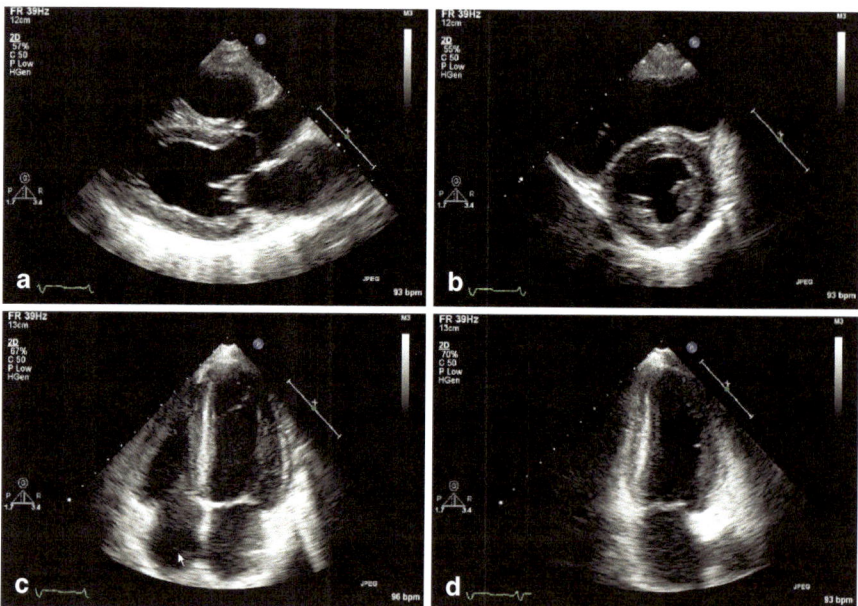

Fig. 2.2 Echocardiographic views. From each window, the transducer is manipulated to obtain multiple views of the heart. The different views are obtained by rotating and/or tilting the transducer without actually moving it to a new window

Fig. 2.3 The parasternal window. The parasternal long axis (PLAX) view is obtained by placing the transducer in the three to four left intercostal spaces close to the sternum with the bean oriented toward the patient's right shoulder. This orientation slices through the heart on a long axis from base to apex (Adapted from Servier Medical Art, www. servier.com, with permission)

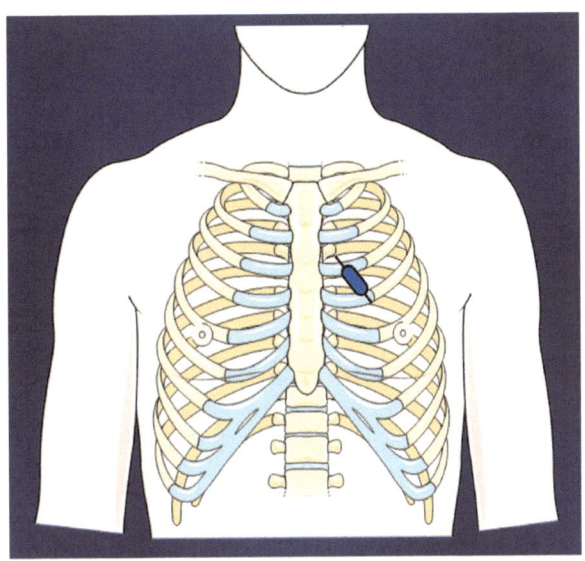

Fig. 2.4 The parasternal window. The parasternal long axis (PLAX) view is obtained by placing the transducer in the third to fourth left intercostal space close to the sternum with the bean oriented toward the patient's right shoulder. This orientation slices through the heart on a long axis from base to apex

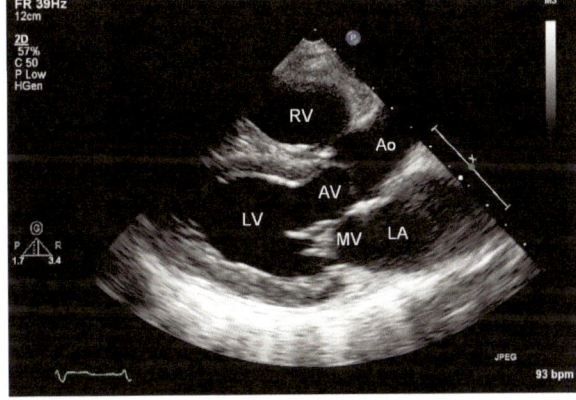

Fig. 2.5 Parasternal long axis – color flow image. Color flow Doppler imaging is used to assess the valves for regurgitation. Pictured here is a systolic still frame demonstrating regurgitation of blood flow back through the mitral valve into the left atrium

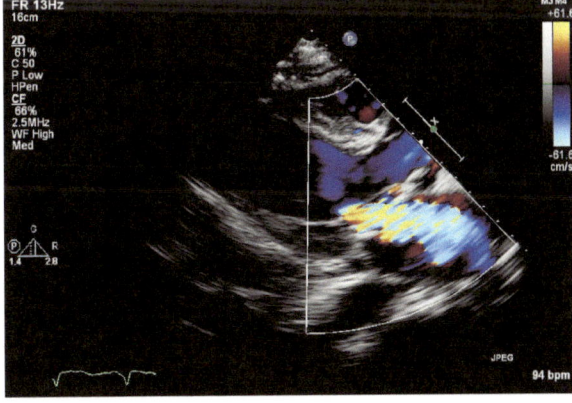

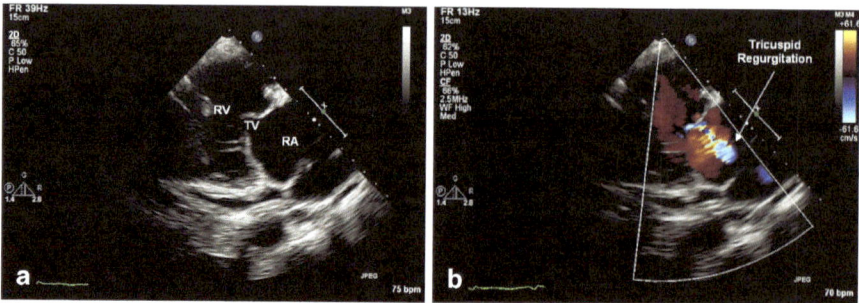

Fig. 2.6 Right ventricular inflow (RVIF) view. The RVIF view is obtained by tilting the transducer toward the left shoulder so the ultrasound beam moves anterior in the chest slicing through the right heart. (**a**) This view is used to assess the right ventricle, tricuspid valve, and right atrium. (**b**) Color flow and spectral Doppler are used to assess the valve for tricuspid regurgitation

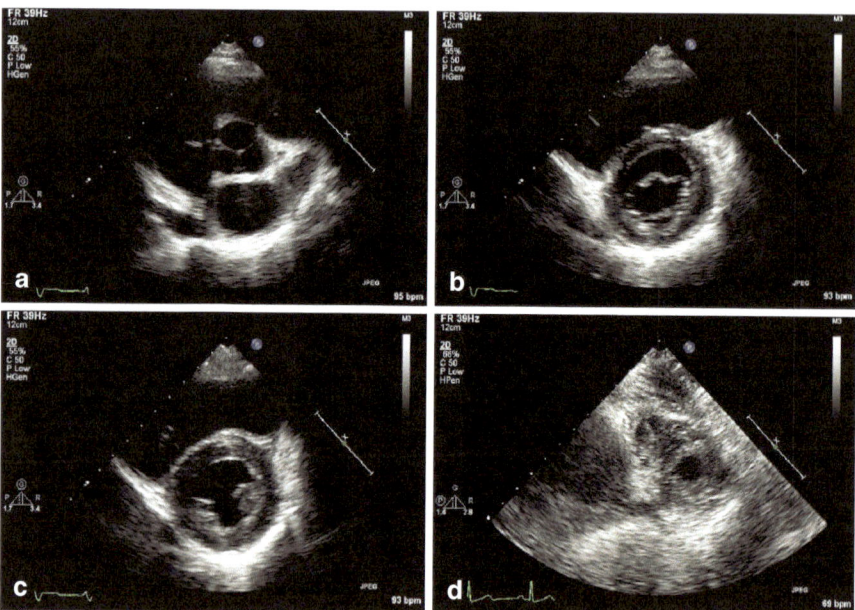

Fig. 2.7 Parasternal short axis (PSAX) view. The PSAX view is obtained by remaining in the parasternal window and rotating the transducer clockwise approximately 90°. Sweeping the transducer from base to apex results in: (**a**) the basal level view, (**b**) the mitral level view, (**c**) the papillary level view, and (**d**) the apical level view. In the basal and mitral level view, color flow Doppler can be used to assess the valves for regurgitation

Fig. 2.8 Apical views. The apical window is usually found in the left lateral portion of the chest at the apex of the heart. This can sometimes be located by placing your hand lightly in the area of the apex and feeling for the point of maximal intensity (PMI). The PMI will serve as your starting point; however, small adjustments will need to be made to the transducer location to maximally optimize your image (Adapted from Servier Medical Art, www.servier. com, with permission)

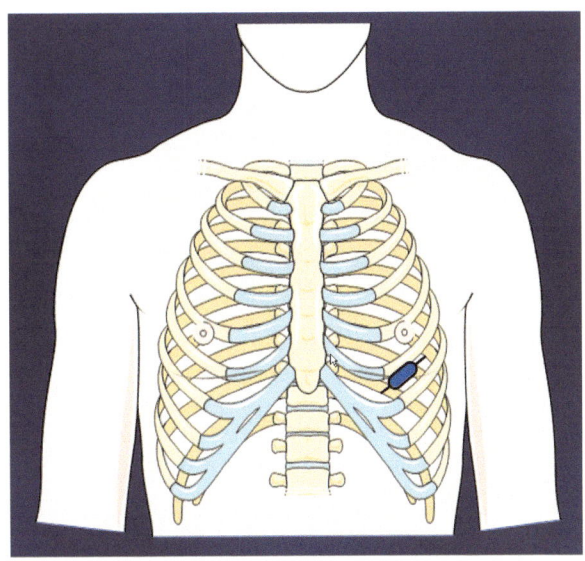

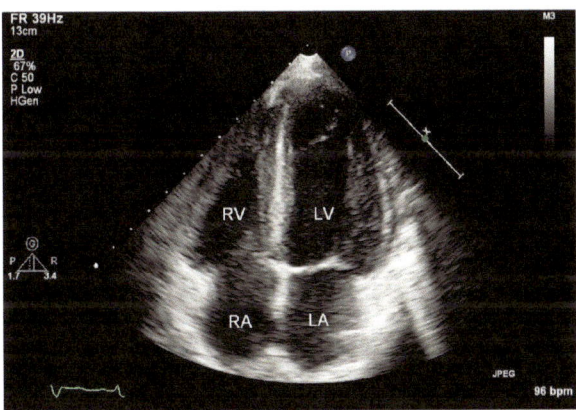

Fig. 2.9 Apical 4 Chamber (4C) view. All four cardiac chambers are visualized in the 4C view along with the mitral and tricuspid valves. Ventricular and atrial size can be assessed using 2D echo. Color flow and spectral Doppler can be used to assess for valvular regurgitation and stenosis. Left ventricular diastolic function can be assessed using pulsed wave Doppler of the mitral valve and pulmonary veins. In this view, the right ventricular freewall, interventricular septum, and left lateral wall can be assessed for systolic motion

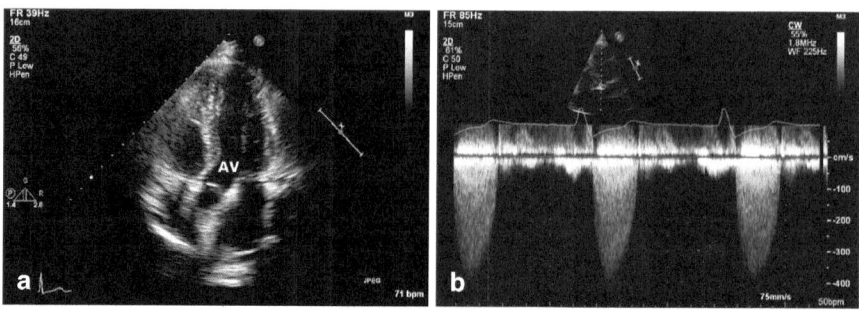

Fig. 2.10 Apical 5 Chamber (5C) view. (**a**) The 5C view is obtained by tilting the transducer slightly so the beam moves anterior in the chest slicing through the left ventricular outflow track (LVOT) and aortic valve. (**b**) Utilizing spectral Doppler, the outflow velocity can be measured. In this example, the high-velocity flow pattern indicates aortic stenosis. The aortic valve area can be calculated by integrating data from the 2D images and Doppler tracings

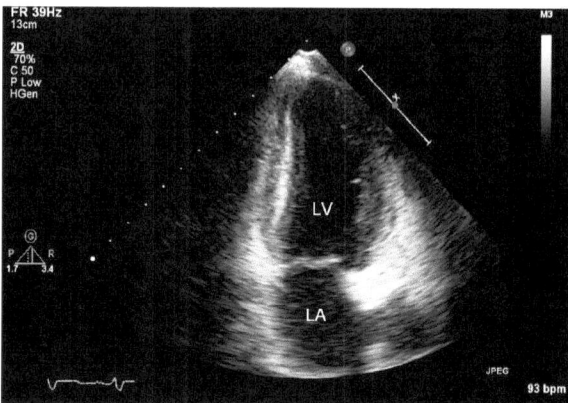

Fig. 2.11 Apical 2 Chamber (2C) view. The 2C view is obtained by starting at the 4C view and rotating the transducer clockwise approximately 90°. In the 2C view, the left ventricle, mitral valve, and left atrium can be seen. The inferior and anterior walls of the left ventricle can be assessed for systolic function. Using color flow and spectral Doppler, the mitral valve can be assessed for regurgitation and stenosis

Fig. 2.12 Apical 3 Chamber (3C) or long axis view. The apical 3C view is also known as the apical long axis view. Structures seen in the 3C view are the same as the parasternal long axis view. The 3C view is utilized to assess chamber size and function as well as aortic and mitral valve function

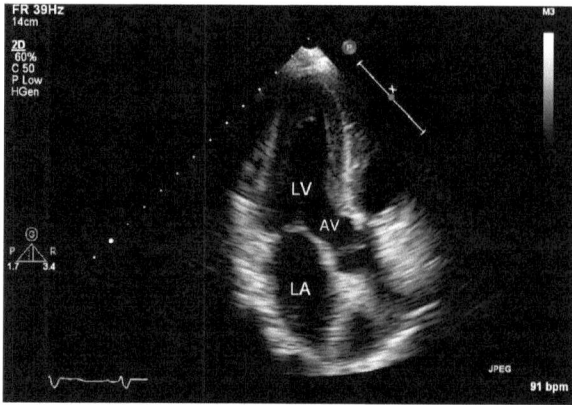

Fig. 2.13 The subcostal window. Subcostal views are obtained by positioning the patient flat on their back and placing the transducer just below the xiphoid process. Asking the patient to bend their knees may help relax the stomach muscles. Having the patient take a deep breath often moves the lungs out of the way and results in better images (Adapted from Servier Medical Art, www.servier.com, with permission)

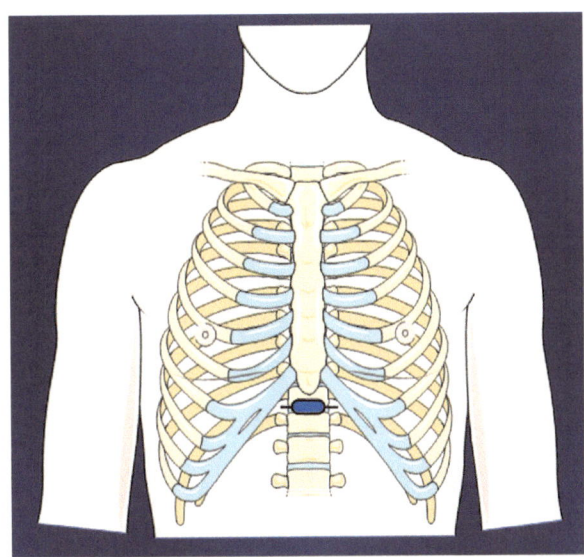

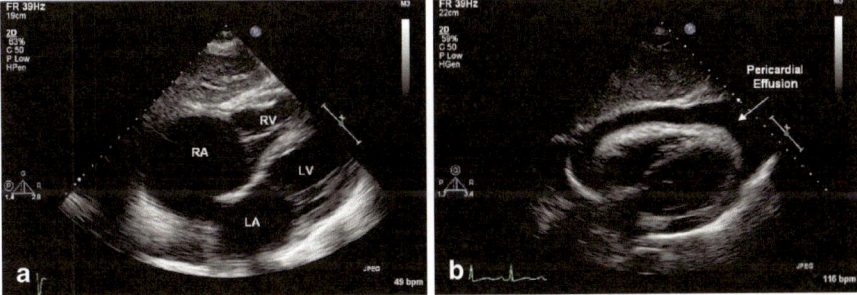

Fig. 2.14 Subcostal 4 Chamber view. (**a**) The subcostal 4C view can be used to assess chamber size and function. Color flow and spectral Doppler imaging can be used to assess valvular function. This is also a good view for assessing for atrial or ventricular septal defects. (**b**) The subcostal view is a good view for assessing the presence and size of a pericardial effusion

Fig. 2.15 Inferior Vena Cava (IVC) view. Beginning in the subcostal 4C view and rotating the transducer counterclockwise 90° and angling toward the liver, the IVC can be seen in long axis. The IVC can be assessed for diameter and collapsibility during respiration. The size and collapsibility of the IVC are used to estimate right atrial pressure

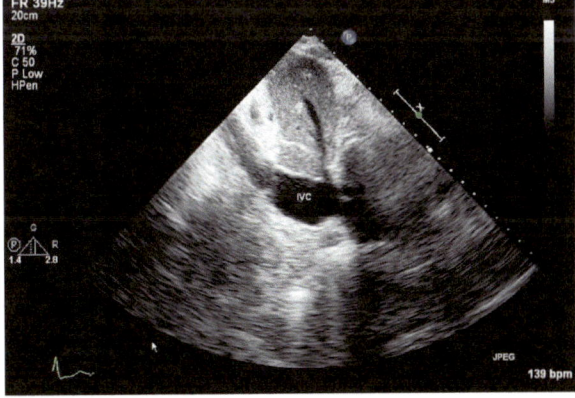

Fig. 2.16 Suprasternal window. The suprasternal window is obtained by placing the transducer in the "notch" at the top of the sternum (the manubrium). This window is used for 2D imaging and also for assessment of aortic flows with a dedicated continuous wave Doppler transducer (Pedoff probe) (Adapted from Servier Medical Art, www.servier.com, with permission)

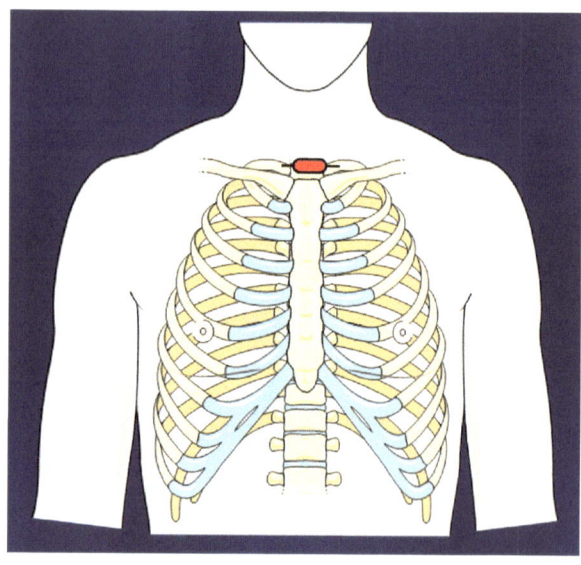

Fig. 2.17 Suprasternal window. The suprasternal 2D image is used to assess the ascending, transverse, and descending aorta and its branches. The inominate, left carotid, and left subclavian arteries can be seen branching off the aorta. The right pulmonary artery can also be seen in short axis

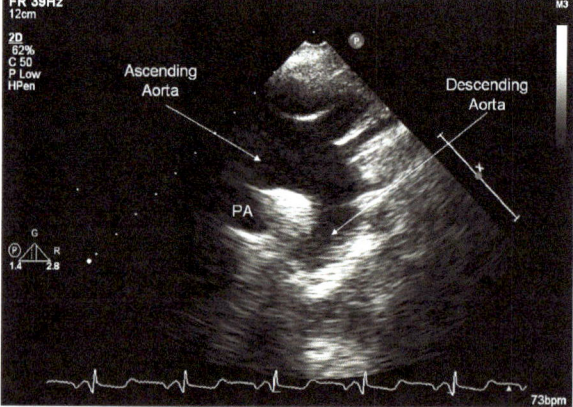

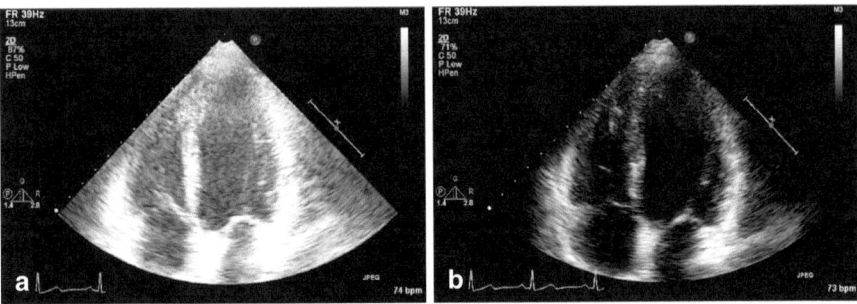

Fig. 2.18 Image optimization – overall gain. The gain controls the brightness of your image. Optimizing the gain will result in better detection of structures and endocardial borders. (**a**) Using excessive gain will result in images that are too bright and may make normal structures appearing calcified. (**b**) Gains should be set at a point that a balance between image brightness and darkness are reached

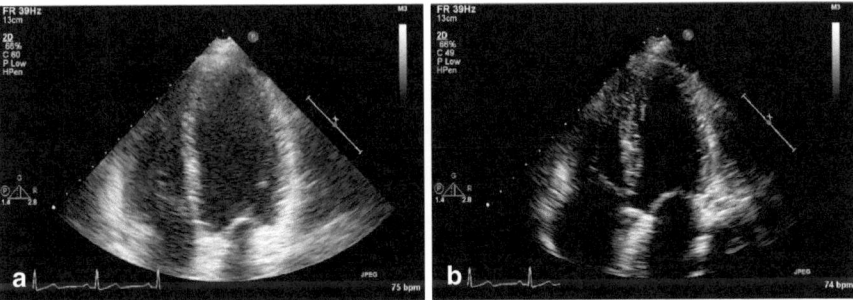

Fig. 2.19 Image optimization – compression or dynamic range. Compression or dynamic range are controls that affect the number of shades of gray that are displayed in the image. (**a**) If these are set too high, the image appears washed out and it may be difficult to visualize endocardial borders. (**b**) The compression or dynamic range should be set so the blood pool is dark and the tissue is bright. This will result in better endocardial border definition

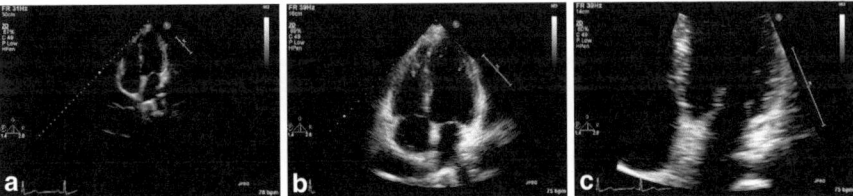

Fig. 2.20 Image optimization – depth and zoom controls. The image depth and zoom controls can be used to optimize the area of interest. In these examples (**a**) the depth is set too deep resulting in a small image that will be difficult to assess, (**b**) the depth is set at the correct level so that all structures can be seen in the apical 4C view, and (**c**) the use of the "zoom" control for better assessment of the mitral valve

Quantification of Left Ventricular Size and Wall Thickness

3

Khaled Bachour and Luis Afonso

Abbreviations

2C	2 chamber
4C	4 chamber
LVIDd	Left ventricular inner dimension during diastole
LVIDs	Left ventricular inner dimension during systole
PWT	Posterior wall thickness
RWMA	Regional wall motion abnormalities
SWT	Septal wall thickness

L. Afonso (✉)
Department of Cardiology, Detroit Medical Centre, Wayne State University, Detroit, MI, USA
e-mail: lafonso@med.wayne.edu

T.P. Abraham (ed.), *Case Based Echocardiography*,
DOI: 10.1007/978-1-84996-151-6_3, © Springer-Verlag London Limited 2011

3.1
LV Wall Thickness and Dimensions

3.1.1
Methods

- Direct 2D
- 2D-guided M-mode (Table 3.1)

Table 3.1 Pros and cons of M-mode and direct 2D methods for assessment of LVIDd, LVIDs, PWT, and SWT

	M-Mode	Direct 2D
Advantages	• Excellent temporal resolution	• Preferred with CAD and asymmetrical LV
	• Higher spatial resolution: separates other structures (trabeculae, false tendons) from LV walls	• Can be used even in oblique parasternal images
Disadvantages	• Cursor has to be perpendicular to the long axis of the LV	• Lower spatial resolution: may not be able to separate other structures (trabeculae, false tendons) from LV walls
	• Assume symmetry of LV	• Lower temporal resolution

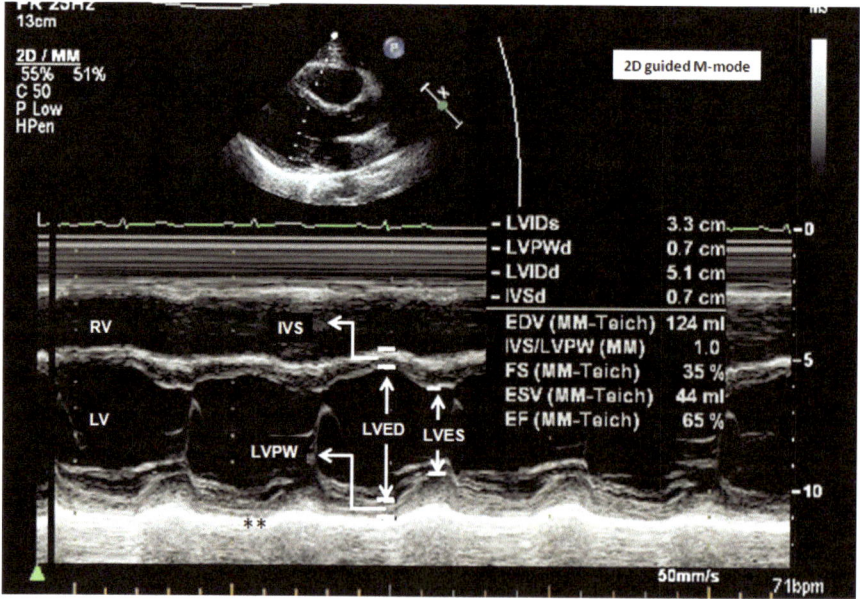

Fig. 3.1 2D guided-linear M-mode dimensions of the left ventricle obtained in end diastole (LVED) and end systole (LVES), along with septal (IVS) and posterior wall (LVPW) thickness, both measured in end-diastole.** Bright posterior echoes represent parietal pericardium

3.1.2
Technical Points

- Always from parasternal long axis view (see Fig 3.1)
- Level: mitral leaflet tips
- Measurement PWT and SWT, LVIDd and LVIDs is done along the LV minor axis, perpendicular to the long axis of the LV
- LVIDd, PWT, and SWT are measured during end diastole when both mitral and aortic valves are closed (direct 2D), or at the end of PR segment (M-mode)
- LVIDs is measured at end systole when both aortic and mitral valves are closed (direct 2D) or at the end of T wave (M-mode)
- LVID is edged by the blood-endocardium interface edge of the septal and posterior wall, i.e., leading edge of the septum to the trailing edge of the posterior wall

3.1.3
Normal Values

- See Table 3.4

3.2
Volumetric Assessment of LV

3.2.1
Methods

- Biplane method of disks (modified Simpson's)
- Unipolar method of disks
- Area-length method
- 3D Volumetric methods: Real-time 3D echocardiography

3.2.2
Biplane Method of Disks

- Using apical 4C and 2C views (Figure 3.2)
- Long axis of LV is longest dimension extending from the apex to the center of mitral annulas
- LV cavity is divided into 20 disks perpendicular to the major long axis of the LV
- Each disk has a height (1/20 of L), and two dimensions (long and short from the two views)
- LV volume is calculated from the summation of volumes of ellipsoid disks along the long axis of LV (Fig. 3.2)

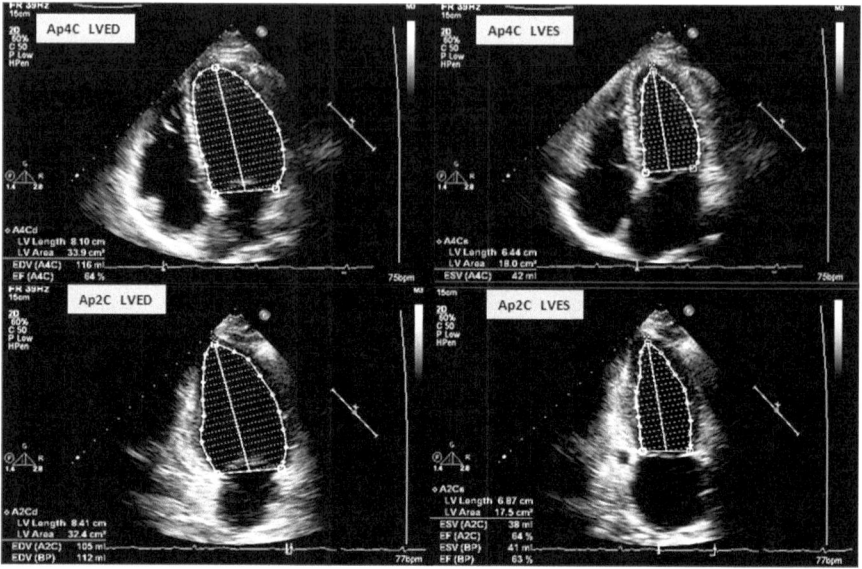

Fig. 3.2 2D end diastolic and end systolic volumes calculated from the apical 4C (Ap4C) and apical 2C (Ap2C) views in end diastole (LVED) and end systole (LVES), respectively, using the biplane method of disks (modified Simpson's rule). The LV cavity endocardium is traced from the mitral annular plane to the apex of the LV cavity and includes the papillary muscles

3.2.3
Uniplane Method of Disks

- Variation of biplane method when two orthogonal apical views are not available
- Utilizes one apical view
- Assumes circular shape of the disks

3.2.4
Length-Area Method

- Assumes a bullet shaped LV
- The long axis of the LV is defined as the longest dimension extending from the apex to the center of the mitral annulus in 4C view.
- The mid-LV cross-sectional area is measured by planimetry at the level of papillary muscles in the parasternal short axis view.
- Volume $= 5 \times$ area $\times$ length$/6$ (Table 3.2)

3.2.5
3D Volumetric methods: Real-time 3D echocardiography

- Semiautomatic border detection of endocardial border (Fig 3.3)
- Unlike 2D techniques, does not rely on geometric assumptions

Table 3.2 Pros and cons of the three methods of evaluation of the LV volumes

	Biplane method of disks	Uniplane method of disks	Area-length method
Advantages	• Recommended whenever possible • Most accurate in ventricles with RWMA	• Require optimal endocardial definition in only one apical view	• Can be used in the absence of optimal endocardial definition
Disadvantages	• Require optimal endocardial definition in two orthogonal apical views	• Assume a regular shape of the LV • Cannot be used in the presence of RWMA	• Assume a regular bullet shape of the LV • Cannot be used in the presence of RWMA

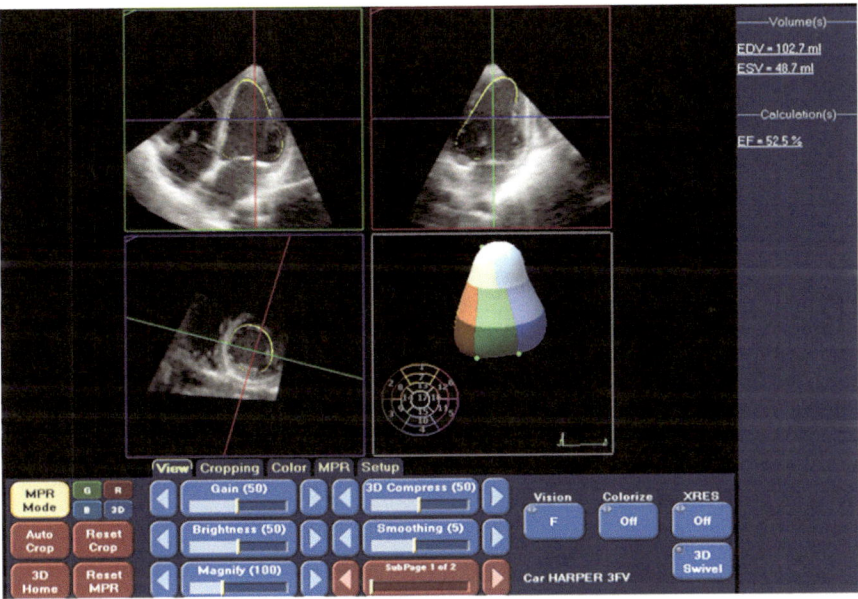

Fig. 3.3 LV volumes and ejection fraction calculated from a real-time 3D echocardiography full volume acquisition. Regional or segmental function can also be assessed from the time–volume curves (not shown)

- Immune from plane-positioning errors (eliminates foreshortening)
- Excellent agreement with cardiac MRI –derived volumes
- Lower interobserver and intraobserver variability compared to 2D echo techniques
- Limited by image quality and irregular cardiac rhythms
- Single beat 3D- volumetric assessment has recently become commercially available

3.3
Calculation of LV Mass

3.3.1
Methods

- Linear measurements
- Volumetric measurements

3.3.2
Linear Method

- LV mass $= 0.8 \times \{1.04\,[(LVIDd + PTW + SWT)^3 - (LVIDd)^3]\} + 0.6$ g

3.3.3
Volumetric Method

- LV mass = LV myocardial volume × cardiac tissue density.
- LV mass = (epicardial LV volume − endocardial LV volume) × 1.05.
- Epicardial and endocardial volumes can be measured using the length-area method or the biplane method of disks.

3.3.4
Technical Points

- Linear method assumes a regular shape of the LV and should not be used in case of geometrical distortions.
- In the presence of RWMA, biplane method should be used.

3.3.5
Relative Wall Thickness (RWT)

- RWT $= 2 \times$ PWT/LVIDd
- Used to differentiate concentric (≥ 0.42) and eccentric (≤ 0.42) remodeling of the LV. See Fig. 3.4 and Tables 3.4.

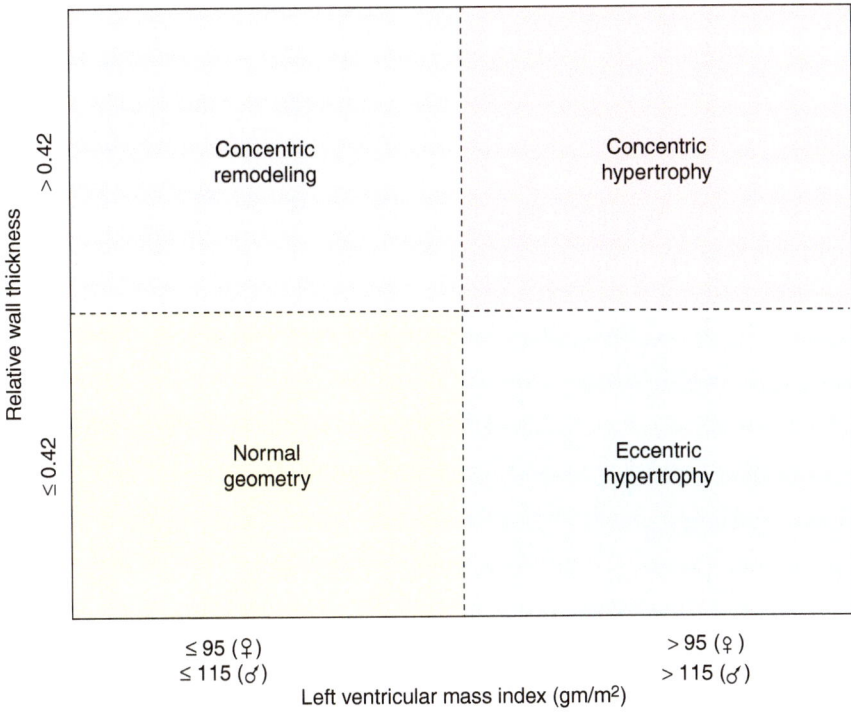

Fig. 3.4 Relative wall thickness in various forms of LV remodeling (With permission from [1])

3.4
Pathologic vs. Physiologic (Athlete's Heart) LVH

Table 3.3 Characteristics of LVH in athlete's heart vs. pathological left ventricular hypertrophy

	Athlete's heart	Pathological hypertrophy
Symmetry	Symmetrical	Symmetrical or asymmetrical
Wall thickness	Rarely > 17 mm	Frequently >17 mm
Systolic function	Normal	Normal or abnormal
LV volume	Increased	Increased, decreased or normal
Diastolic function	Normal with E' > 7 cm/s	Abnormal with E' < 7 cm/s
Strain	Homogenous and normal	Abnormal and can be paradoxical

E'= medial mitral annular tissue Doppler velocity

3.5
Normal and Abnormal Values of LV Dimensions, Wall Thickness, and Mass

Table 3.4 The reference values and classification of abnormal values of LV dimensions, wall thickness and volumes in men and women based on the guidelines of the American society of echocardiography

	Women				Men			
	Normal	Mildly abnormal	Moderately abnormal	Severely abnormal	Normal	Mildly abnormal	Moderately abnormal	Severely abnormal
Dimensions								
LVIDd, cm	3.9–5.3	5.4–5.7	5.8–6.1	>6.1	4.2–5.9	6.0–6.3	6.4–6.8	>6.8
LVIDd/BSA, cm/m²	2.4–3.2	3.3–3.4	3.5–3.7	>3.7	2.2–3.1	3.2–3.4	3.5–3.6	>3.6
PWT, cm	0.6–0.9	1.0–1.2	1.3–1.5	>1.5	0.6–1.0	1.1–1.3	1.4–1.6	>1.6
SWT, cm	0.6–0.9	1.0–1.2	1.3–1.5	>1.5	0.6–1.0	1.1–1.3	1.4–1.6	>1.6
LV volume								
Diastolic, mL	56–104	1.5–117	118–130	>130	67–155	156–178	179–201	>201
Diastolic/BSA, mL/m²	35–75	76–86	87–96	>96	35–75	76–86	87–96	>96
Systolic, mL	19–49	50–59	60–69	>69	22–58	59–70	71–82	>82
Systolic/BSA, mL/m²	12–30	31–36	37–42	>42	12–30	31–36	37–42	>42
LV mass								
Linear, g	67–162	163–186	187–210	>210	88–224	225–258	259–292	>292
Linear/BSA, g/m²	43–95	96–108	109–121	>121	49–115	116–131	132–148	>149
Volumetric, g	66–150	151–171	172–182	>182	96–200	201–227	228–254	>255
Volumetric/BSA, g/m²	44–88	89–100	101–112	>112	50–102	103–116	117–130	>130
RWT	0.22–0.42	0.43–0.47	0.48–0.52	>0.52	0.24–0.42	0.43–0.46	0.47–0.51	>0.51

BSA body surface area, *LV* left ventricle, *LVIDd* left ventricular inner dimension in diastole, *PWT* posterior wall thickness, *RTW* relative wall thickness, *SWT* septal wall thickness

Adapted from [1]

Recommended Reading

Lang RM et al. Recommendations for chamber quantification: a report from the American Society of Echocardiography's Guidelines and Standards Committee and the Chamber Quantification Writing Group, developed in conjunction with the European Association of Echocardiography, a branch of the European Society of Cardiology *J Am Soc Echocardiogr.* 2005;18(12):1440-1463.

Quantification of Left Ventricular Systolic Function

4

Yasuhiko Takemoto and Minoru Yoshiyama

4.1
Introduction

The assessment of left ventricular (LV) systolic function is an essential part of all echocardiographic examinations and provides crucial and indispensable information for diagnosis, treatment, and prognosis of almost all cardiac conditions.

4.2
Global LV Systolic Function

The most commonly used expression of global LV systolic function is LV ejection fraction (LVEF). LVEF is preferably calculated from two-dimensional (2D) volume measurements using the following formula:

$$\text{LVEF}(\%) = \left(\text{LVEDV}(\text{ml}) - \text{LVESV}(\text{ml})\right) / \text{LVEDV}(\text{ml}) \times 100$$

$$\text{(LVEDV; left ventricular end-diastolic volume,}$$
$$\text{LVESV; left ventricular end-systolic volume)}$$

The biplane Simpson method is most commonly used for measuring 2D LV volumes (LVEDV, LVESV) and LVEF.

Y. Takemoto ($\boxtimes$)
Department of Internal Medicine and Cardiology, Osaka City University School of Medicine, Osaka, Japan
e-mail: yatakemoto@med.osaka-cu.ac.jp

T.P. Abraham (ed.), *Case Based Echocardiography*,
DOI: 10.1007/978-1-84996-151-6_4, © Springer-Verlag London Limited 2011

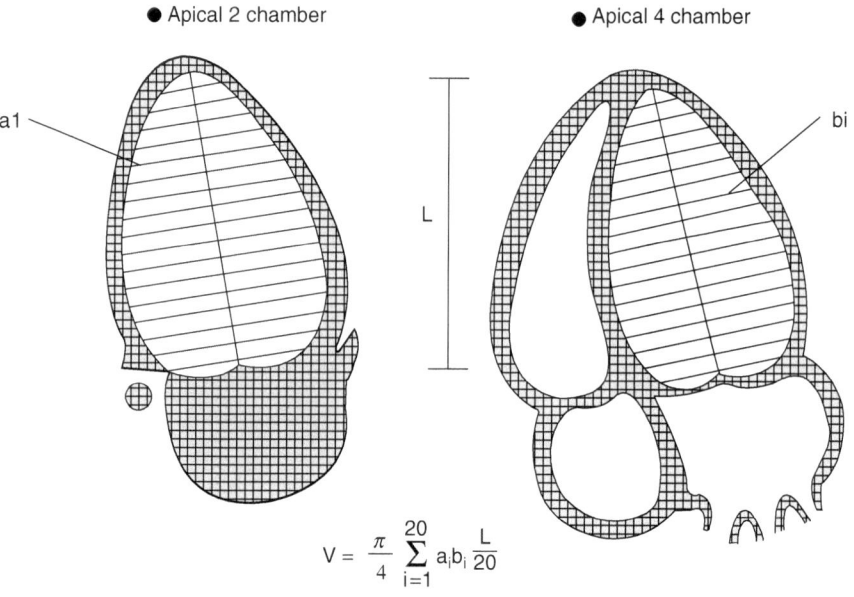

$$V = \frac{\pi}{4} \sum_{i=1}^{20} a_i b_i \frac{L}{20}$$

4.3
Limitations of the Biplane Simpson Method

Myocardial dropout, especially at the apex, is a potential problem. The transducer must be at the true apex and the ultrasonic beam must be through the center of the LV.

4.4
Regional LV Systolic Function

Regional LV systolic function is assessed by dividing the LV into segments using a 16-segment model recommended by the American Society of Echocardiography.

A numeric scoring system is adopted based on the contractility of the individual segments.

16-segment model

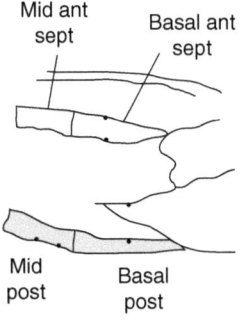
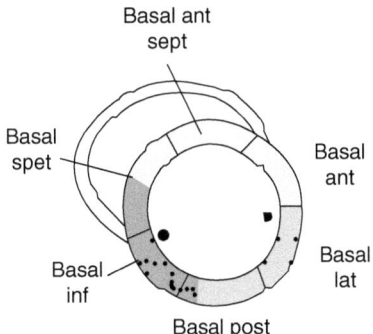
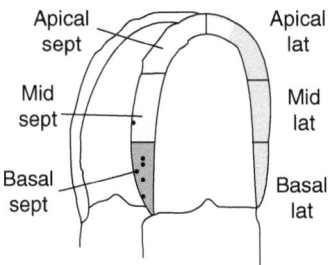
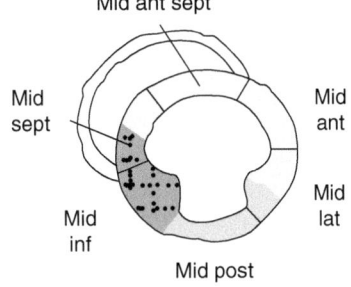
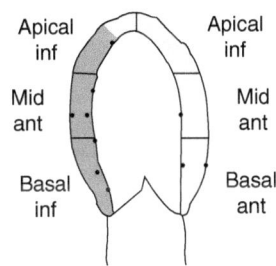
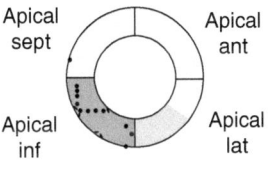

Scoring system

1. Normal
2. Hypokinesis
3. Akinesis
4. Dyskinesis
5. Aneurysmal

Noninvasive Hemodynamic Assessment

5

Jacob Abraham and Kimberly Chadwell

Hemodynamic assessment is one of the oldest applications of echocardiography (echo). With the increasing prevalence of patients with heart failure, the need to accurately measure hemodynamics is growing. Although cardiac catheterization remains the gold standard, it is invasive and expensive. With standard two-dimensional imaging and Doppler techniques, qualitative and quantitative estimation of cardiac output, ventricular filling pressures, and vascular resistances is possible. Because echo measurements correlate strongly with invasively measured values, echo can be a surrogate for catheterization in a variety of settings. This chapter will review the methods for determining some of the most commonly employed hemodynamic parameters (Fig. 5.1).

J. Abraham (✉)
Department of Medicine, Johns Hopkins Hospital, Baltimore, MD, USA
e-mail: ja@jhmi.edu

T.P. Abraham (ed.), *Case Based Echocardiography*,
DOI: 10.1007/978-1-84996-151-6_5, © Springer-Verlag London Limited 2011

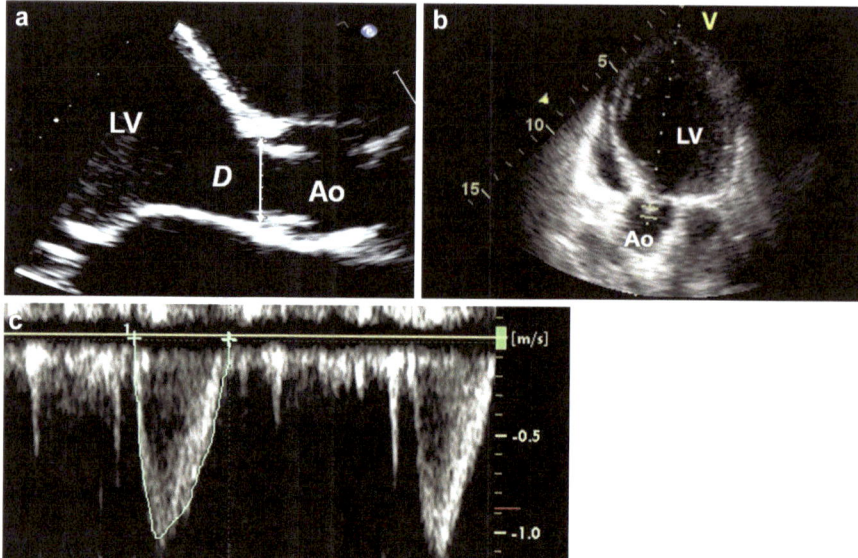

Fig. 5.1 (**a**) Calculation of stroke volume (SV) involves careful measurement of the LVOT diameter in systole at the level of the aortic annulus from the parasternal long axis view. An inner-edge to inner-edge method should be employed. The aortic annulus is the most accurate location for stroke volume measurements. (**b**) Pulse wave Doppler interrogation of LVOT or ascending aorta from the apical five chamber view. The sample volume is placed at the same location as where the diameter was measured. (**c**) Measurement of the LVOT velocity time integral.

$$SV \;=\; \tfrac{1}{4}^{*}\pi * (D)^{2^{*}}(LVOT\ VTI).$$

Cardiac output equals SV multiplied by heart rate

5.1
Cardiac Output (Figs. 5.2–5.8)

- Caveats
  - If using PW Doppler, measure aortic diameter at aortic annulus. If using CW Doppler, measure diameter at sinotubular junction.
  - Aortic valve disease, including bicuspid valve or aortic stenosis/sclerosis, will render the measurement inaccurate.
  - Velocity and diameter measurements should be made at the same site and under the same heart rate and loading conditions.
  - Best beam alignment is critical to avoid underestimation of stroke volume.

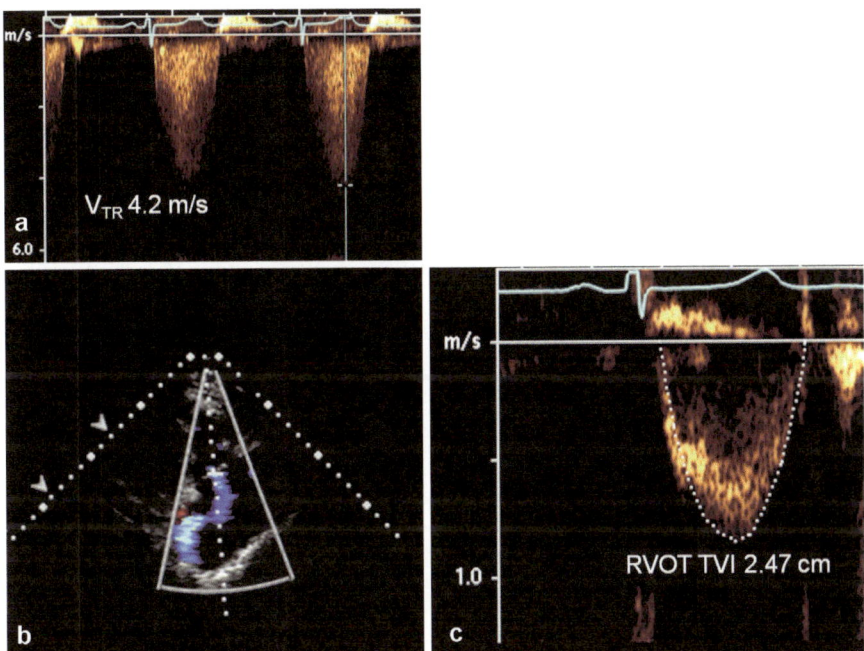

Fig. 5.2 The pulmonary vascular resistance (PVR) is related to the peak velocity of tricuspid regurgitation (V_{TR}) and right ventricular time–velocity integral (RVOT TVI) through the following equation:

$$PVR = (V_{TR} / RVOT\ TVI \times 10) + 0.16.$$

(a) Measurement of VTR. To avoid underestimation of PVR, tricuspid regurgitation jet should be interrogated from multiple views to obtain the peak velocity.
(b) The basal short axis is the best view for determining the RVOT TVI using pulse Doppler.
(c) RVOT TVI measurement. Note that RVOT TVI is expressed in units of centimeters, rather than meters.
In this example, $V_{TR} = 4.2$ m/s and RVOT TVI = 2.47 cm. Therefore, PVR = $(4.2/2.47 \times 10) + 0.16$, or 17.2 Woods Units

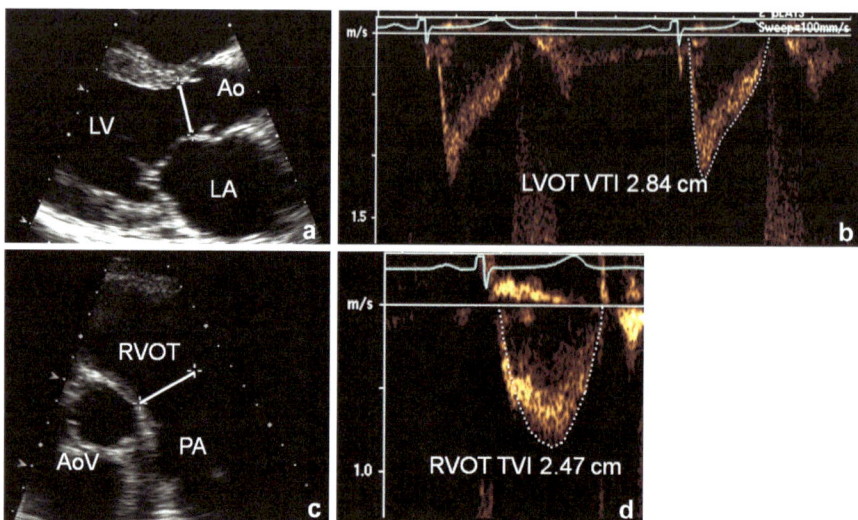

Fig. 5.3 Calculation of the ratio of pulmonary to system blood flow (Qp/Qs) uses the preceding principles to measure stroke volumes for both right and left ventricles. Although stroke volume calculations can be made at any level, it is generally preferable to use the pulmonic valve and the aortic valve for stroke volume measurement. (**a**) Measurement of LVOT diameter from parasternal long-axis view. (**b**) Pulse Doppler of the LVOT from an apical four chamber view. (**c**) Measurement of RVOT diameter from basal short axis view. (**d**) Pulse Doppler of the RVOT. In this example,

LVOT D = 2.26 cm

$$Qs = 1/4^{*}(\pi)^{*}(2.26)^{2^{*}}(2.84) = 11.38 \text{ cm}^{3}$$

RVOT D = 2.96 cm

$$Qp = 1/4^{*}(\pi)^{*}(2.96)^{2^{*}}(2.47) = 16.98 \text{ cm}^{3}$$

$$Qp/Qs = 16.98/11.38$$

$$= 1.5.$$

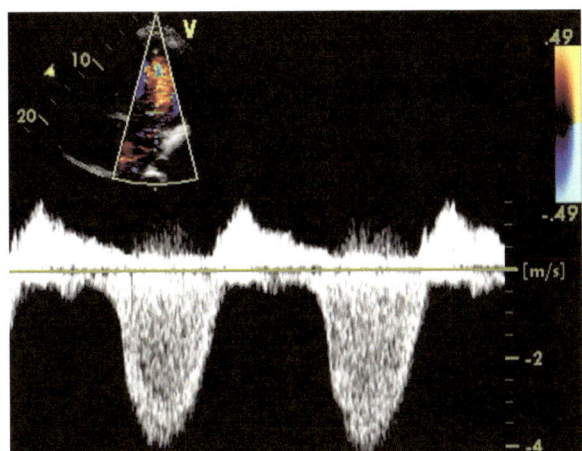

Fig. 5.4 The mitral regurgitation velocity (V_{MR}) reflects the pressure gradient between the LA and LV in systole. In the absence of outflow obstruction, the systolic blood pressure (SBP) equals the left ventricular systolic pressure. Application of the Bernoulli equation allows calculation of the left atrial systolic pressure from the mitral regurgitation velocity (V_{MR}). In this patient with severe left ventricular dysfunction, severe MR, and SBP 95:

$$\text{LA systolic pressure} = \text{SBP} - 4(V_{MR})^2$$
$$= 95 - 4\,(4)^2$$
$$= 31 \text{ mmHg.}$$

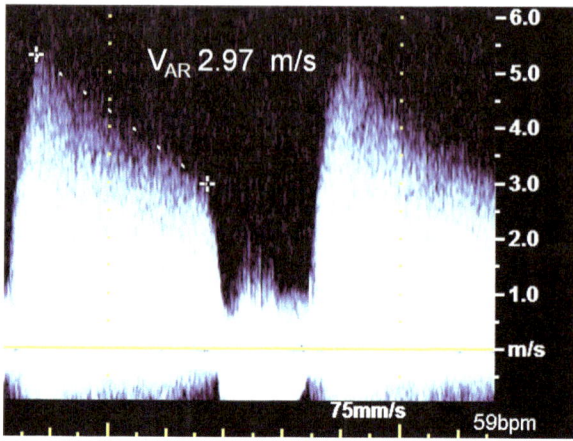

Fig. 5.5 Pulse Doppler of aortic valve in patient with severe aortic regurgitation (AR). The jet velocity at end-diastole (V_{AR}) is 2.97 m/s. From the Bernoulli equation,

Aortic diastolic pressure – LV diastolic pressure = $4(V_{AR})^2$

Therefore, LVEDP = Aortic diastolic pressure $4(V_{AR})^2$

Diastolic pressure can be used as an estimate of aortic diastolic pressure. In this patient with blood pressure of 110/65, the estimated LVEDP is

$$LVEDP = 65 - 4(2.97)^2$$
$$= 30 \text{ mmHg.}$$

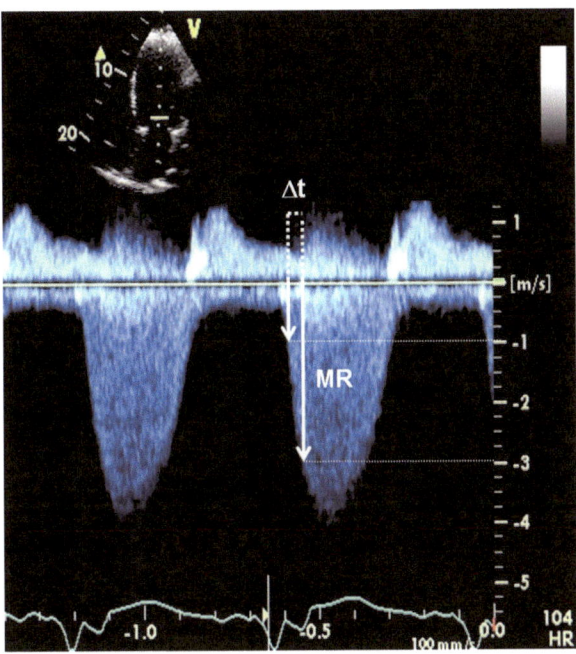

Fig. 5.6 dP/dt is estimated from the time interval (dt) required for the mitral regurgitation jet velocity to increase from 1 to 3 m/s. The LV pressure rise is derived from the Bernoulli equation $(4v_1^2 - 4v_2^2)$ and assumes that left atrial pressure does not change significantly during systole. The latter assumption makes this equation invalid in the setting of acute mitral regurgitation. In this patient with systolic dysfunction,

$$dt = 0.04 \text{ s}$$

$$dP/dt = (4^*3^2 - 4^*1^2)(mmHg)/dt(s)$$

$$= 32/0.04$$

$$= 800 \text{ mmHg}/s.$$

Normal dP/dt $> 1,000$ mmHg/s.

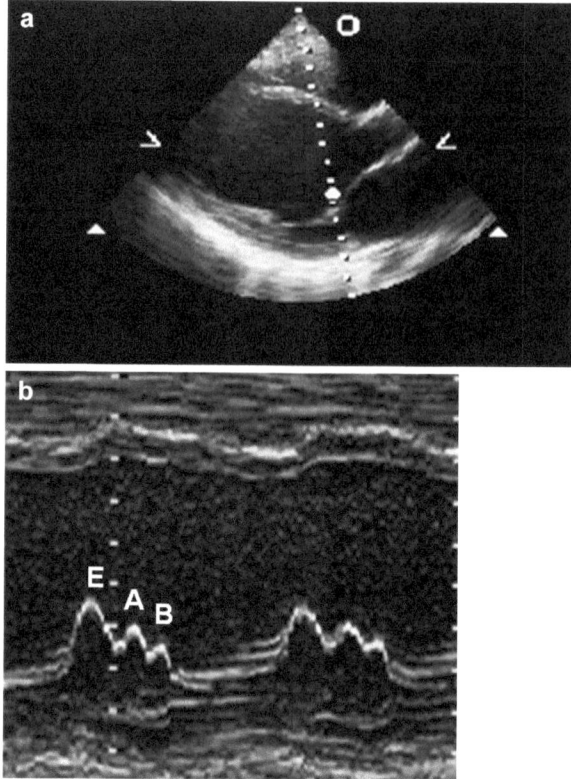

Fig. 5.7 (**a**) M-mode cursor is placed through the mitral valve leaflets in the parasternal long-axis view. (**b**) Anterior mitral leaflet motion entails early diastolic motion (E) and late diastolic motion (A). In this patient with systolic dysfunction, a third movement, the B hump (B), is seen, indicating elevated LVEDP. The sign has low sensitivity but high specificity for LVEDP>20 mmHg

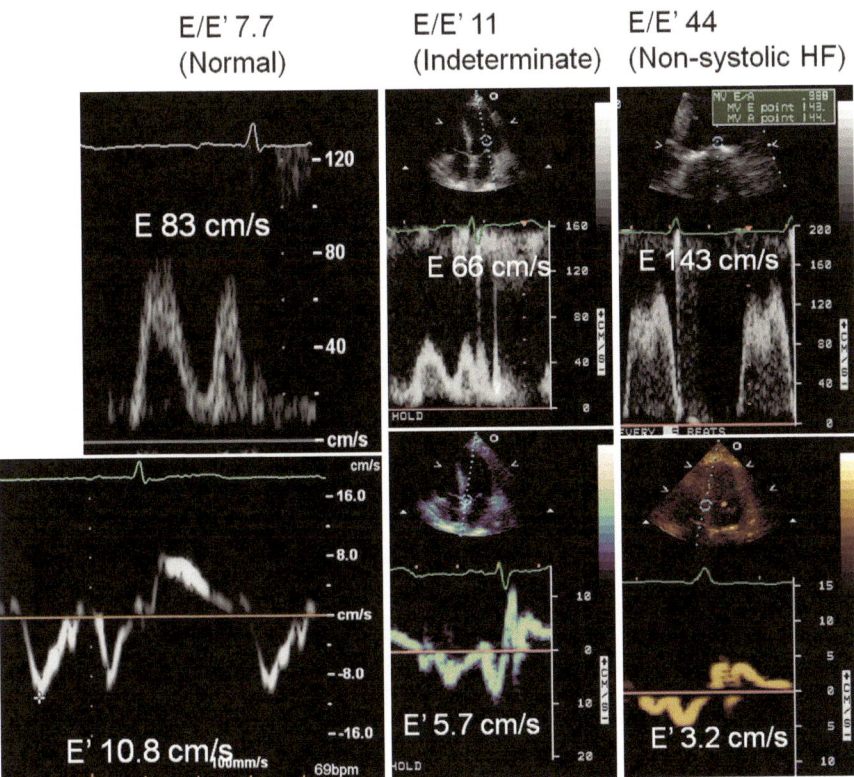

Fig. 5.8 Demonstration of normal and abnormal relaxation patterns based on mitral inflow velocity and tissue Doppler imaging of the septal mitral annulus (E′). Mitral inflow velocity obtained by placing sample volume at mitral valve leaflet tips. (*Left*) Normal E/A ratio and normal E′ velocity in a normal subject. Note that E/E′ in patients with normal EF the correlation with wedge pressure is weaker due to the lower correlation of E to filling pressures. (*Middle*) Reduced E′ and indeterminate E/E′ in patient with reduced ejection fraction. (*Right*) Markedly elevated E and reduced E′ in patient with non-systolic heart failure.

- E/E′ caveats
  - E/E′ 8–15 indeterminate for prediction of PCWP
  - Does not predict PCWP if normal relaxation
  - Not reliable in setting of severe mitral regurgitation
  - Falsely low in setting of constrictive pericarditis (annulus paradoxus) (Table 5.1)

Summary

Table 5.1 Quantitative hemodynamic measurements

Hemodynamic parameter	Echocardiographic correlate	Comment
Right atrial pressure (RAP)	IVC diameter and respirophasic variation	Not valid in positive pressure ventilation except to exclude high RAP
Pulmonary artery systolic pressure	$4(V_{TR})^2 + RAP$	
Pulmonary capillary wedge pressure (PCWP)	E/E′	E/E′ > 12 predicts PCWP > 15 mmHg in patients with reduced EF
Left ventricular end-diastolic pressure (LVEDP)	Aortic diastolic pressure $- 4(V_{AR})^2$	
Left atrial pressure (LAP)	$SBP - 4(V_{MR})^2$	Exclude patients with acute MR, prosthetic MV, and LVOT obstruction or peripheral arterial disease of the arm
Cardiac output (Q)	$HR \times VTI \times Area$	Accurate measure of LVOT diameter is critical
dP/dt	$32/\Delta t$	Δt measured from continuous wave Doppler of MR jet
Pulmonary vascular resistance (PVR)	$10 \times (V_{TR}/RVOT\ VTI) + 0.16$	

Recommended Reading

Abbas AE, Fortuin FD, Schiller NB, Appleton CP, Moreno CA, Lester SJ. A simple method for non-invasive estimation of pulmonary vascular resistance. *J Am Coll Cardiol*. 2003;41(6):1021-1027.

Abraham J, Abraham TP. The role of echocardiography in hemodynamic assessment in heart failure. *Heart Fail Clin*. 2009;5(2):191-208.

Lewis JF, Kuo LC, Nelson JG, Limacher MC, Quinones MA. Pulsed Doppler echocardiographic determination of stroke volume and cardiac output: clinical validation of two new methods using the apical window. *Circulation*. 1984;70:425-431.

Nagueh SF, Middleton KJ, Kopelen HA, Zoghbi WA, Quinones MA. Doppler tissue imaging: a noninvasive technique for evaluation of left ventricular relaxation and estimation of filling pressures. *J Am Coll Cardiol*. 1997;30:1527-1533.

Xie GY, Berk MR, Smith MD, Gurley JC, DeMaria A. Prognostic value of Doppler transmitral flow patterns in patients with congestive heart failure. *J Am Coll Cardiol*. 1994;24:132-139.

Echocardiographic Assessment of Diastolic Dysfunction (DD) and Heart Failure with Normal EF (HFnlEF)

6

Anil Mathew and Luis Afonso

6.1
Physiology

A. About half of patients with new diagnoses of heart failure have normal or near normal global ejection fractions (EF). These patients are diagnosed with diastolic heart failure or heart failure with preserved/normal EF(HFnlEF).

B. *Elevated filling pressures* are the main physiologic consequence of diastolic dysfunction.

C. *Diastolic function* is modulated by myocardial relaxation and myocardial tone but is mainly determined by myocardial stiffness (filling and passive properties of the LV wall).

D. *Myocardial relaxation* is determined by:
   a. Load – increased afterload, late systolic load and/or elevated preload → delays myocardial relaxation → elevated filling pressures
   b. Myocardial inactivation – in cardiac myocyte, cross bridge detachment caused by calcium exit from cell
   c. Nonuniformity (of relaxation in cardiac muscle)

E. *Myocardial stiffness* is determined by
   a. Intrinsic factors (ex: titin within myocardial cell fibrosis in interstitial, matrix)
   b. Extrinsic factors (ex: pericardial constraint and ventricular interaction)

F. Four phases of diastole (Fig. 6.1)
   First Phase – Isovolumetric Relaxation (IR)
   Rapid decline in LV pressure due to LV relaxation
   Second Phase – Rapid Filling
   a. First pressure crossover – end of isovolumic relaxation and mitral valve opening
   b. LA–LV pressure gradient – acceleration of mitral flow
   c. Second pressure crossover – Peak mitral E
      (Thereafter, left ventricular pressure exceeds left atrial pressure, decelerating mitral flow)

L. Afonso (✉)
Department of Cardiology, Detroit Medical Centre, Wayne State University, Detroit, MI, USA
e-mail: lafonso@med.wayne.edu

T.P. Abraham (ed.), *Case Based Echocardiography*,
DOI: 10.1007/978-1-84996-151-6_6, © Springer-Verlag London Limited 2011

Fig. 6.1 The Four
phases of diastole

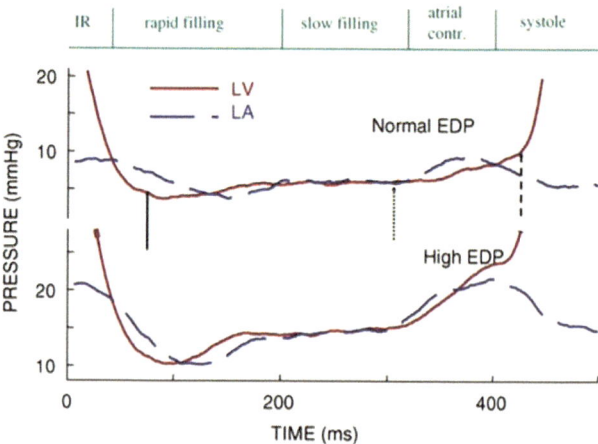

Nagueh et al. Journal of the American Society of Echocardiography, February 2009

Third Phase – Slow Filling
No pressure differences between LA and LV
Fourth Phase – Atrial Contraction
LA–LV pressure gradient from atrial contraction, resulting in another acceleration of
mitral flow

6.2
Echocardiographic Parameters of Diastolic Dysfunction

6.2.1
Morphologic and Functional Correlates of Diastolic Dysfunction

1. Left ventricular hypertrophy
   - Concentric vs. eccentric hypertrophy: Concentric hypertrophy is generally associated with preserved EF and DD. Eccentric hypertrophy is generally associated with reduced EF and DD.
   - LV thickness: measure this to determine if (concentric) LV hypertrophy is present.
2. LA volume/area
   - LA volume/area: reflects the cumulative effects of filling pressure over time and therefore a potential indicator for the presence of diastolic dysfunction.
3. Pulmonary artery pressures
   - Patients with diastolic dysfunction who are symptomatic usually have increased pulmonary artery pressures.
   - In the absence of pulmonary or valvular disease, increased PA pressures indicates the presence of elevated LV filling.

- Tricuspid regurgitation jets and pulmonic regurgitation jets can be used to estimate PA systolic and diastolic pressures, respectively:

$$PASP = 4\,(TR\ peak)^2 + RA\ pressure$$

$$PADP = 4\,(PR\ end\ diastole)^2 + RA\ Pressure$$

$$(RA\ pressure\ estimated\ from\ IVC)$$

- PA diastolic pressure usually correlates well with invasively measured PCWP (LVEDP) and may be used as its surrogate but this estimation is dependent on quality of PR signal and accuracy of RA pressure estimate.

4. Mitral annular motion
   - Reduced apical motion of the mitral valve during diastole may be a visual clue to reduced e' velocity as seen on tissue Doppler (discussed later).

6.2.2
Mitral Inflow Velocities

Technical tips – PW Doppler

In the apical four chamber view, using a 1–3 mm sample volume, PW Doppler cursor is placed between the mitral leaflet tips during diastole.

Measurements: Peak E velocities, Peak A velocities, E/A ratio

Deceleration time (DT) – time from peak velocity of E wave to termination of E wave

1. Mitral hemodynamics
   - Mitral E velocity reflects the LA–LV pressure gradient during early diastole and is affected by preload and alterations in LV relaxation.
   - Mitral A velocity reflects the LA–LV pressure gradient during late diastole and is affected by LV compliance and LA contractile function.
   - DT (of E wave) reflects the rate of decline in the early LA–LV pressure gradient and is affected by LV relaxation, LV diastolic pressures post-MV opening and LV compliance.

2. Mitral inflow patterns
   Four Mitral Filling Patterns based on E:A ratio and DT (Fig. 6.2):

Normal	E/A: 1–2	DT: 160–200 ms
Impaired Relaxation	E/A<0.8	DT>200 ms
Pseudonormal	E/A: 0.8–1.5	DT: 160–200 ms
Restrictive	E/A≥2	DT<160 ms

3. Normal values (see Table 6.1)
   - Definition of normal depends on age of patient: increasing age → decrease in mitral E velocity, E/A ratio, increase in DT and A velocity
   - Variables which affect mitral inflow (other than diastolic function and filling): HR and rhythm, PR interval, cardiac output, mitral annular size, LA function

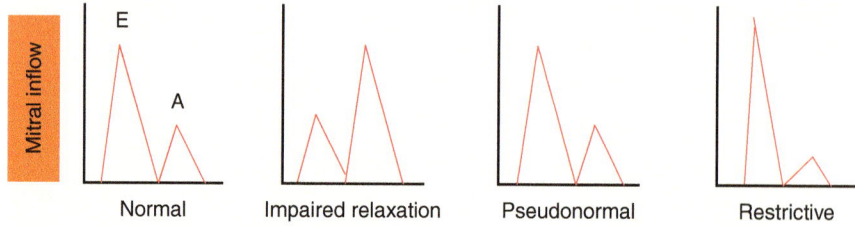

Fig. 6.2 Mitral inflow profiles across spectrum of diastolic dysfunction

Table 6.1 Normal values for Doppler-derived diastolic parameters partitioned according to age

Measurement	Age group (y)			
	16-20	21-40	41-60	>60
IVRT (ms)	50 ± 9 (32-68)	67 ± 8 (51-83)	74 ± 7 (60-88)	67 ± 7 (73-101)
E/A ratio	1.88 ± 0.45(0.98-2.78)	1.53 ± 0.40 (0.73-2.33)	1.28 ± 0.25 (0.78-1.78)	0.96 ± 0.18 (0.6-1.32)
DT (ms)	142 ± 19 (104-180)	166 ± 14 (138-194)	181 ± 19 (143-219)	200 ± 29 (142-258)
A duration (ms)	113 ± 17 (79-147)	127 ± 13 (101-153)	133 ± 13 (107-159)	138 ± 19 (100-176]
PV S/D ratio	0.82 ± 0.18 (0.46-1.18)	0.98 ± 0.32 (0.34-1.62)	1.21 ± 0.2 (0.81-1.61)	1.39 ± 0.47 (0.45-2.33)
PV Ar (cm/s)	16 ± 10 (1-36)	21 ± 8 (5-37)	23 ± 3 (17-29)	25 ± 9 (11-39)
PV Ar duration (ms)	66 ± 39 (1-144)	96 ± 33 (30-162)	112 ± 15 (82-142)	113 ± 30 (53-173)
Septal e' (cro/s)	14.9 ± 2.4 (10.1-19.7)	15.5 ± 2.7 (10.1-20.9)	12.2 ± 2.3 (7.6-16.8)	10.4 ± 2.1 (6.2-14.6)
Septal e'/a' ratio	2.4'	1.6 ± 0.5 (0.6-2.6)	1.1 ± 0.3 (0.5-1.7)	0.85 ± 0.2 (0.45-1.25)
Lateral e' (cm/s)	20.6 ± 3.8 (13-28.2)	19.8 ± 2.9 (14-25.6)	16.1± 2.3 (11.5-20.7)	12.9 ± 3.5 (5.9-19.9)
Lateral e'/a' ratio	3.1'	1.9 ± 0.6 (0.7-3.1)	1.5 = 0.5 (0.5-2.5)	0.9 ± 0.4 (0.1-1.7)

From Nagueh et al Journal of the American Society of Echocardiography Feb 2009

4. Clinical application to patients with depressed and normal EFs
   - Dilated cardiomyopathies – filling patterns correlate well with filling pressures functional class and prognosis – better than LV EF
   - Coronary artery disease and hypertrophic cardiomyopathy (EF ≥ 50%) – filling patterns correlate poorly with hemodynamics

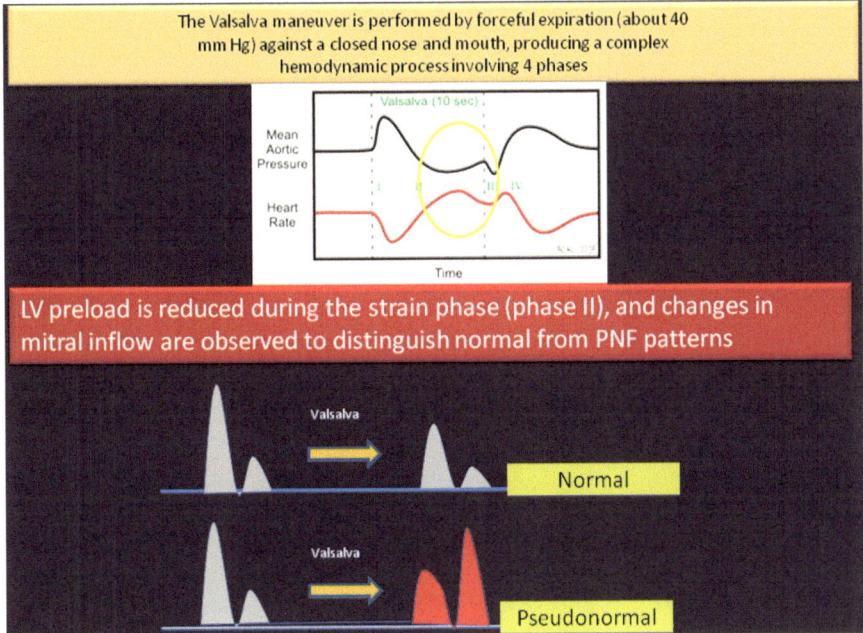

Fig. 6.3 Discriminatory utility of the Valsalva maneuver

5. Valsalva maneuver and mitral inflow: distinguishing normal from PNF (Fig. 6.3)
   - LV preload is reduced during the strain phase (phase II) and changes in mitral inflow can be used to distinguish normal from PNF
   - Valsalva maneuver results in decreased preload during the strain phase. Mitral filling pattern changes to impaired relaxation in patients with PNF post-Valsalva
6. Caveats
   - LV filling patterns have a "U-shaped" relation with LV diastolic function with similar patterns in healthy subjects and patients with Grade II (Pseudonormal) dysfunction.
   - Arrhythmias make filling patterns difficult to interpret sinus tachycardia, first degree AV block: partial or complete fusion of E and A waves, atrial flutter: LV filling heavily influenced by atrial contractions.

6.2.3
Pulmonary Vein Inflow Velocities

Technical tips – PW Doppler
- Color Doppler is used to localize area of inflow of right upper pulmonary vein (RUPV) in the apical four chamber view.
- In this view, using a 2–3 mm sample volume, PW Doppler cursor is placed at (RUPV) >0.5 cm into RUPV.

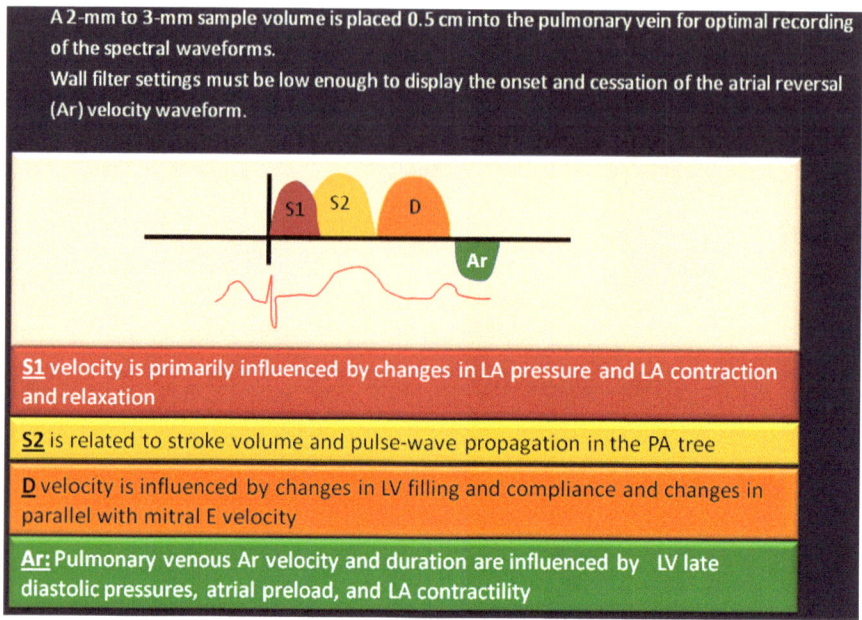

A 2-mm to 3-mm sample volume is placed 0.5 cm into the pulmonary vein for optimal recording of the spectral waveforms.
Wall filter settings must be low enough to display the onset and cessation of the atrial reversal (Ar) velocity waveform.

S1 velocity is primarily influenced by changes in LA pressure and LA contraction and relaxation

S2 is related to stroke volume and pulse-wave propagation in the PA tree

D velocity is influenced by changes in LV filling and compliance and changes in parallel with mitral E velocity

Ar: Pulmonary venous Ar velocity and duration are influenced by LV late diastolic pressures, atrial preload, and LA contractility

Fig. 6.4 Schematic illustrating various components of pulmonary venous flow

- Measurements: systolic (S) velocity and components (S1, S2), peak anterograde diastolic (D) velocity, S/D ratio, atrial reversal (Ar) wave (Ar wave duration, peak Ar velocity in late diastole)
1. Pulmonary vein inflow waveforms
   Reflect phases of LA function during cardiac cycle(see Fig. 6.4)
   Reduction in LA compliance and increase in LA filling pressure result in:
   - Decrease in S velocity, increase in D velocity → decrease in S/D velocity ratio
   - Increase in Ar velocity, duration and increase in Ar amplitude and duration
2. Normal values
   Definition of normal depends on age of patient:
   Increasing age → S/D ratio increases, Ar velocity increases (not greater than 35 cm/s)
3. Clinical application to patients with depressed and normal EFs
   In patients with depressed EFs, reduced systolic filling fractions (<40%) are related to decreased LA compliance and increased mean LA pressure.
   - Ar duration – Mitral A duration difference >30 ms indicates elevated LVEDP and can reliably distinguish those with high LVEDP but normal filling pressures in both normal and reduced EFs.
4. Limitations
   Difficulty in obtaining high quality recordings suitable for measurements
   - Tachycardia and arrhythmias make filling patterns difficult to interpret
   - Atrial fibrillation – loss of atrial contraction and relaxation reduces pulmonary systolic venous flow velocities regardless of filling pressures

6.2.4
Tissue Doppler Annular Early and Late Diastolic Velocities

Technical tips

Tissue Doppler velocities are a measure of the speed of movement of myocardial tissue in comparison to the inflow velocities, which measure the speed of movement of blood cells. In the apical four chamber view, using a 5–10 mm sample volume, tissue Doppler cursor is placed at or 1 cm within septal and/or lateral insertion sites of mitral valve leaflets (Figs. 6.5 and 6.6)

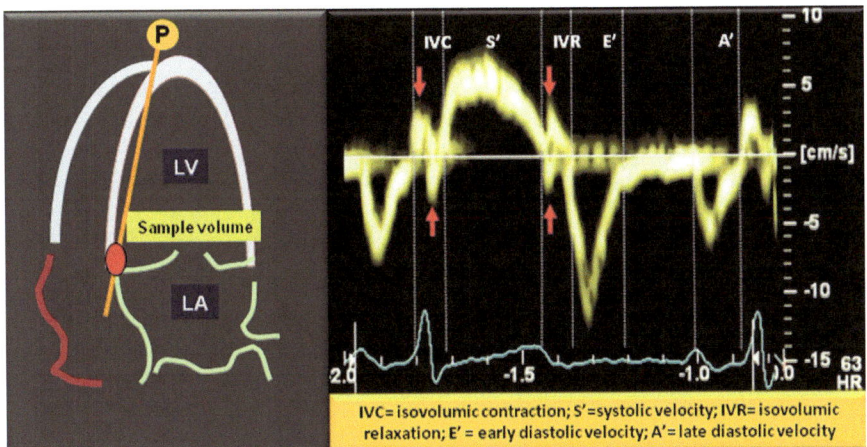

IVC = isovolumic contraction; S' = systolic velocity; IVR = isovolumic relaxation; E' = early diastolic velocity; A' = late diastolic velocity

Fig. 6.5 Mitral annular tissue Doppler velocity acquisition and waveforms

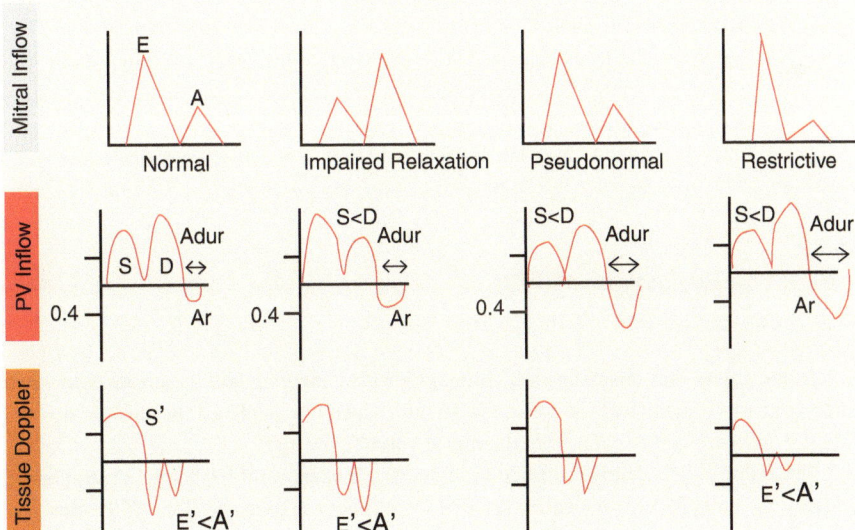

Fig. 6.6 Spectrum of pulmonary flow and mitral annular tissue Doppler velocities in diastolic dysfunction

Measurements: Early diastolic (e′) and late diastolic (a′) velocities

Additional value computed from velocities – E (mitral inflow)/e′ (see below)

1. Hemodynamic determinants
   - e′ is determined by LV relaxation, preload (minimally), systolic function and LV minimal pressure
   - a′ is determined by LA systolic function and LVEDP
2. Normal values
   - Definition of normal depends on age of patient: increasing age → e′ decreases, a′ and E/e′ increases
3. Clinical application

   E/e′ ratio:

   As diastolic dysfunction progressively worsens, LV filling pressures increase.

   As diastolic dysfunction progressively worsens, the LA–LV pressure gradient (E) increases and e′ velocity declines.

   Thus, E/e′ ratio is useful as an estimate of LV filling pressures in patients with LV dysfunction.
   - E/e′ < 8 = normal filling pressures, E/e′ > 15 = elevated filling pressures
   - If E/e′ ratio = 8–14, other echocardiographic indices should be used to estimate LV filling pressures
4. Caveats
   - In normal subjects, e′ is positively related to preload and therefore E/e′ may not always accurately reflect filling pressures.
   - e′ velocity is reduced in patients with mitral annular calcification, surgical rings, mitral stenosis and prosthetic mitral valves.
   - e′ velocity is increased in patients with moderate to severe primary MR and normal relaxation due to increased flow across the mitral valve.
   - Constrictive pericarditis.
     — Septal e′ velocity is increased with constrictive pericarditis due to preserved LV longitudinal expansion compensating for limited lateral and anteroposterior diastolic excursion.
     — Lateral e′ velocity may be less than septal e′ in constrictive pericarditis

6.2.5
Color M-Mode Flow Propagation Velocity

Technical tips

In the apical four chamber view, using color flow imaging with a narrow color sector and gain adjustment to avoid noise, the M-mode scan line is placed through the center of the LV inflow blood column from the mitral valve to the apex.

The color flow baseline is shifted to lower the Nyquist limit so that the central highest velocity is blue. Flow propagation velocity (Vp) is measured as the slope of the first aliasing velocity during early filling, measured from mitral valve plane to 4 cm distally into the LV cavity (Fig. 6.7).

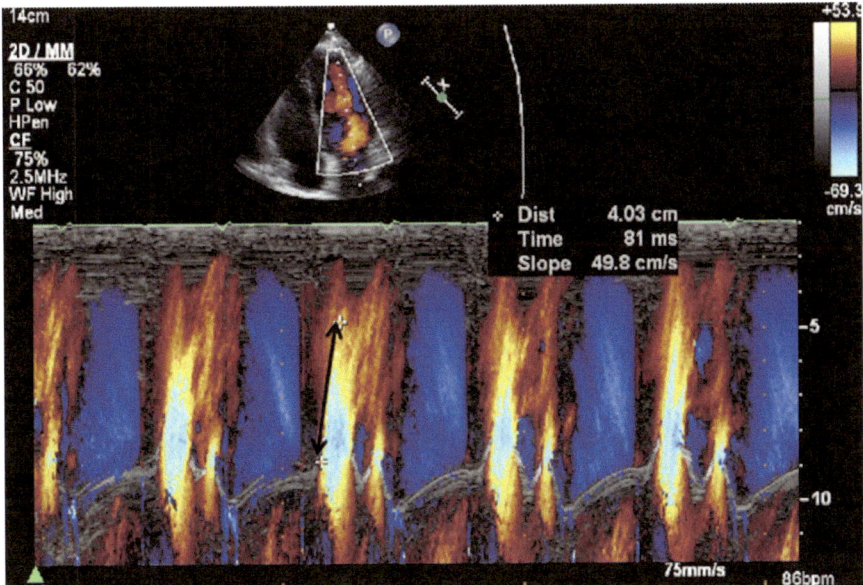

Fig. 6.7 Color M-mode obtained from the Ap-4C view. Velocity of flow propagation (Vp or slope) estimated at 49.8 cm/s (*arrow*) in this patient with normal diastolic function

1. Hemodynamic determinants
   Vp is a measure of the early diastolic filling gradient and is determined by pressure gradient between LV base and apex
   - Normal Values: Vp>50 cm/s is considered normal.
2. Clinical application
   - Slowing of Vp is a semiquantitative marker of LV diastolic dysfunction.
   - E/Vp may be used to predict LV filling pressures –E/Vp≥2.5 predicts PCWP >15 mmHg.
3. Caveats
   - E/Vp may not be reliable if EF is normal.

6.3
Estimation of Left Ventricular Filling Pressures and Diastolic Dysfunction in Special Populations (see Fig 6.8)

1. Atrial fibrillation
   Variability in cycle length, absence of organized atrial activity and LA enlargement limits the assessment of LV filling pressures in atrial fibrillation if LV EF is depressed, mitral DT (≤150 ms) is reasonably accurate as a predictor of increased filling pressures and adverse clinical outcome

ATRIAL FIBRILLATION	Peak acceleration rate of mitral E velocity (≥1,900 cm/s2), IVRT (<65 ms), DT of pulmonary venous diastolic velocity (<220 ms), E/Vp ratio (≥1.4), and septal E/e= ratio (≥11)
SINUS TACHYCARDIA	Mitral inflow pattern with predominant early LV filling in patients with EFs 50%, IVRT 70 ms is specific (79%), systolic filling fraction <40% is specific (88%), lateral E/e= > 10 (a ratio >12 has highest the specificity of 96% (valid with E:A fusion)
HYPERTROPHIC CARDIOMYOPATHY	Lateral E/e= (≥10), PA pressure (≥35 mm Hg), and LA volume (≥34 mL/m2)
RESTRICTIVE CARDIOMYOPATHY	DT (<140 ms), mitral E/A (>2.5), IVRT (<50 ms has high specificity), and septal E/e= (>15)
NON CARDIAC PULMONARY EDEMA	Lateral E/e= can be applied to determine whether a cardiac etiology is the underlying reason for the increased PA pressures (cardiac etiology: E/e ≥ 10; noncardiac etiology: E/e≤ 8
MITRAL STENOSIS	IVRT (<60 ms has high specificity), mitral A velocity(>1.5 m/s)
MITRAL REGURGITATION	IVRT (<60 ms has high specificity)may be applied for the prediction of LV filling pressures in patients with MR and normal EFs, whereas average E/e= (>15) is applicable only in the presence of a depressed EF

Nagueh et al Journal of the American Society of Echocardiography Feb 2009

Fig. 6.8 Diastolic dysfunction assessment in special populations

Other measurements that may be used include deceleration time (DT) and E/e′ and E/Vp Given variation in cycle length, three nonconsecutive beats with cycle lengths within 10–20% of average heart rate or measurements from one cardiac cycle with an RR interval corresponding to HR of 70–80 bpm should be used to obtain measurements of diastolic function.

2. Sinus tachycardia

If E and A wave are fused, measure the peak velocity of the fused wave as the E wave velocity, do likewise for the e′ velocity. E/e′ correlates well with filling pressure

3. Restrictive cardiomyopathy

In restrictive cardiomyopathy, regardless of whether idiopathic or infiltrative, mitral, pulmonary venous and tissue Doppler variables are all good indicators of elevation in filling pressures.

4. Hypertrophic cardiomyopathy
   - E/A ratio and DT have weak to no correlations with LV filling pressures.
   - E/e′ ratio correlates fairly well w/LV pre-A pressure.
   - Ar – (A duration)≥30 ms may be used in this population as in other populations.

5. Mitral stenosis (MS)

Mitral stenosis patients will have elevated left atrial pressures due to valvular restriction of LV inflow. However the LV diastolic pressures will be normal or low (unless there is coexisting myocardial disease).

Determining LA pressures is more difficult in MS but the following can be used as semiquantitative measures of mean LA pressures:
   - IVRT interval – shorter interval → higher early diastolic LA pressure

6. Mitral regurgitation (MR)

Determining LA pressures is more difficult in MR but the following can be used as semi quantitative measures of mean LA pressures:

- IVRT interval – shorter interval → higher early diastolic LA pressure
- E/e′ ratio – is only useful in patients w/depressed ejection fractions

6.4
Other Causes of Heart Failure Symptoms in Patients with Normal EF

6.4.1
Differentiating Constrictive Pericarditis from Restrictive Cardiomyopathy (Diastolic Dysfunction)

a. Mitral annular velocities
   - Constrictive Pericarditis
   Pericardium restricts movement of the lateral annulus → myocardial relaxation preserved BUT lateral annular vertical excursion impaired → SEPTAL e′ normal or increased (≥7 cm/s), lateral e′ reduced
b. Septal motion
   - Restrictive cardiomyopathy (diastolic dysfunction) –septal motion is normal
   - Constrictive pericarditis – septal motion shows respiratory shift – inspiration → left, expiration → right
c. Mitral inflow pattern with respiration
   - Restrictive cardiomyopathy (diastolic dysfunction): no variation in mitral inflow pattern
   - Constrictive pericarditis: ≥25% increase in mitral inflow E velocity with expiration
d. Hepatic flow vein pattern
   - Restrictive cardiomyopathy (diastolic dysfunction): Diastolic forward flow reversal is augmented during *inspiration*
   - Decrease in intrapleural pressures → increase in diastolic filling
   - Constrictive Pericarditis: Diastolic forward flow reversal is augmented during *expiration*
   - Ventricular interdependence → increase in LV filling results in reduction in RV filling

6.5
Left Atrium

The size and volume of the left atrium (LA) increase with increasing grades of diastolic dysfunction.
Mitral inflow parameters and E/e′ reflect instantaneous filling pressure.
LA volume, in comparison reflects chronicity of elevated filling pressure.
Normal LA volume rules out clinically significant diastolic dysfunction.
Normal-appearing mitral inflow likely reflects PNF if the LA volume is increased.

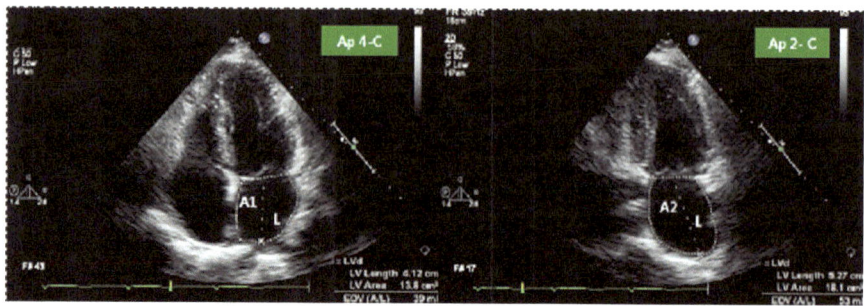

Fig. 6.9 Estimation of left atrial volume using the area-length method, from the apical-4C (A1) and apical-2C (A2) views, at end-systole. Left atrial volume (ml) = 8/3π [(A1)(A2)/ (L*)], where L*= shortest vertical length between Ap-4C and Ap-2C views, measured from back wall to line across hinge points of mitral valve. LA volume may be indexed to body surface area and expressed as LA volume index (ml/m2)

Technical tips

LA size is measured in end systole (end of T-wave or the frame prior to mitral valve opening). Recommended methodology is the area–length method, using the apical −4C and 2C views (Fig. 6.9)

Caveats

LA dilation should be interpreted with caution in high flow states such as anemia, pregnancy.

Afib and MR can cause atrial enlargement not related to diastolic dysfunction

LA dilation in the setting of mitral stenosis occurs due to inflow obstruction

Anteroposterior measurement of LA diameter can be misleading and may underestimate

LA size as the LA enlarges asymmetrically in the lateral and infero-superior direction

Normal values: LA volume/BSA (mL/m²): Normal reference range: 22±6 mL/m²
LA area: normal<20 cm²; 20–30 cm² (mild dilation); 30–40 (moderate); >40 cm² (severely dilation)

6.6
Evaluation of Patient with Diastolic Dysfunction (DD) or Heart Failure with Normal EF (HFnlEF)

6.6.1
Evaluation, Differential Diagnosis and Subtypes of the DD/HFnlEF Patient

The first step in evaluation of a patient with dyspnea due to diastolic dysfunction is to exclude noncardiogenic causes through history, physical and appropriate medical testing.

The second step is to evaluate for cardiogenic causes of dyspnea by echocardiography. Evaluating ejection fraction, looking for structural abnormalities and evaluation for the presence of valvular disease.

Once these have been excluded, in the third step the presence of signs of diastolic dysfunction must be confirmed which are left atrial enlargement or the presence of diastolic function abnormalities.

The final step in the evaluation of DD/HFnlEF is to evaluate wall motion, chamber geometry and pulmonary artery pressures to define the subtype of DD/HFnlEF that is present.

6.6.2
Estimation of Elevated Filling Pressures in Normal EF (Refer to algorithm outlined in Fig. 6.10)

The E/e' ratio should be used to determine if filling pressures are elevated.

- E/e' ratios <8 indicate the presence of normal filling pressures.
- E/e' ratios >12 (if lateral e' is measured), 15 (if septal e' is measured) or 13 (if the average of septal and lateral e' are obtained) indicate the presence of elevated filling pressures.
- E/e' ratios between 9 and 14 require the use of additional Doppler parameters.

The most commonly used parameters are LA volume and pulmonary artery systolic pressures (PAS) as estimated by peak TR velocities.

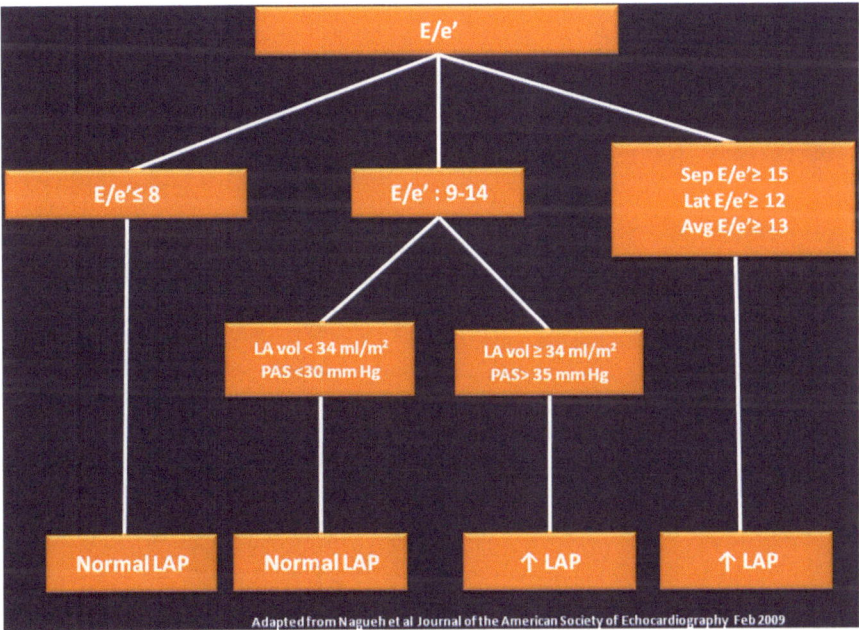

Fig. 6.10 Estimation of LV filling pressure in patients with normal systolic function

6.6.3
Estimation of Elevated Filling Pressures in Reduced EF (Refer to algorithm outlined in Fig. 6.11)

The mitral inflow pattern is very useful in determining left atrial filling pressures in this subset of patients.

- E/A ratios of <1 and E velocities <50 cm/s indicate the presence of normal filling pressures.
- E/A ratios of >2 and DT <150 ms indicate the presence of restrictive filling and elevated filling pressures.
- E/A ratios between 1 and 2 require the use of additional Doppler parameters.

The most commonly used are E/e′ or pulmonary artery systolic pressures (PAS) as estimated by peak TR velocities. PAS may be used only in the absence of pulmonary disease.

- Other measures also may be used to determine normal or elevated filling pressures.
- LA volume should NOT be used to estimate LV filling pressures in this population because some LA dilatation may occur even when LV filling pressures are still normal.

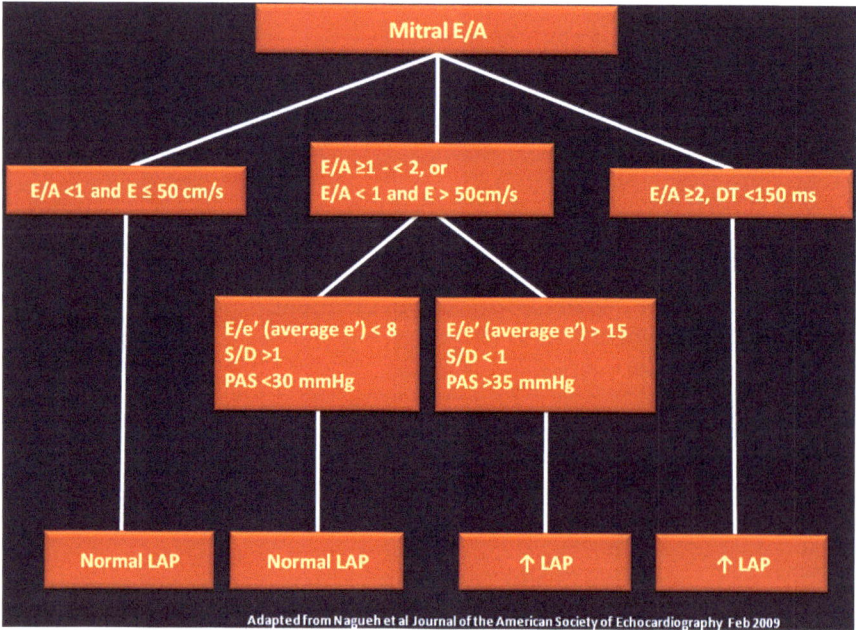

Fig. 6.11 Estimation of LV filling pressure in patients with depressed systolic function

6.6.4
Grading Diastolic Dysfunction (Refer to Fig 6.12)

The grading scheme is Grade I (mild), Grade II (moderate), or Grade III (severe).

This scheme was an important predictor of all cause mortality in a large epidemiology study

Aside from the parameters mentioned in the figure, age and heart rate should be taken into account in grading diastolic dysfunction

- Age – in elderly individuals without cardiovascular disease, grade I diastolic dysfunction is commonly seen and may be considered normal in this population.
- Heart rate – increasing heart rate→reduction in mitral E, E/A ratio, and annular e'velocities.
- *Grade I Diastolic Dysfunction*
  These patients have reduced diastolic reserve that can be uncovered with stress testing.
  Volume depleted subjects may have reduced E/A ratios but normal tissue Doppler velocities.
  Therefore E/A ratio<0.8 should not alone determine the presence of diastolic dysfunction.
  LA pressures in these patients are not elevated (exceptions: hypertension, hypertrophic cardiomyopathy).
  LA volume may be normal

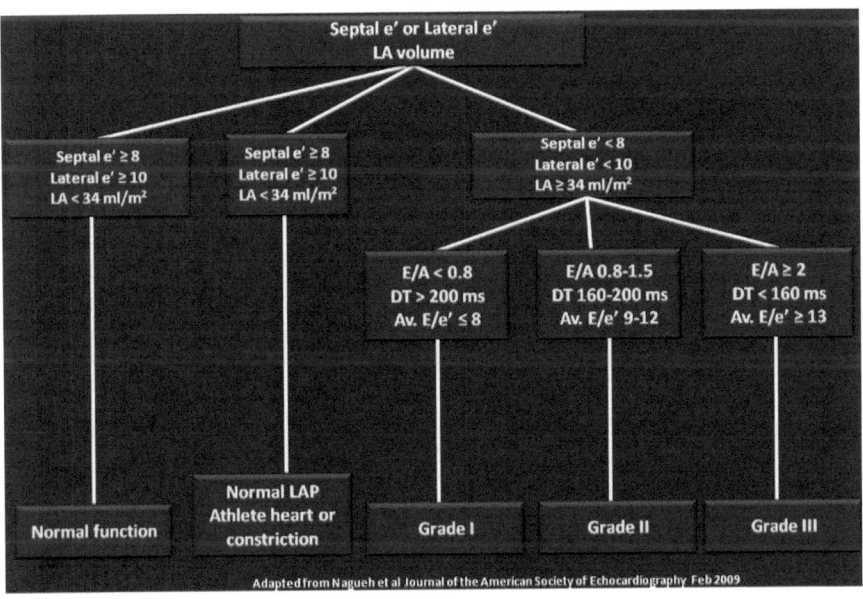

Fig. 6.12 Practical approach to grading diastolic dysfunction

- *Grade II Diastolic Dysfunction*

  LA pressures in these patients are elevated

  LA volume is increased

- *Grade III Diastolic Dysfunction*

  LV filling may revert to impair relaxation with successful treatment

  Response to treatment indicates a subtype of grade III with the more favorable prognosis (Grade IIIa) compared with those who do not respond, indicating the subtype of grade III with a high risk of cardiac morbidity and mortality (Grade IIIb/restrictive filling).

Tissue Doppler Imaging and Strain Echocardiography

7

Veronica Lea J. Dimaano

Doppler principle has been routinely used in echocardiography to provide hemodynamic data to the anatomical information offered by two-dimensional (2D) examination. It measures *high-frequency, low-amplitude* signals from rapidly moving red blood cells enabling quantification of blood flow velocities. Recently, modifications have been applied to the filter settings on pulsed Doppler to allow imaging *low-velocity, high-intensity* myocardial signal, thereby selectively calculating and displaying on-line myocardial velocity information derived from Doppler shifts created by cardiac motion. This technique referred to as tissue Doppler imaging (TDI) or Doppler myocardial imaging (DMI) provides segmental velocity information utilizing three principal approaches: spectral pulsed-Doppler (PW), color-coded M-mode Doppler display, and 2D color-coded Doppler approach. PW and 2D color-coded TDI are more commonly used in clinical settings. While both techniques provide the same mechanical information, data acquired via each method may differ and may not be interchangeable requiring appropriate labeling to avoid confusion (Figs. 7.1 and 7.2). Pulsed Doppler technique yields peak tissue velocity that is 20–30% higher than the mean velocity provided by color-coded Doppler approach; a difference that should be considered when estimating left ventricular filling pressures using the E/E' ratio.

Tissue velocity depicts myocardial motion at specific locations in the heart and indicates the rate at which a particular point in the myocardium is displaced *relative to an external transducer*. Integration of velocity over time yields displacement or the absolute distance traversed by that particular point. Longitudinal cardiac motion is such that the base descends toward the generally immobile apex during systole and moves away from it during diastole. A triphasic tissue velocity display represents the magnitude of myocardial motion as the heart contracts and relaxes during systole and diastole, respectively. Because assessment of tissue velocity has its reference on a point outside the heart (transducer), a velocity gradient exists between a more basal and a more apical segment of interest. (Fig. 7.3). As with the classical Doppler technique, tissue velocity assessment is greatly influenced by the angle of insonation and the translational motion of the heart. It is limited

V.L.J. Dimaano
Divison of Cardiology, Johns Hopkins University School of Medicine,
Baltimore, MD, USA
e-mail: vdimaan1@jhmi.edu

T.P. Abraham (ed.), *Case Based Echocardiography*,
DOI: 10.1007/978-1-84996-151-6_7, © Springer-Verlag London Limited 2011

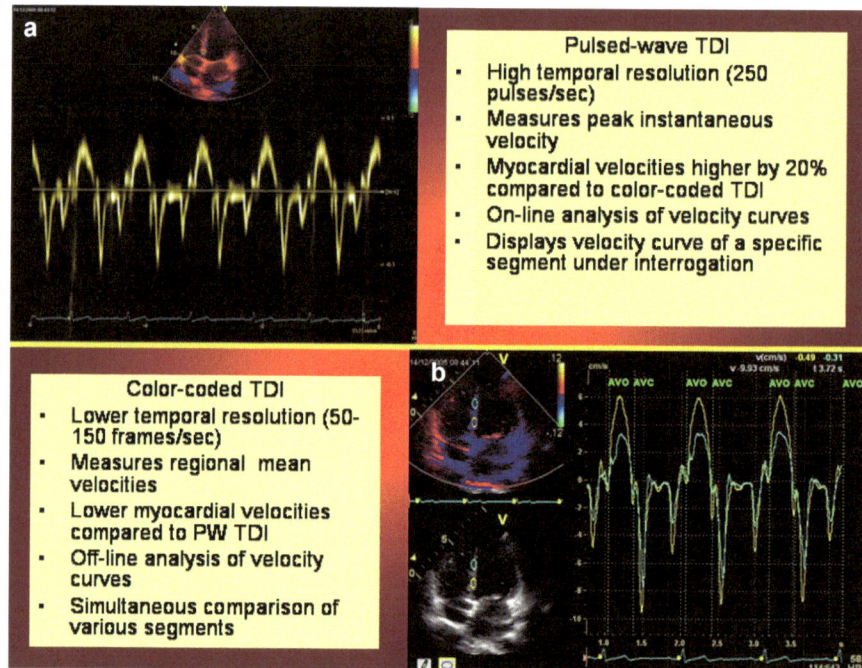

Pulsed-wave TDI
- High temporal resolution (250 pulses/sec)
- Measures peak instantaneous velocity
- Myocardial velocities higher by 20% compared to color-coded TDI
- On-line analysis of velocity curves
- Displays velocity curve of a specific segment under interrogation

Color-coded TDI
- Lower temporal resolution (50-150 frames/sec)
- Measures regional mean velocities
- Lower myocardial velocities compared to PW TDI
- Off-line analysis of velocity curves
- Simultaneous comparison of various segments

Fig. 7.1 Tissue Doppler imaging (TDI) provides segmental velocity information, which can be displayed by (**a**) pulsed wave or (**b**) color Doppler technique. While both methods yield the same mechanical information, differences inherent to each technique exist. Velocities obtained via pulsed-wave TDI are higher than that obtained using the color-coded TDI. This difference is of prime importance when estimating left ventricular filling pressures using the E/E′ ratio

by its inability to differentiate passive from active myocardial motion consequent to the "tethering effect" wherein a normal more apical segment of the myocardium drags an abnormal basal segment toward the apex.

Doppler-derived strain rate (SR) and strain measure the speed of myocardial deformation derived from velocity gradient and is expressed in s^{-1} (Fig. 7.4). SR profile is a triphasic display of the magnitude of myocardial deformation rate as the heart contracts in systole and relaxes in diastole (Fig. 7.5). Integration of SR yields strain. Strain is a measure of myocardial deformation defined as the change in length normalized to the original length and is expressed in percent (Fig. 7.6). Understanding tissue velocity-SR-strain relationship (Fig. 7.7 and 7.8) and the limitations (Fig.7.9-7.12) inherent to the Doppler technique are essential in the analysis and interpretation of these studies.

Speckle tracking is a relatively angle-independent method of quantifying strain. It enables measurement of myocardial deformation in basically all regions of the myocardium in the longitudinal, radial, and circumferential directions (Fig.7.13-7.15). As it utilizes 2D images, it operates on a lower frame rate and may be inferior to Doppler-derived

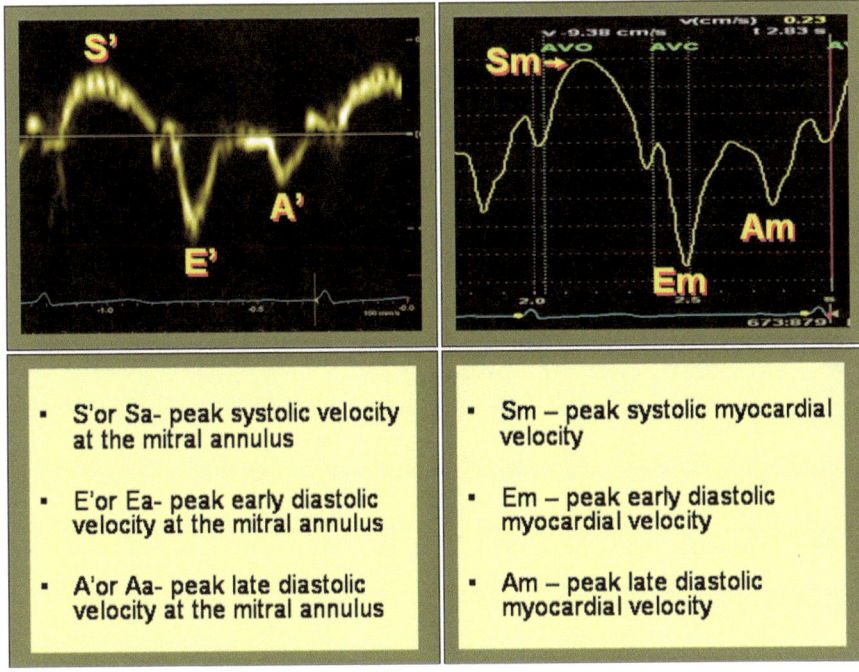

- **S'or Sa-** peak systolic velocity at the mitral annulus

- **E'or Ea-** peak early diastolic velocity at the mitral annulus

- **A'or Aa-** peak late diastolic velocity at the mitral annulus

- **Sm –** peak systolic myocardial velocity

- **Em –** peak early diastolic myocardial velocity

- **Am –** peak late diastolic myocardial velocity

Fig. 7.2 Tissue velocity nomenclature. Relative to an external transducer, a triphasic wave form characterizes the typical tissue velocity curve. Depending on the location of sample volume (mitral annulus vs. myocardium), each wave form is identified by its timing relative to the phase of the cardiac cycle. Following a positive wave representing ventricular systole, two negatively directed waves corresponding to early and late diastole appear as a mirror image of the early (E) late and (A) left ventricular filling velocities. Mitral annular velocity has been frequently interrogated using pulsed wave TDI. Its combination with mitral inflow velocity (E/E' or E/Ea) can predict LV filling pressure

strain where temporal resolution is concerned. With speckle-tracking, SR is derived from strain, while with Doppler-based technique, it is integrated to yield strain.

Myocardial deformation is the result of the complex interaction of intrinsic contractile force and extrinsic loading conditions applied to a tissue with variable elastic properties. Therefore, changes in preload and afterload, and the changes in myocardial stiffness, are important determinants of the pattern and the magnitude of myocardial deformation. Thus, SR and strain indices are not direct measures of contractility. However, peak systolic strain rate (SRs) was found to correlate best with dP/dt (an index of contractile function). On the other hand peak systolic strain was found to correlate best with changes in stroke volume and, therefore, was more closely related to changes in global hemodynamics than changes in contractility.

Some of the clinical applications of the TDI and strain imaging include assessment of global and regional left ventricular systolic and diastolic function, differentiating

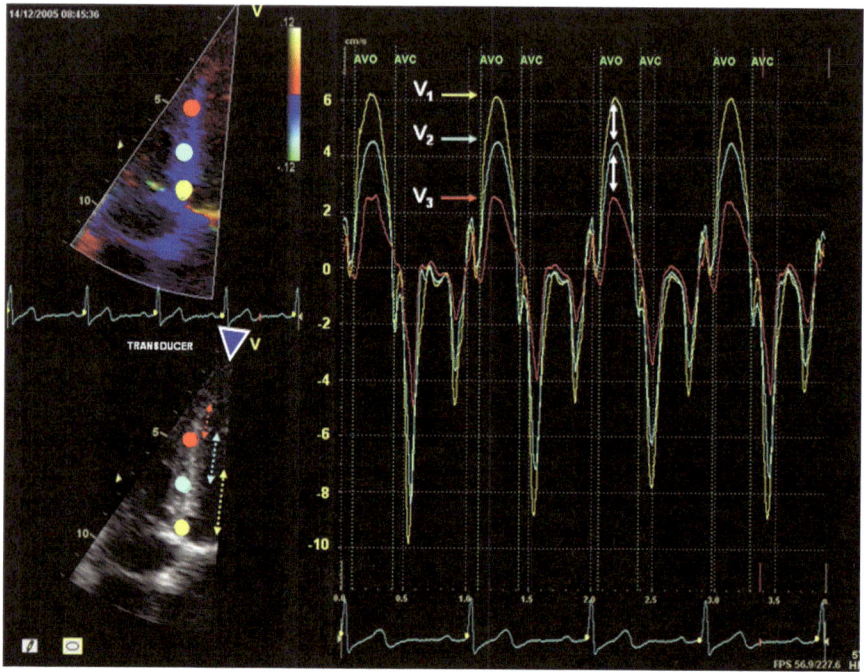

Fig. 7.3 Tissue velocity interrogation has been almost exclusively performed in the longitudinal direction in which the base descends toward the generally immobile apex during systole and moves away from it during diastole. Because assessment of tissue velocity has its reference on a point outside the heart (transducer) a velocity gradient (*white arrows*) exists between a more basal and a more apical segment of the myocardium. Thus, tissue velocity is maximum at the base (V_1), lower in the mid (V_2), and least at the apex (V_3)

constrictive pericarditis and restrictive cardiomyopathy, ischemia detection and evaluation of viability, early detection of cardiomyopathies, and evaluation of mechanical dyssynchrony (Fig.7.16-7.18). Application of TDI and strain imaging in the evaluation of right ventricular (RV) function is more challenging because of the ventricle's complex shape and its marked load dependence.Fig. 7.19

There exists a significant variability in TDI-derived parameters due to lack of standardized guidelines on data acquisition, partly resulting from the differences in the machine design, and standardized guidelines on post-processing analysis and interpretation. Thus it is difficult to recommend one. It is, however, important to have an insight on the mechanics by which each technique operates and interpret the results in the light of the limitations inherent to each technique.

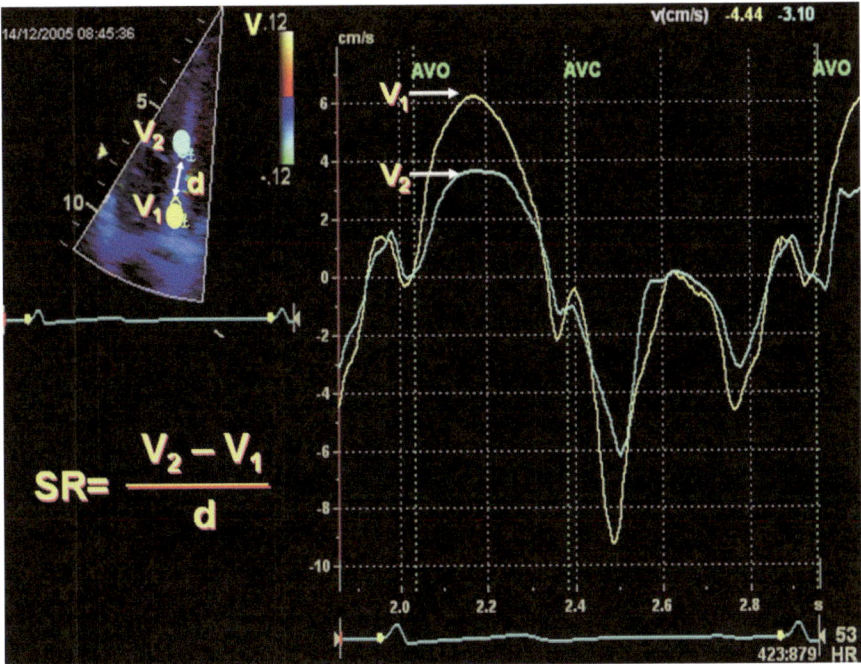

Fig. 7.4 Velocity gradient is used to calculate strain rate. With tissue Doppler, differential velocity of two adjacent segments in myocardium along the ultrasound beam normalized to the distance between these velocities (V_1 and V_2) yields strain rate. Strain rate measures the speed at which myocardial deformation occurs and is expressed as s^{-1}

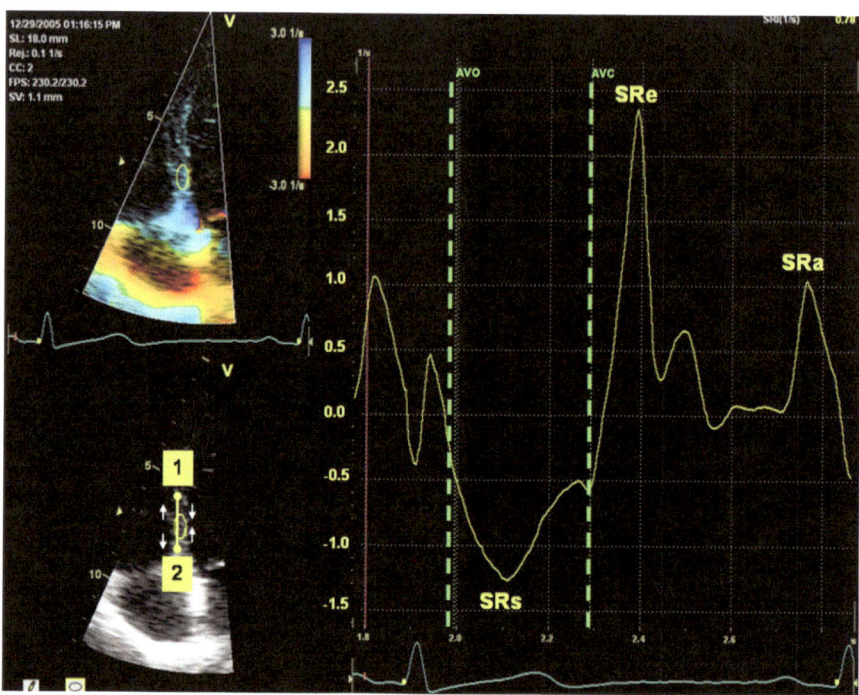

Fig. 7.5 Doppler-derived strain rate is a *spatial* derivation of the velocity gradient. In contrast to tissue velocity, the points of reference reside within the segment under interrogation. While both entities define the rate at which a particular change occurs (location for tissue velocity and length for strain rate) the triphasic curve depicting the timing of events in one cardiac cycle is displayed on an *opposite* magnitude. To illustrate, a sample volume is placed at the base of the left ventricular septum using a strain length of 18 mm (distance between points 1 and 2). The speed by which the two reference points (1 and 2) in the myocardium move closer to each other during systole (myocardial contraction) is termed systolic strain rate (SRs). Since the distance between these two reference points becomes progressively shorter, the resulting SRs amplitude is directed negatively. SRs normally peaks at early to mid-systole. The rate by which the reference points in the myocardium move away from each other during relaxation is termed diastolic strain rate. Since the distance between these reference points becomes longer, the resulting early (SRe) and late (SRa) diastolic amplitudes are directed positively

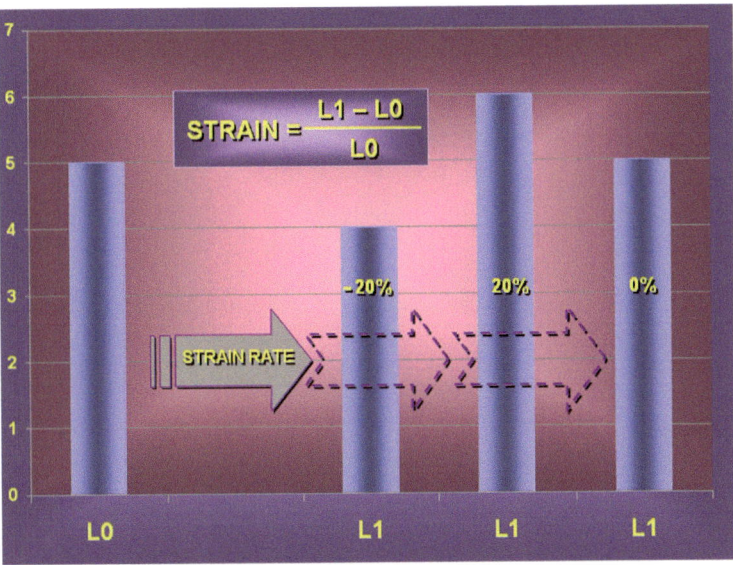

Fig. 7.6 Strain denotes myocardial deformation and is defined as the change in length normalized to the initial length. In a one-dimensional object, the only possible deformation of the object is lengthening or shortening. The relative amount of deformation is defined as strain and is expressed in percent. The equation is defined in such a way that lengthening is represented as a positive value for strain while shortening is represented by a negative value (13). Hence, if the initial length is noted to be 5 cm and it shortens to 4 cm, the strain will be −20%. However, if from 5 cm it lengthens to 6 cm, the strain will be 20%

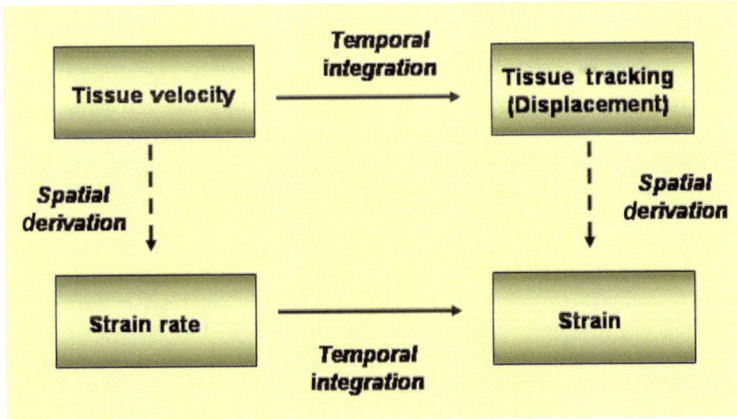

Fig. 7.7 Using velocity gradient technique, strain and strain rate are derived from the tissue velocity data. Knowledge of the relationship between these Doppler-derived measures of myocardial function play an important role in the analysis and interpretation of a strain/strain rate curve

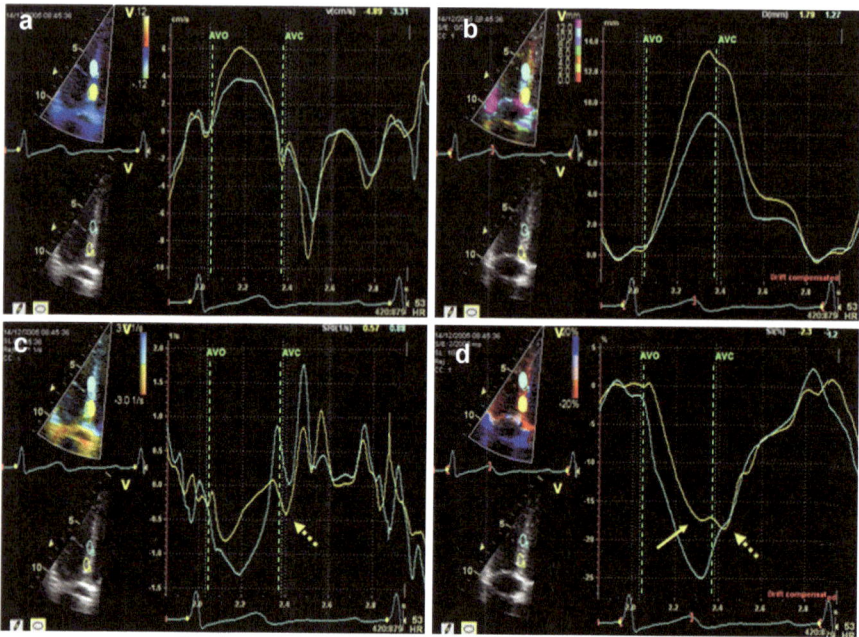

Fig. 7.8 To elucidate on tissue velocity–SR–strain relationship, a narrow sector color Doppler image of interventricular septum using the apical 4-chamber view was acquired from a normal volunteer. Timing of aortic valve opening (AVO) and (AVC) closure (*vertical green dashed lines*) was measured from the spectral Doppler display of left ventricular outflow tract. Sample volumes were placed at the base and mid-septum. (*yellow* and *green circles*, respectively, in the upper *left panel* of all sets of images). (**a**) Velocity profile is extracted over one cardiac cycle. Motion during systole, early and late diastole can be identified by the triphasic display. (**b**) Time-integration of the velocity curve results in the displacement curve. In the longitudinal direction, there is motion toward the transducer during systole and away from the transducer during diastole. The displacement of the more apical segment (*green curve*) is smaller than that of more basal one (*yellow curve*). (**c**) Strain rate curve extracted from the same velocity color-Doppler data in (a). Calculation of the spatial gradient in the myocardial velocities yields an estimate of strain rate. During systole, longitudinal shortening of the ventricle is identified by a negative strain rate value while the two lengthening phases during diastole (passive and active LV filling) are depicted by positive strain rate phases. Presence of multiple peaks may interfere with identification of the true peak diastolic strain rates (*yellow* curves corresponding to the basal septum tracing). (**d**) Time integration of strain rate curves yields regional strain curves. It is evident that the wall shortens during systole and lengthens during diastole. In this particular example, the strain curve is characterized by two peaks marked by *yellow arrows*. Cross-checking with the strain rate curve, a second negatively directed curve appears near the AVC (*broken yellow arrow* in c). This curve corresponds to the second peak in the strain curve (*broken yellow arrow* in d) and, therefore, is *not* the true peak systolic strain

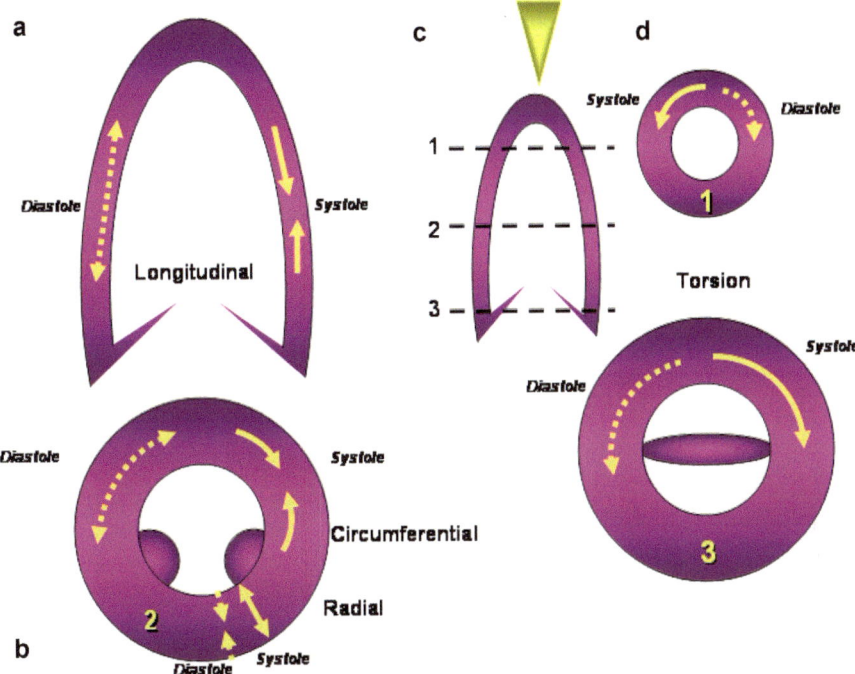

Fig. 7.9 Local coordinates of strain measurement. Using the heart coordinate system (13) myocardial strain can be measured in three directions. The heart shortens and lengthens in the longitudinal direction (**a**), thickens and thins in radial direction, and shortens and lengthens in circumferential direction (**b**). (**c**) When the heart is viewed from the apex, the base (3) and the apex (1) rotate in opposite direction effecting a wringing motion or torsion. (**d**) During systole (*solid yellow arrow*), the apex rotates counterclockwise and the base, clockwise (twisting). The heart untwists in diastole (*yellow broken arrow*)

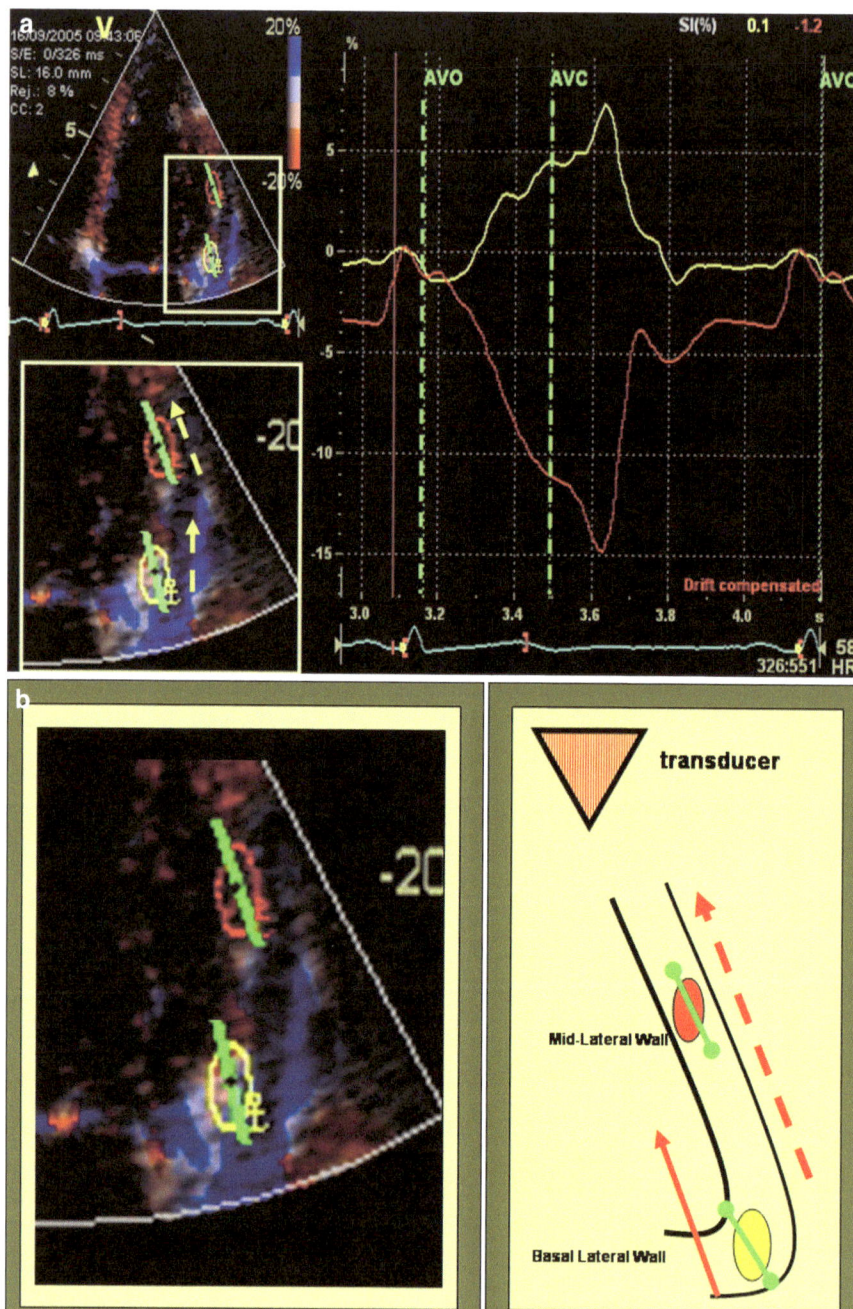

Fig. 7.10 (**a**) The magnitude of the Doppler-derived strain curve is influenced by the angle of insonation. The *line of deformation* of a particular myocardial segment should be parallel to the Doppler beam. Thus myocardial wall should be kept parallel to the beam when longitudinal strain is being assessed and perpendicular to it when measuring radial strain. The translational motion of the heart exists in a multi-plane coordinate and myocardial deformation is not unidimensional. In this example of a Doppler-derived strain curve taken from a normal volunteer, sample volumes were placed at the base (*yellow circle*) and the mid segment (*red circle*) of the lateral wall in the apical 4-chamber view. The longitudinal strain profile is displayed as two strain curves in opposite magnitudes typical of dyskinesis or dyssynchrony. Lower left panel, inset: A closer look at the position of the strain bars (*solid green lines*) in relation to the myocardial fiber orientation would reveal that the Doppler beam is approaching a perpendicular relationship to the basal segment and a more parallel relationship to the mid-segment where the respective sample volumes were placed. Hence, during systole, the predominant pattern of myocardial deformation at the base is thickening rather than shortening, resulting in a positively directed strain curve. A *schematic diagram* is presented in the right panel (**b**). To address this problem, movement of the sample volume around the basal segment should be performed. During image acquisition, narrow sector images should be taken in addition to proper positioning of the transducer to ensure alignment of wall with the Doppler beam

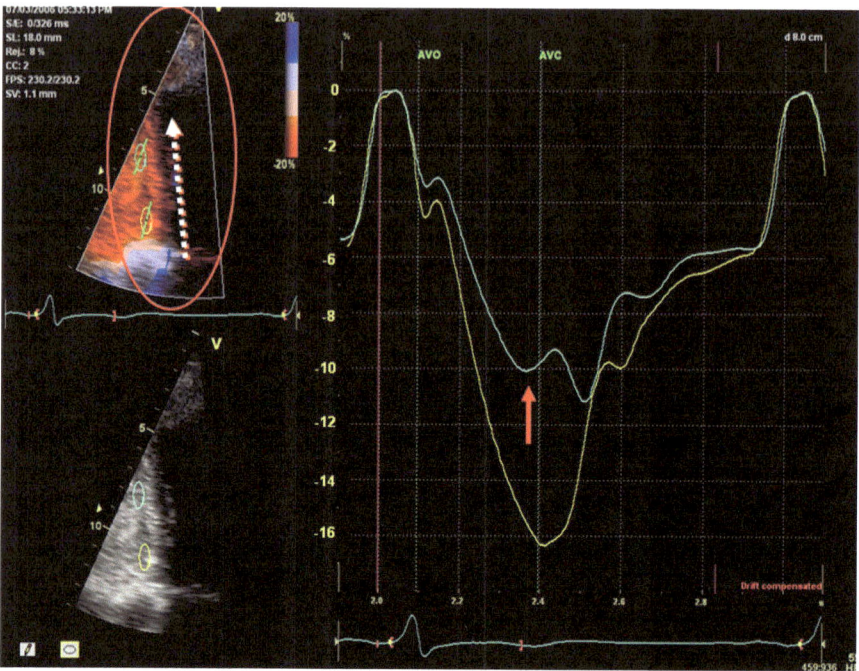

Fig. 7.11 The amplitude of the Doppler-derived velocity, strain rate, or strain curve is influenced by the insonation angle. When the Doppler beam obliquely impinges on the myocardial wall, the resultant vector (strain) corresponds to a combination of radial, longitudinal, and circumferential strains. When the regions of interest are both parallel to the Doppler beam, as with interventricular septum interrogation, the strain value should normally be approximately the same. It is not uncommon to register a "numerically" abnormal value when interrogating left ventricular walls that would normally create an angle with the Doppler beam. In this example from a normal volunteer, sample volumes are placed at the base (*yellow*) and mid-inferior (aqua) segments in a narrow sector image from apical 2-chamber view. The longitudinal deformation profile displays a peak strain value of 10% (identified by *red arrow*) in the mid-segment and approximately 16% in the basal segment. Poor alignment of the ultrasound beam (approximated by the direction of the *strain length bar in green line*) with the inferior wall (longitudinal deformation is marked by *white broken arrow*) is evident in the images on the *left panel* with the mid-segment creating a more oblique angle with the ultrasound beam. The low numerical longitudinal strain value in the mid-inferior can be explained by the "hybrid effect" of the longitudinal (negative magnitude) and radial (positive magnitude) strain. Thus, care should be taken during acquisition of data sets when interrogating myocardial deformation using this technique. AVO, aortic valve opening; AVC, aortic valve closure

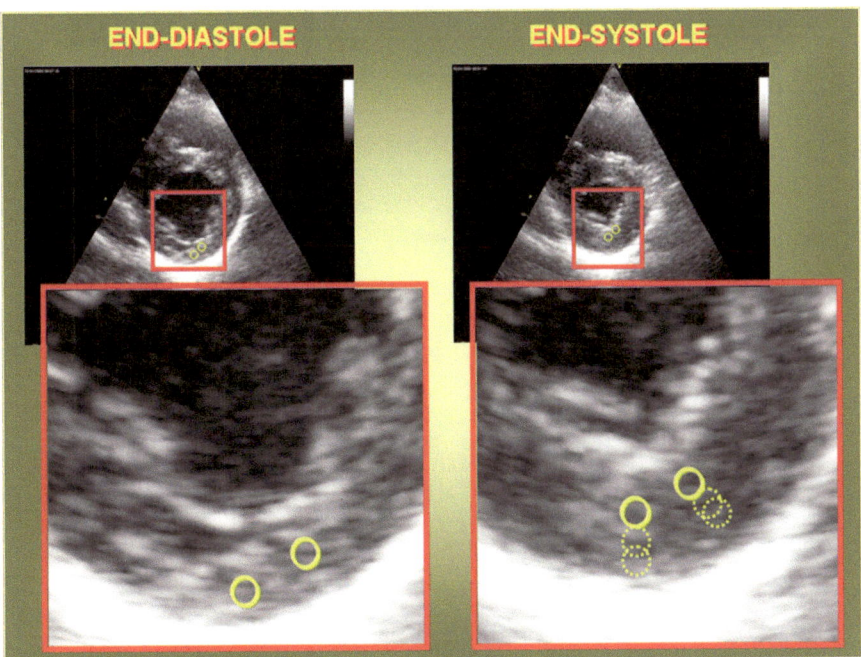

Fig. 7.12 Two-dimensional speckle tracking-derived strain measurement. The interaction of ultrasound with the myocardium produces unique acoustic patterns, or "speckles." These speckles can be tracked overtime and speckle displacement used to calculate tissue velocity and strain. Initial speckle locations (*yellow circles*) are recorded at end-diastole (*left panel*) and tracked over time (*dotted yellow circles*) to their final locations at end-systole (*solid yellow circles in the right panel*). Integration of displacement yields strain where, in turn, strain rate is derived. This technique is relatively *angle-independent* because it is not based on the Doppler principle. However, the technique is inferior to Doppler-based imaging in terms of temporal resolution and may not be accurate in timing mechanical events. Speckle-tracking is performed on B-mode images with a much lower frame rate (40–90 fps) compared to the Doppler-derived imaging where frame rates are high (100–250 fps)

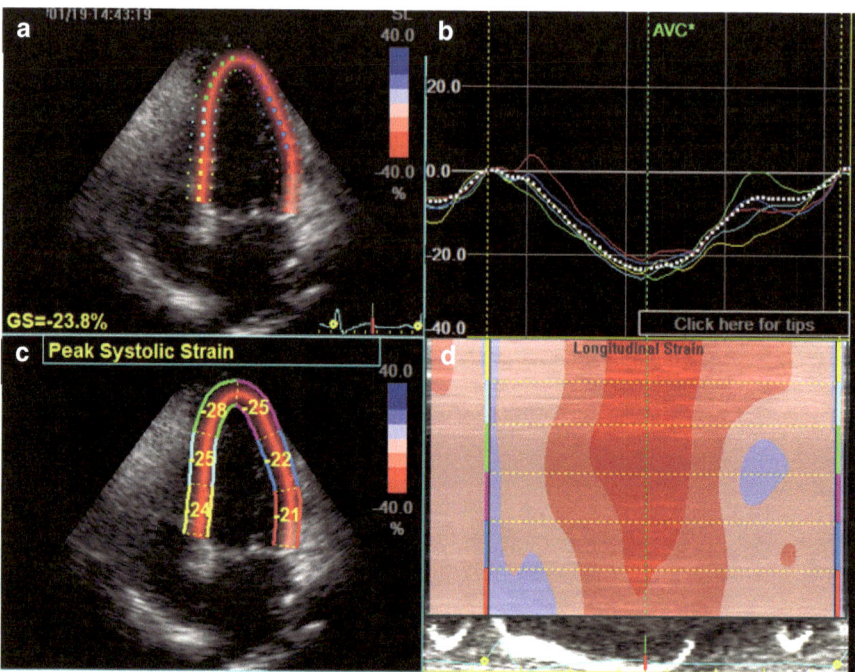

Fig. 7.13 Quad-view of longitudinal strain by speckle-tracking in the LV septum and lateral wall using apical 4-chamber view. Speckle tracking method utilizes automated tracking of the region of interest (ROI). All points in the myocardium are included in the analysis. (**a**) Automated tracking of septum and lateral wall in the apical 4-chamber view. Each segment of the myocardium is color-coded (*dotted line*). The color overlay indicates peak systolic strain along the longitudinal direction per color scale on the right upper corner. (**b**) Longitudinal strain tracings resulting from the analysis of the tracked myocardium in (a). (**c**) Numerical strain values of the corresponding segments. (**d**) Colored M-mode display of the strain analysis. *Dotted lines* (a) and corresponding tracings in (b) *yellow*, basal septum; aqua, mid-septum; green, apical septum; pink, apical lateral wall; blue, mid-lateral wall; red, basal lateral wall. *White dotted line* in (b) corresponds to the global strain

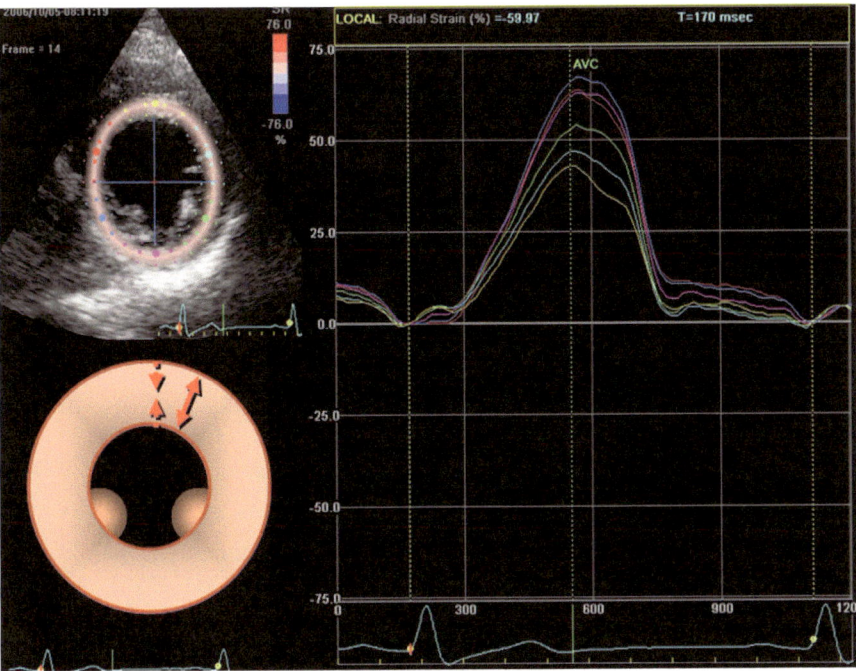

Fig. 7.14 Speckle-tracking allows measurement of radial strain in all LV segments, a great contrast to the Doppler-based technique where only the posterior wall can be interrogated due to issues on insonation angle. Radial strain profile is displayed on a positively directed curve that peaks around end-systole heralded by aortic valve closure (AVC). The schematic diagram on the lower *left panel* indicates the direction of myocardial deformation in systole (*solid arrow*) and diastole (*broken arrows*)

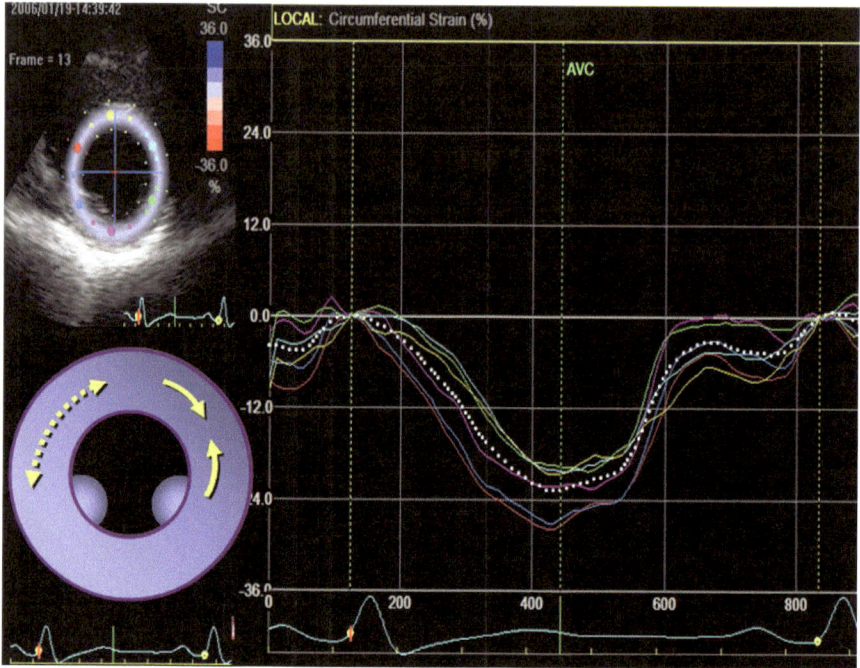

Fig. 7.15 Circumferential strain profile is displayed on a negatively directed curve that peaks around end-systole heralded by aortic valve closure (AVC). The schematic diagram on the *lower left panel* indicates the direction of myocardial deformation in systole (*solid arrow*) and diastole (*broken arrows*). Measurement of circumferential strain via Doppler-based imaging can only be performed on the lateral wall. Speckle-tracking allows measurement of circumferential strain in all LV segments

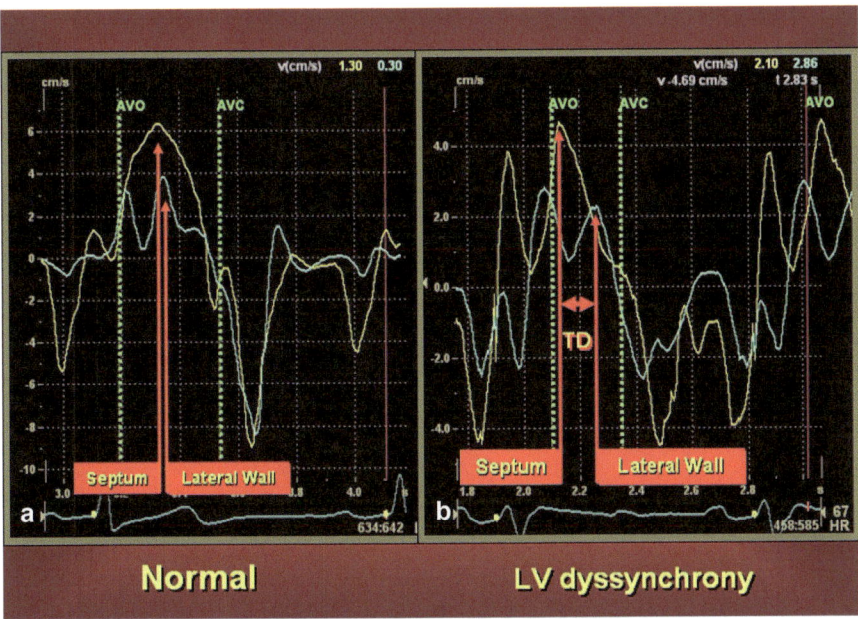

Fig. 7.16 TDI has been routinely applied in dyssynchrony analysis to identify candidates for cardiac resynchronization therapy (CRT) and is found to be superior to strain rate and strain in predicting response. The intraventricular mechanical delay between the early and late segments predicts response to resynchronization. Two criteria more commonly used in the clinical practice are (1) septal to lateral wall delay >65 ms and (2) standard deviation of the time to peak systolic velocity of 12 segments >33 ms. (**a**) In a normal synchronous heart, regional systolic velocities peak almost simultaneously. Here, the timing of the peak systolic velocity of the septum occurred 20 ms earlier than that of the lateral wall. (**b**) In failing hearts with left bundle branch block, the lateral/posterior segment systolic velocity peaks later than septum. Time delay (TD) can be quantified by measuring the difference in the timing of peak systolic velocity between the two opposite walls. In this figure, the septum to lateral wall TD was measured at 110 ms. Alternatively, if one is working on dedicated narrow-sector images (single-wall), TD can be assessed by taking the difference between the time to peak systolic velocities of the basal septum and lateral wall as measured from the onset of electrocardiographic QRS complex

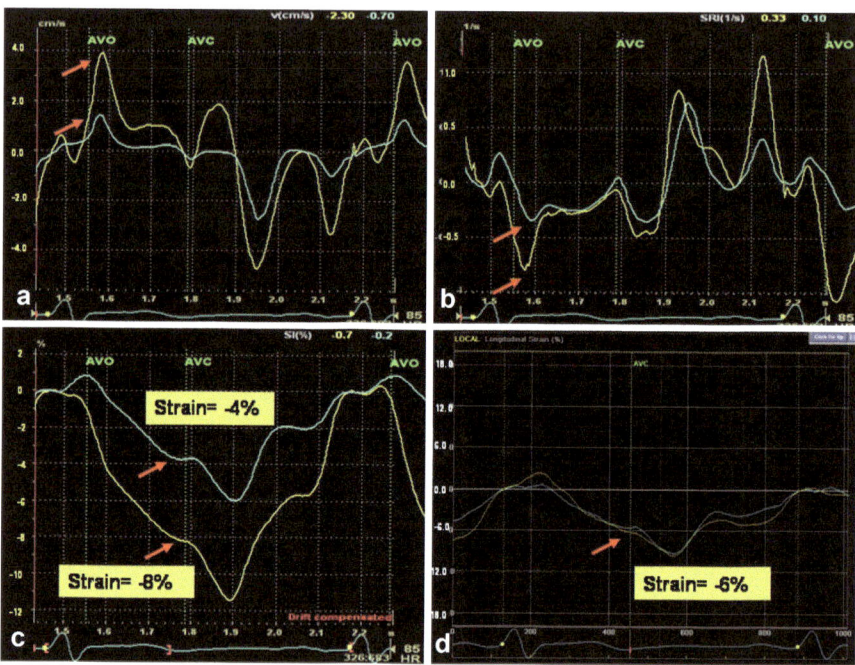

Fig. 7.17 Wall motion can be quantified by TDI or strain echocardiography. Tissue velocities, strain rates and strain are reduced in ischemia and infarction. However, tissue velocity may not accurately reflect regional function due to tethering. Strain and strain rate identify infarcted segment and correlate with the extent of transmural infarction. Both are less susceptible to cardiac translational motion and tethering. It is encouraged to perform multiple mode of regional analysis to confirm findings that may be confounded by some technical limitations set by the method employed. In this representative TDI curve from a patient with anterior MI, (**a**) tissue velocity profile may fail to detect hypokinetic/akinetic segments for reasons explained above. Reduction in the measured Doppler-derived systolic strain rate (**b**) and strain (**c**) may be more reflective of regional wall motion abnormalities. Even so, Doppler-derived indices are dependent on the angle of insonation, and this factor may operate on providing a similar reduction in the numerical values of the respective indices. (**d**) Performing strain analysis by speckle-tracking may eliminate the effect of angle issues and may confirm a true reduction in the myocardial deformation reflected by the Doppler-derived indices

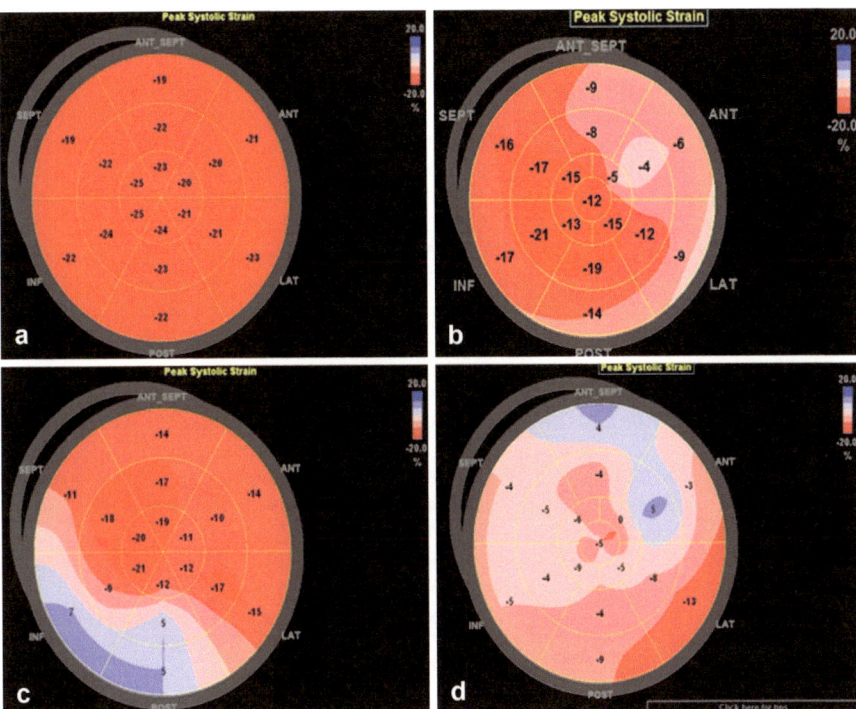

Fig. 7.18 Semiautomated measurements of strain by speckle-tracking allows generation of a color-coded image display such as bull's eye plot of the longitudinal segmental strain. The *strain color code* is depicted in the *upper right-hand* corner of each image. (**a**) Normal volunteer with normal strain (*shades of red*) in all segments. (**b**) Patient with a myocardial infarction related to proximal left-anterior descending artery lesion demonstrating reduced strain in the anterior septum and anterior and lateral LV free walls. (**c**) A patient with inferior–posterior myocardial infarction who demonstrated reduced and abnormal (*shades of blue*) systolic strain in the inferior and posterior walls and preserved strain elsewhere. (**d**) Patient with nonischemic cardiomyopathy demonstrating reduced strain in all segments and abnormal systolic strains in the anterior septum and anterior LV free wall (*shades of blue*)

Recommended Reading

Abraham TP, Dimaano VL, Liang HY. Role of tissue doppler and strain echocardiography in current clinical practice. *Circulation.* 2007;116(22):2597-2609.

Amundsen BH, Helle-Valle T, Edvardsen T, et al. Noninvasive myocardial strain measurement by speckle tracking echocardiography: validation against sonomicrometry and tagged magnetic resonance imaging. *J Am Coll Cardiol.* 2006;47(4):789-793.

Bax JJ, Bleeker GB, Marwick TH, et al. Left ventricular dyssynchrony predicts response and prognosis after cardiac resynchronization therapy. *J Am Coll Cardiol.* 2004;44(9):1834-1840.

Bountioukos M, Schinkel AF, Bax JJ, et al. Pulsed-wave tissue doppler quantification of systolic and diastolic function of viable and nonviable myocardium in patients with ischemic cardiomyopathy. *Am Heart J.* 2004;148(6):1079-1084.

Derumeaux G, Loufoua J, Pontier G, et al. Tissue doppler imaging differentiates transmural from nontransmural acute myocardial infarction after reperfusion therapy. *Circulation.* 2001; 103(4):589-596.

Derumeaux G, Ovize M, Loufoua J, et al. Assessment of nonuniformity of transmural myocardial velocities by color-coded tissue doppler imaging: characterization of normal, ischemic, and stunned myocardium. *Circulation.* 2000;101(12):1390-1395.

Derumeaux G, Ovize M, Loufoua J, et al. Doppler tissue imaging quantitates regional wall motion during myocardial ischemia and reperfusion. *Circulation.* 1998;97(19):1970-1977.

D'hooge J, Heimdal A, Jamal F, et al. Regional strain and strain rate measurements by cardiac ultrasound: principles, implementation and limitations. *Eur J Echocardiogr.* 2000;1(3):154-170.

Garcia MJ. Echocardiographic assessment of left ventricular function. *J Nucl Cardiol.* 2006; 13(2):280-293.

Gilman G, Khandheria BK, Hagen ME, et al. Strain rate and strain: a step-by-step approach to image and data acquisition. *J Am Soc Echocardiogr.* 2004;17(9):1011-1020.

Gorcsan J 3rd, Strum DP, Mandarino WA, et al. Quantitative assessment of alterations in regional left ventricular contractility with color-coded tissue doppler echocardiography. Comparison with sonomicrometry and pressure-volume relations. *Circulation.* 1997;95(10):2423-2433.

Haddad F, Hunt S, Rosenthal D, et al. Right ventricular function in cardiovascular disease, part I: anatomy, physiology, aging, and functional assessment of the right ventricle. *Circulation.* 2008;117(12):1436-1448.

Kukulski T, Voigt JU, Wilkenshoff UM, et al. A comparison of regional myocardial velocity information derived by pulsed and color doppler techniques: An in vitro and in vivo study. *Echocardiography.* 2000;17(7):639-651.

Leitman M, Lysyansky P, Sidenko S, et al. Two-dimensional strain-a novel software for real-time quantitative echocardiographic assessment of myocardial function. *J Am Soc Echocardiogr.* 2004;17(10):1021-1029.

Madler CF, Payne N, Wilkenshoff U, et al. Non-invasive diagnosis of coronary artery disease by quantitative stress echocardiography: optimal diagnostic models using off-line tissue doppler in the MYDISE study. *Eur Heart J.* 2003;24(17):1584-1594.

Marwick TH, Case C, Leano R, et al. Use of tissue doppler imaging to facilitate the prediction of events in patients with abnormal left ventricular function by dobutamine echocardiography. *Am J Cardiol.* 2004;93(2):142-146.

McCulloch M, Zoghbi WA, Davis R, et al. Color tissue doppler myocardial velocities consistently underestimate spectral tissue doppler velocities: Impact on calculation peak transmitral pulsed doppler velocity/early diastolic tissue doppler velocity (E/Ea). *J Am Soc Echocardiogr.* 2006;19(6):744-748.

McDicken WN, Sutherland GR, Moran CM, et al. Colour doppler velocity imaging of the myocardium. *Ultrasound Med Biol.* 1992;18(6–7):651-654.

Miyatake K, Yamagishi M, Tanaka N, et al. New method for evaluating left ventricular wall motion by color-coded tissue doppler imaging: in vitro and in vivo studies. *J Am Coll Cardiol.* 1995;25(3):717-724.

Nagueh SF, Middleton KJ, Kopelen HA, et al. Doppler tissue imaging: a noninvasive technique for evaluation of left ventricular relaxation and estimation of filling pressures. *J Am Coll Cardiol.* 1997;30(6):1527-1533.

Ommen SR, Nishimura RA, Appleton CP, et al. Clinical utility of doppler echocardiography and tissue doppler imaging in the estimation of left ventricular filling pressures: a comparative simultaneous doppler-catheterization study. *Circulation.* 2000;102(15):1788-1794.

Pauliks LB, Vogel M, Madler CF, et al. Regional response of myocardial acceleration during iso-volumic contraction during dobutamine stress echocardiography: a color tissue doppler study and comparison with angiocardiographic findings. *Echocardiography.* 2005;22(10):797-808.

Perk G, Tunick PA, Kronzon I. Non-doppler two-dimensional strain imaging by echocardiogra-phy–from technical considerations to clinical applications. *J Am Soc Echocardiogr.* 2007;20(3): 234-243.

Rushmere RF, Crystal DK, Wagner C. The functional anatomy of ventricular contraction. *Circ Res.* 1953;1(2):162-170.

Sutherland GR, Bijnens B, McDicken WN. Tissue doppler echocardiography: historical perspec-tive and technological considerations. *Echocardiography.* 1999;16(5):445-453.

Sutherland GR, Di Salvo G, Claus P, et al. Strain and strain rate imaging: a new clinical approach to quantifying regional myocardial function. *J Am Soc Echocardiogr.* 2004;17(7):788-802.

Urheim S, Edvardsen T, Torp H, et al. Myocardial strain by Doppler echocardiography. Validation of a new method to quantify regional myocardial function. *Circulation.* 2000;102(10):1158-1164.

Weidemann F, Wacker C, Rauch A, et al. Sequential changes of myocardial function during acute myocardial infarction, in the early and chronic phase after coronary intervention described by ultrasonic strain rate imaging. *J Am Soc Echocardiogr.* 2006;19(7):839-847.

Wilkenshoff UM, Sovany A, Wigstrom L, et al. Regional mean systolic myocardial velocity esti-mation by real-time color doppler myocardial imaging: a new technique for quantifying regional systolic function. *J Am Soc Echocardiogr.* 1998;11(7):683-692.

Yu CM, Zhang Q, Chan YS, et al. Tissue doppler velocity is superior to displacement and strain mapping in predicting left ventricular reverse remodelling response after cardiac resynchroni-sation therapy. *Heart.* 2006;92(10):1452-1456.

Van de Veire N, De Sutter J, Bax JJ et al. Technological advances tissue doppler imaging echocar-diography. Heart. 2008;Aug;94(8):1065-1074

Transesophageal Echocardiography

8

Julie A. Humphries, Christopher J. Kramer, Partho P. Sengupta, and Bijoy K. Khandheria

Transesophageal echocardiography (TEE) involves ultrasound imaging of cardiovascular system from the confines of the gastroesophageal track. This helps reduce signal attenuation and permits the use of higher ultrasound frequencies, thereby providing an enhanced spatial resolution. TEE is currently used in approximately 5–10% of patients being evaluated in the cardiovascular ultrasound imaging and hemodynamic laboratory.

8.1
Protocol for TEE

Fasting based on conscious sedation guidelines, an intravenous access, careful history to rule out presence of laryngeal or gastroesophageal diseases, and removal of dentures are prerequisites.

- Absolute contraindications to TEE include esophageal stricture, diverticulum, tumor, and recent esophageal or gastric surgery.
- Topical spray, intravenous sedation, a drying agent to minimize oral secretion, and use of appropriate lubrication are helpful.
- Before the introduction of the scope into the esophagus, the array is rotated to 0° to place the transducer into a conventional transverse plane. A bite guard is used always unless the patient is edentulous. The tip of the transducer is advanced into the esophagus gently without force and stopped if any resistance is encountered. After moving the transducer into the desired location, the probe is manipulated to orient the imaging planes for obtaining the desired cross-sectional images.
- Although each of the views represents echocardiographic image in cross section, moving the probes through the entire extent of a structure permits a rapid three-dimensional evaluation of cardiac structures.

J.A. Humphries (✉)
Department of Cardiology, Heart Care Partners, Greenslopes, Queensland, Australia
e-mail: jhumphries@heartcarepartners.com.au

T.P. Abraham (ed.), *Case Based Echocardiography*,
DOI: 10.1007/978-1-84996-151-6_8, © Springer-Verlag London Limited 2011

Procedural risks are low in trained hands. However, they need to be explained clearly to the patient. These include transient throat pain, laryngospasm, aspiration, hypotension, hypertension, tachycardia, mucosal bleeding, esophageal rupture, and rare risk of death. Benzocaine topical spary can cause toxic methemoglobinemia. The treatment is administration of methylene blue in addition to supportive measures. Being semi-invasive, appropriate training requirements are needed and have been laid down by both, the American Society of Echocardiography and the British Society of Echocardiography.

8.2
Standard TEE views

Normal cardiac structures seen on different transesophageal views (Table 8.1) are shown in Figs. 8.1–8.20. Figure 8.21 shows maneuvers utilized for delineation of flow across inter-atrial septum. Transgastric views are shown in Figs. 8.22–8.28.

8.3
Application of TEE

In addition to the usual indications for TEE (suspected endocarditis, source of embolus, and suspected aortic dissection), there are several indications that are unique to critical care patients. These include:

1. Assessment of unexplained hypotension
2. Suspected massive pulmonary embolism
3. Unexplained hypoxemia
4. Complications of cardiothoracic surgery

Less common indications for TEE in the critical care unit include continuous hemodynamic monitoring, evaluation of potential transplant donors, and guidance of central-line placement. The recent development of transnasal TEE probes may allow for monitoring in the awake patient. The potential benefits of the transnasal probe include less risk for esophageal trauma in patients with varices or coagulopathies and less need for sedation in those with compromised respiratory or hemodynamic status. Figures 8.29–8.35 show clinical examples where incremental use of advanced techniques in TEE has been illustrated.

Table 8.1 Transesophageal echocardiography cross sections (Reproduced with permission from the recommendations of American Society of Echocardiography)

Window (depth from incisors)	Cross section	Multiplane angle range	Structures imaged
Upper esophageal (20–25 cm)	Aortic arch long axis (s)	0°	Aortic arch, left brachio v
	Aortic arch short axis	90°	Aortic arch, PA, PV, left brachio v
Mid-esophageal (30–40 cm)	Four-chamber	0°–20°	LV, LA, RV, RA, MV, TV, IAS
	Mitral commissural	60°–70°	MV, LV, LA
	Two-chamber	80°–100°	LV, LA, LAA, MV, CS
	Long axis	120°–160°	LV, LA, AV, LVOT, MV, asc aorta
	RV inflow-outflow	60°–90°	RV, RA, TV, RVOT, PV, PA
	AV short axis	30°–60°	AV, IAS, coronary ostia, LVOT, PV
	AV long axis	120°–160°	AV, LVOT, prox asc aorta, right PA
	Bicaval	80°–110°	RA, SVC, IVC, IAS, LA
	Asc aortic short axis	0°–60°	Asc aorta, SVC, PA, right PA
	Asc aortic long axis	100°–150°	Asc aorta, right PA
	Desc aorta short axis	0°	Desc thoracic aorta, left pleural space
	Desc aorta long axis	90°–110°	Desc thoracic aorta, left pleural space
Transgastric (40–45 cm)	Basal short axis	0°–20°	LV, MV, RV, TV
	Mid short axis	0°–20°	LV, RV, pap mm
	Two-chamber	80°–100°	LV, MV, chordae, pap mm, CS, LA
	Long axis	90°–120°	LVOT, AV, MV
	RV inflow	100°–120°	RV, TV, RA, TV chordae, pap mm
Deep transgastric (45–50 cm)	Long axis	0°–20° (anteflexion)	LVOT, AV, asc aorta, arch

Brachio v Brachiocephalic vein, *PA* pulmonary artery, *PV* pulmonic valve, *LV* left ventricle, *LA* left atrium, *RV* right ventricle, *RA* right atrium, *MV* mitral valve, *TV* tricuspid valve, *IAS* inter atrial septum, *LAA* left atrial appendage, *CS* coronary sinus, *AV* aortic valve, *LVOT* left ventricular outflow tract, *prox* proximal, *RVOT* right ventricular outflow tract, *SVC* superior vena cava, *IVC* inferior vena cava, *RPA* right pulmonary artery, *asc* ascending, *desc* descending, *pap mm* papillary muscles

Fig. 8.1 Four chamber
mid-esophageal view.
LA left atrium, *LV* left
ventricle, *RA* right atrium,
RV right ventricle

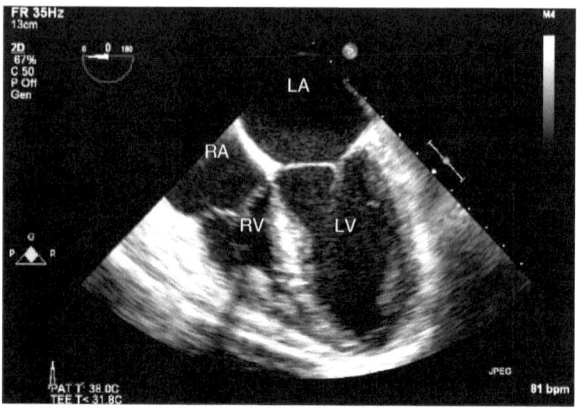

Fig. 8.2 Two chamber
mid-esophageal view.
LA left atrium, *LV* left
ventricle

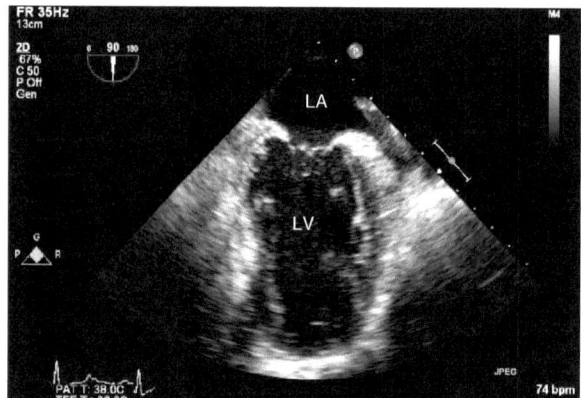

Fig. 8.3 Long axis mid-
esophageal view. *LA* left
atrium, *LV* left ventricle,
AO aorta

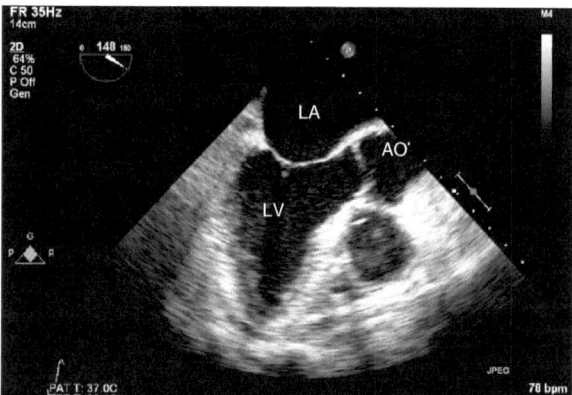

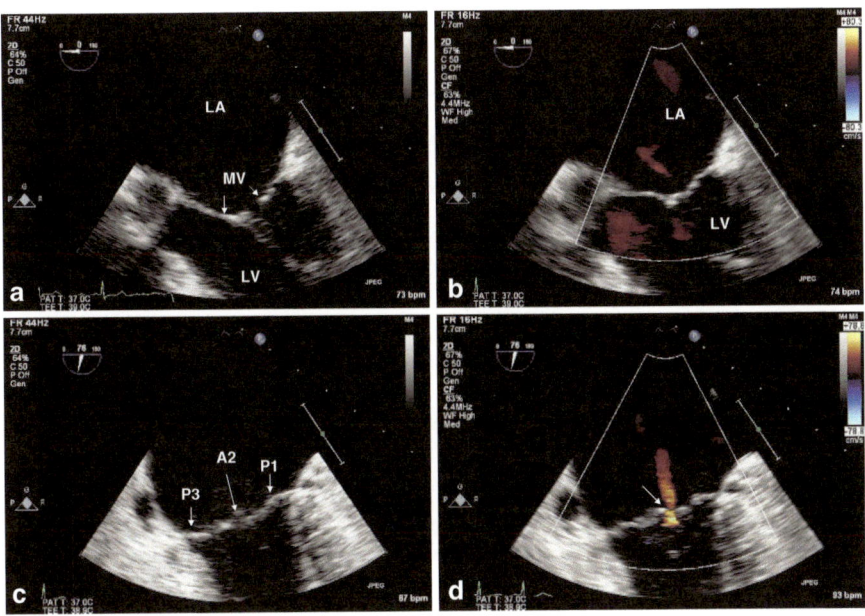

Fig. 8.4 (**a**) Mitral valve 0° view. *LA* left atrium, *LV* left ventricle, *MV* mitral valve. (**b**) Mitral valve at 0 degrees with color Doppler. (**c**) Mitral valve "drop out" view at 76° (usually best seen 60–80°) and shows P3, A2 and P1 segments of the mitral valve leaflets. (**d**) "Drop out" view of mitral valve showing mid A2 segment regurgitation

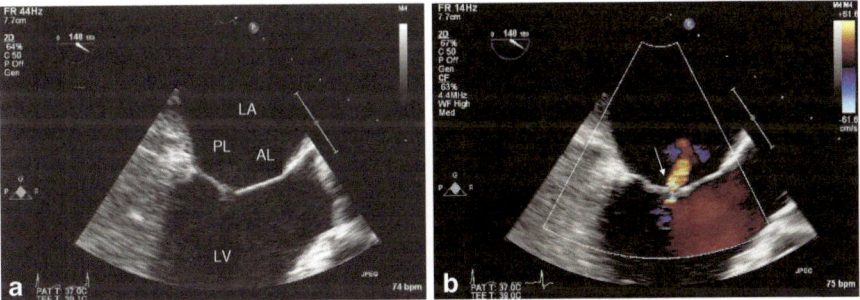

Fig. 8.5 (**a**) Long axis view of the mitral valve. *AL* anterior leaflet, *PL* posterior leaflet. (**b**) Long axis mitral valve view shows mild mitral regurgitation on color flow Doppler

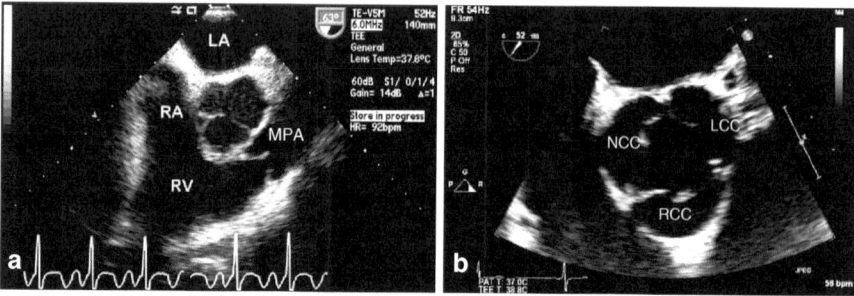

Fig. 8.6 (**a**) Short axis mid-esophageal view at approximately 60°. The trileaflet aortic valve (center) and pulmonary valve (arrow) are both seen. *MPA* main pulmonary artery, *RV* right ventricle, *RA* right atrium, *LA* left atrium. (**b**) Zoomed up view of the open trileaflet aortic valve. The left main coronary artery (*arrow*) arises from the left coronary cusp (*LCC*). *RCC* right coronary cusp, *NCC* non-coronary cusp

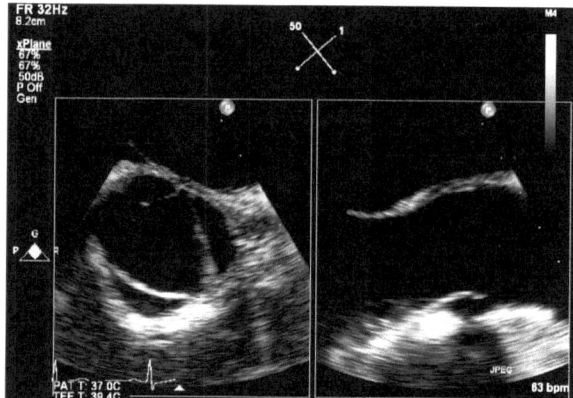

Fig. 8.7 Two-dimensional biplane view of the open trileaflet aortic valve. Views are at 90° orthogonal to each other using the 3D tranesophageal probe

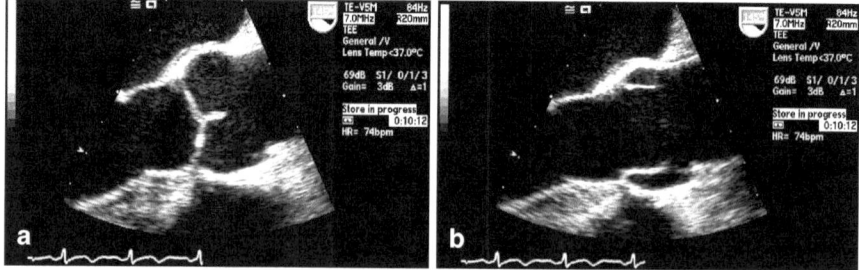

Fig. 8.8 (**a**) Long axis view at 145° showing closed aortic valve in long axis. (**b**) Long axis view at 145° showing open aortic valve

Fig. 8.9 Aortic root and
ascending aorta. This view
is achieved by withdrawing
the probe and reducing the
multiplane angle to
110–120°

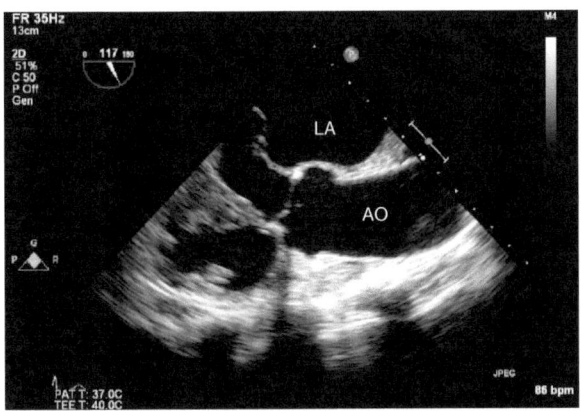

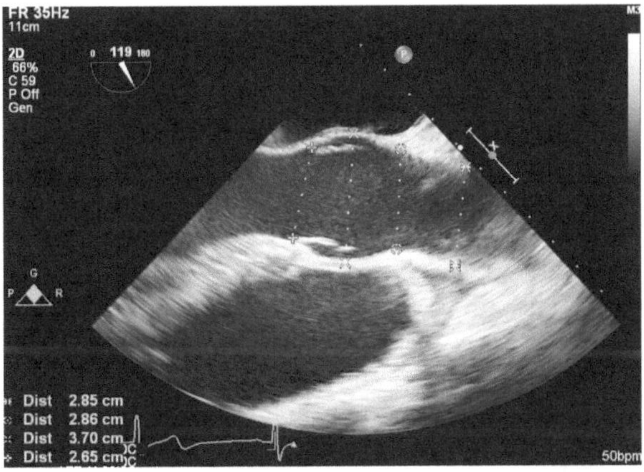

Fig. 8.10 Aortic root
dimensions (from left
to right): aortic annulus,
trans-sinus diameter,
sino-tubular junction,
proximal ascending aorta

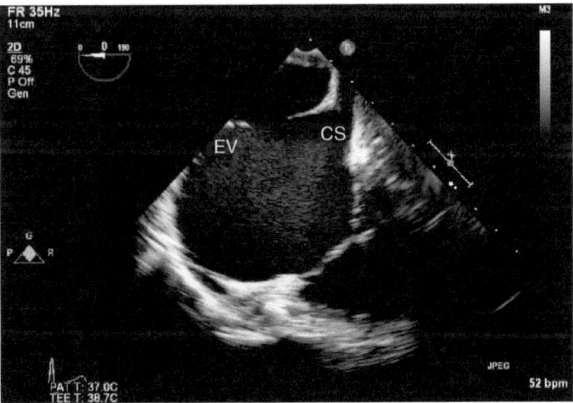

Fig. 8.11 Standard lower-
esophageal view of the
tricuspid valve (at 0°). There
is a Eustachian valve (*EV*)
seen here. The coronary
sinus (*CS*) is also seen

Fig. 8.12 Tricuspid valve
(*arrows*) seen at 52°. This
is often a good position for
color Doppler tricuspid
regurgitation signal

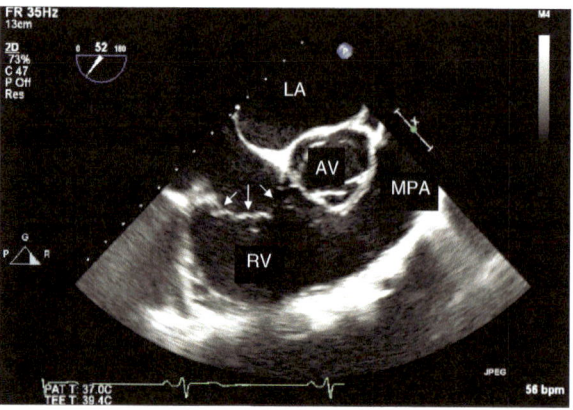

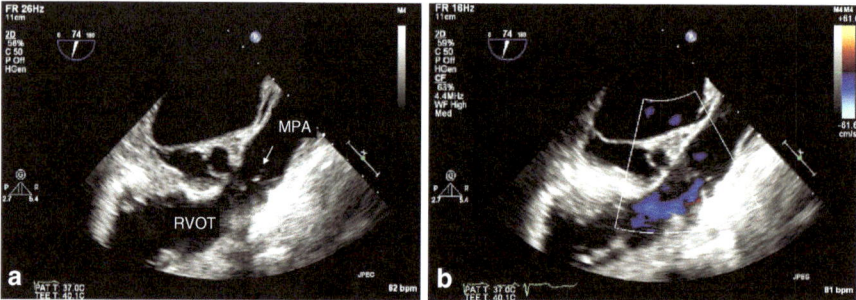

Fig. 8.13 (**a**) Mid-esophageal view of right ventricular outflow tract, pulmonary valve (*arrow*) and
main pulmonary artery seen at 74°. (**b**) Pulmonary regurgitation color Doppler in the same view

Fig. 8.14 Biplane imaging
through the pulmonary valve
with color Doppler shows
the pulmonary valve in short
axis (*right panel*) with
central regurgitation

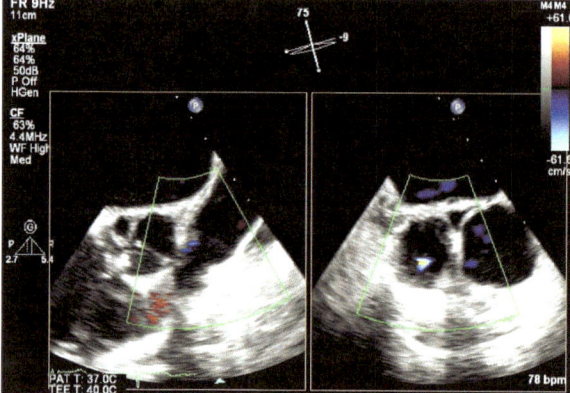

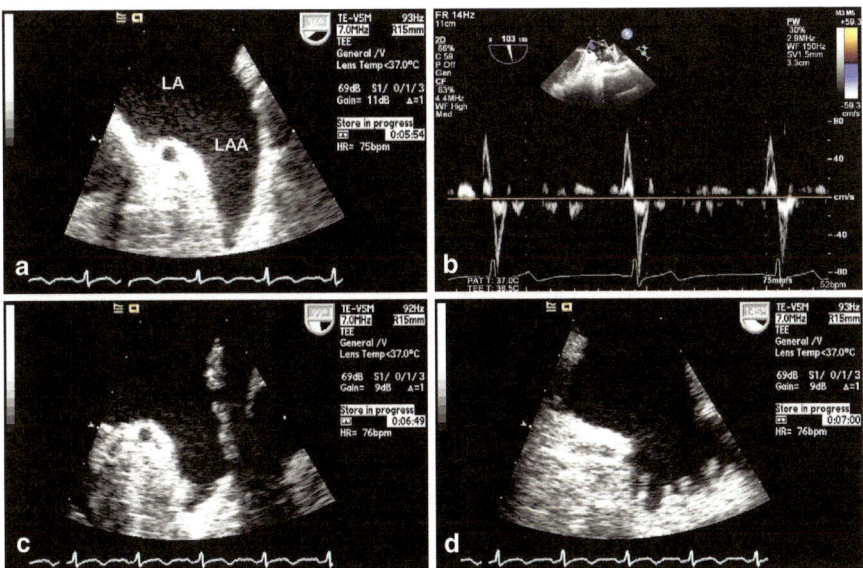

Fig. 8.15 (**a**) Left atrial appendage seen in the mid-esophageal view (36°). This is an optimal view for Pulse Wave Doppler sample placement. No thrombus seen. The coronary sinus (*arrow*) is seen coursing between the left atrial appendage and the annulus of the mitral valve. (**b**) Pulse wave Doppler signal approximately 1 cm into the mouth of the left atrial appendage demonstrating normal velocities. Signals above the line and corresponding with the P wave are ejection velocities, and below the line are filling velocities. Velocities above 0.35m/s are less likely to develop thrombus. (**c**) Further left atrial appendage views on multiplane imaging. It is important to image the left atrial appendage in multiple planes as multilobed left atrial appendage can have thrombus in a lobe not seen in other planes. This example is free of thrombus. (**d**) Left atrial appendage multiplane view at 145° shows prominent pectinate muscles which can sometimes be confused with thrombus

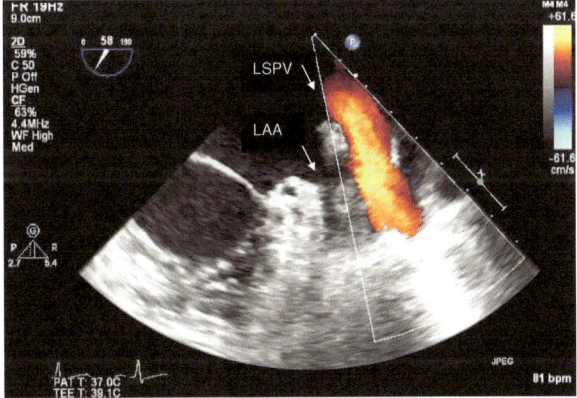

Fig. 8.16 Left superior pulmonary vein seen with color flow Doppler. It lies adjacent to the left atrial appendage separated by the "Q tip"

Fig. 8.17 Biplane color imaging of the left superior pulmonary vein orifice allows for easy identification of the left inferior pulmonary vein (*LIPV*) seen in the *right panel*

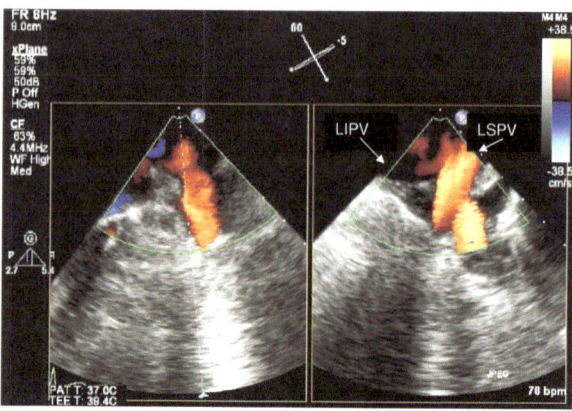

Fig. 8.18 Right superior, middle and inferior pulmonary veins seen on color flow imaging

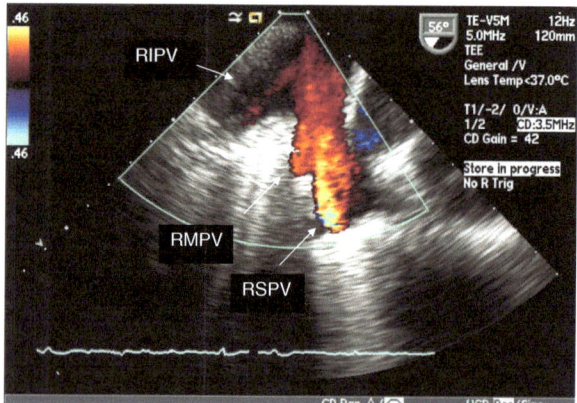

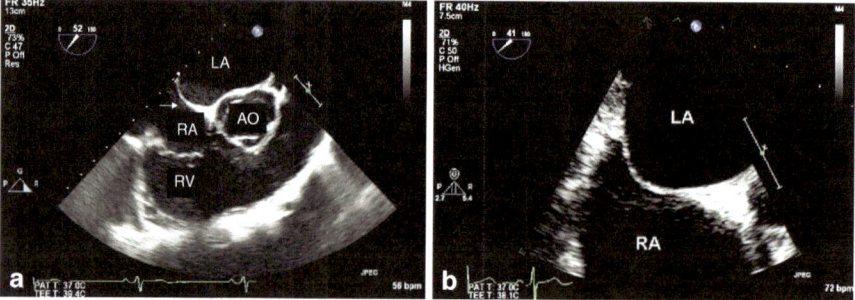

Fig. 8.19 (**a**) Interatrial septum (*arrow*). This view demonstrates the retroaortic part of the interatrial septum which represents the most superior aspect. (**b**) Interatrial septum (zoomed up view from previous image)

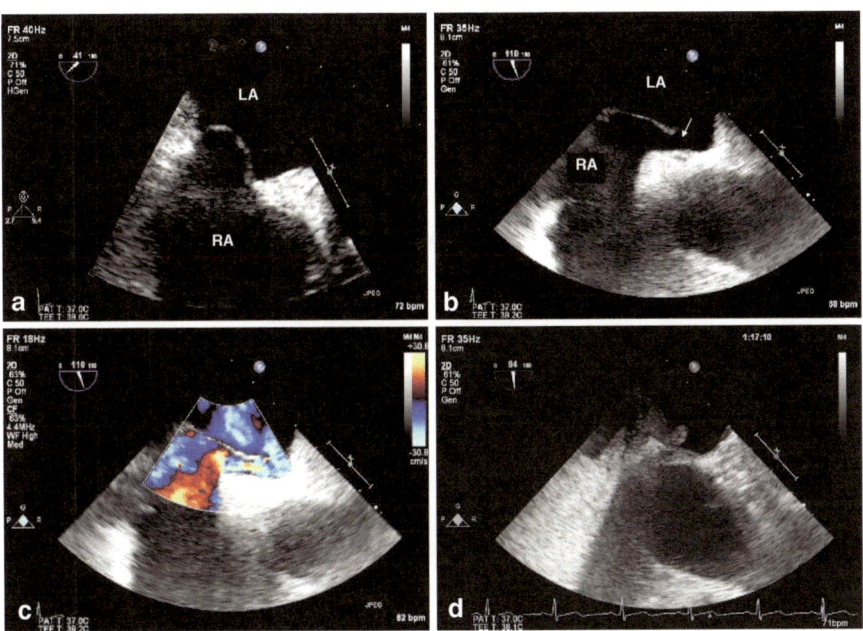

Fig. 8.20 (**a**) Interatrial septum seen bowing towards the left atrium in the setting of raised right atrial pressure during inspiration. (**b**) Large patent foramen ovale (*arrow*). (**c**) Left to right color flow seen through large patent foramen ovale. (**d**) Bubble contrast seen coming through patent foramen ovale during valsalva demonstrating right to left shunting

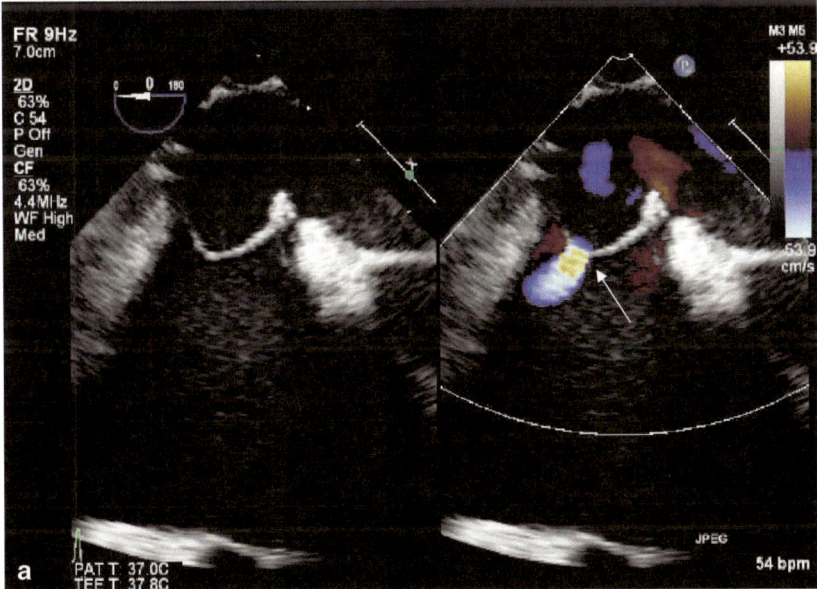

Fig. 8.21 (**a**) Small secundum ASD with and without color flow Doppler. Color imaging shows small left to right shunt (*arrow*) (**b**) Patient with a PFO and an ASD which is very posterior. Separate communications and shunting can be seen on the two images (a) and (b)

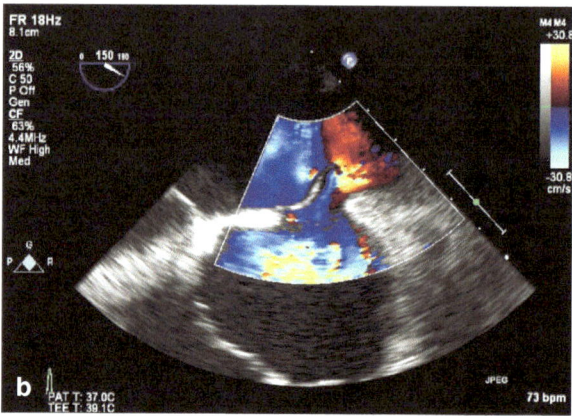

Fig. 8.21 (continued)

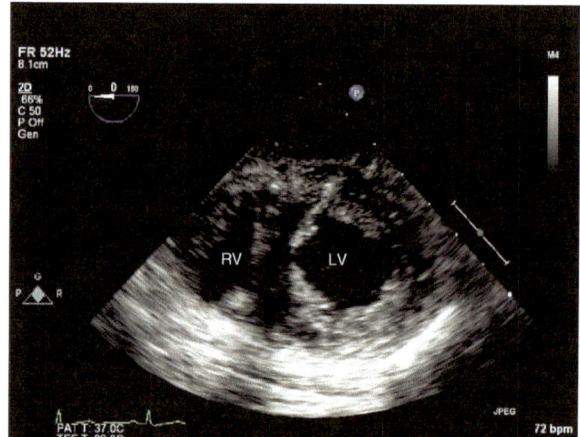

Fig. 8.22 Standard transesophageal transgastric view showing the left ventricle in short axis at the mid ventricular level

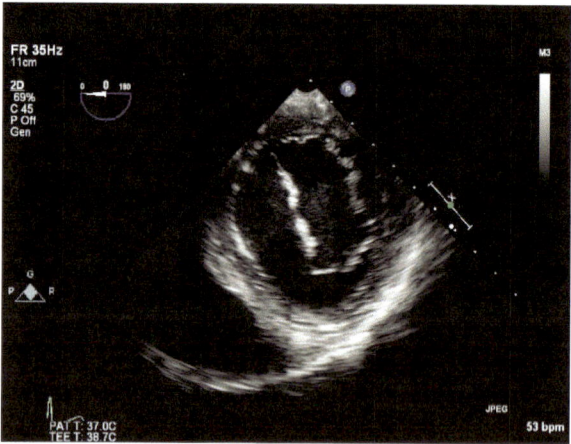

Fig. 8.23 Transgastric view of the left ventricle at the level of the mitral valve seen in short axis (valve open)

Fig. 8.24 Transgastric view of the left ventricle in the long axis (87°). This view gives good information about the subvalvular apparatus

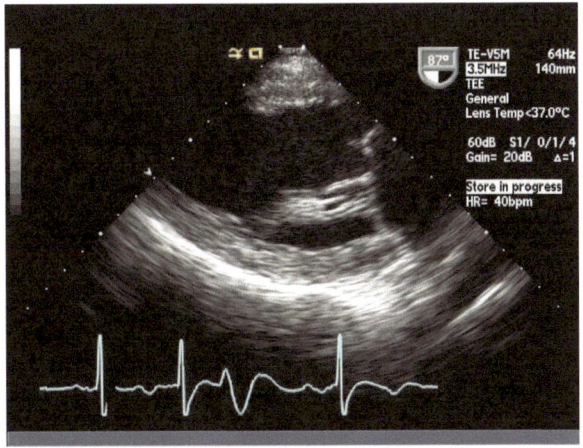

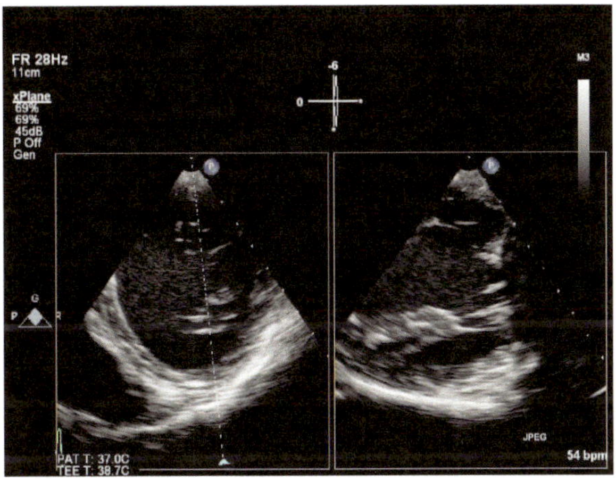

Fig. 8.25 Transgastric biplane view through the mitral valve which shows the valve in short and long axis simultaneously, with detailed subvalvular apparatus examination

Fig. 8.26 Transgastric view of the open tricuspid valve (*arrows*) in the short axis (*left panel*) and long axis (*right panel*)

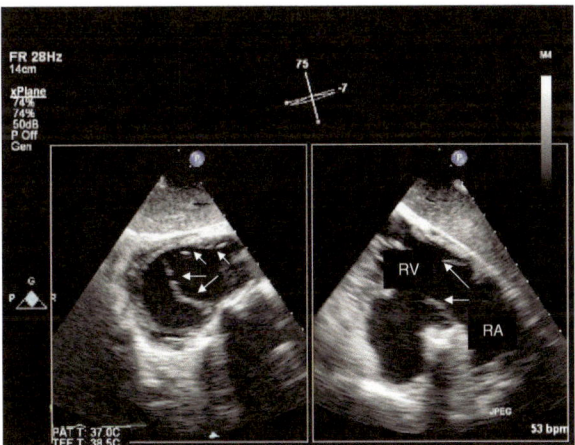

Fig. 8.27 Transgastric view of right ventricular inflow and outflow. *RA* right atrium, *RV* right ventricle, *AO* aorta, *MPA* main pulmonary artery

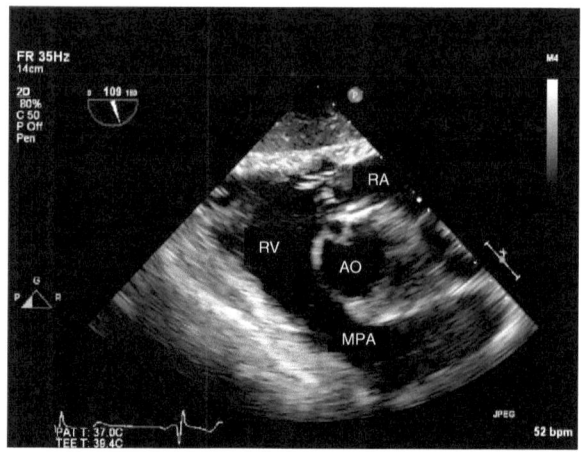

Fig. 8.28 Inferior vena cava (*IVC*) in long axis seen via the deep transgastric view at 48°. *HV* hepatic vein

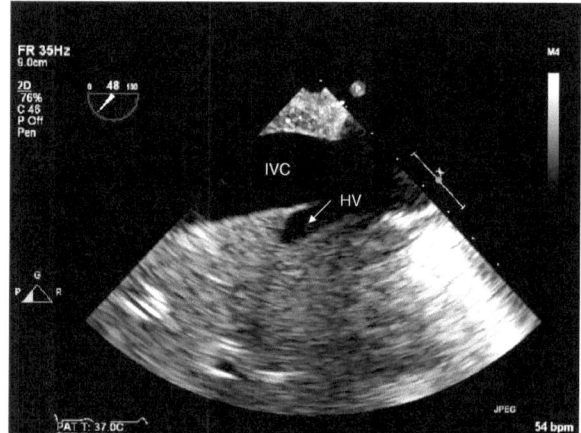

Fig. 8.29 52 year old male for routine kidney transplant workup. Incidental finding of mass on mitral valve anterior leaflet. Histological surgical specimen showed non-bacterial thrombotic endocarditis

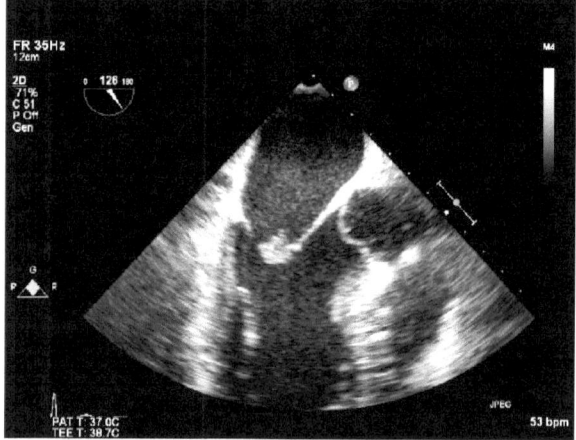

Fig. 8.30 Biplane imaging of the anterior leaflet mass

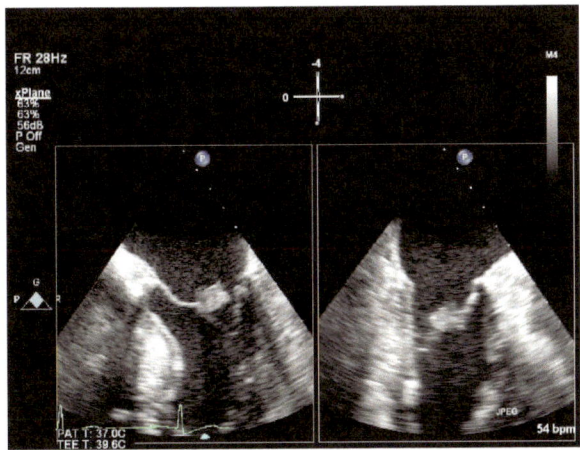

Fig. 8.31 Color imaging showing mitral regurgitation around the mass

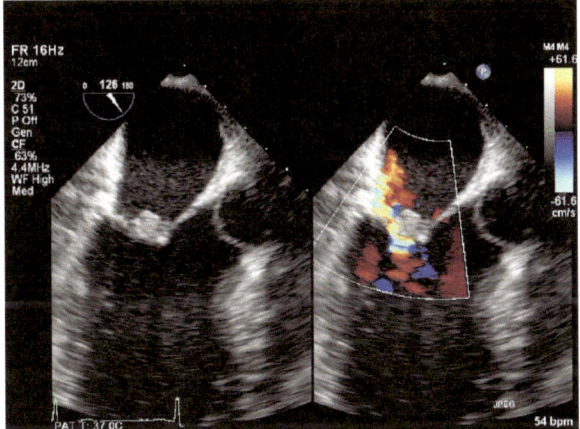

Fig. 8.32 Three-dimensional imaging of the anterior mitral valve leaflet mass from the left atrial perspective at valve closure

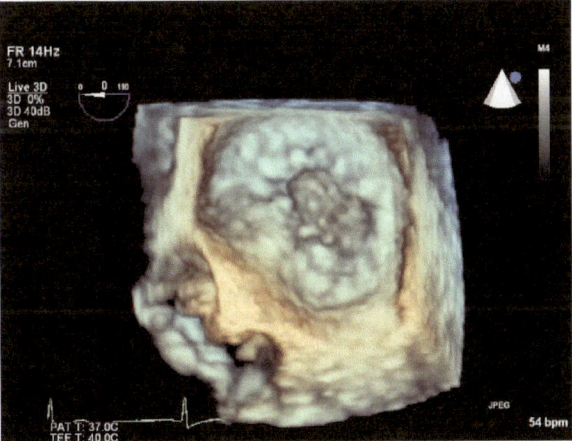

Fig. 8.33 Three-dimensional transesophageal imaging of the anterior mitral valve leaflet mass from the left ventricular perspective, showing involvement of the atrial surface on the leaflet

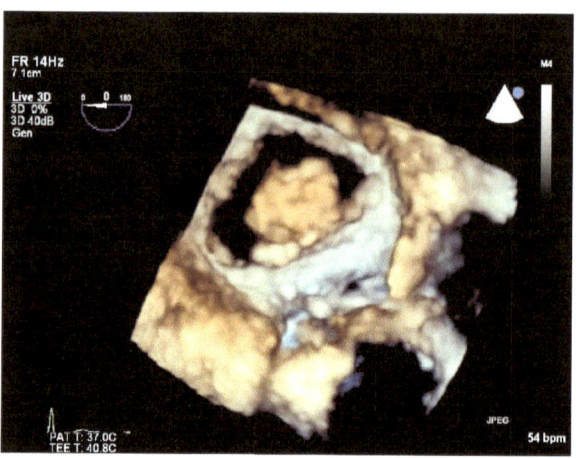

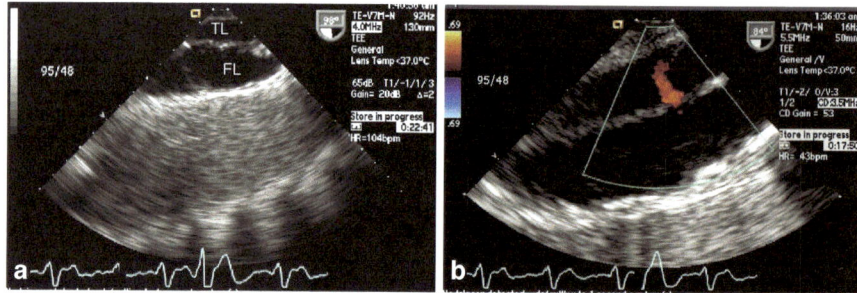

Fig. 8.34 (**a**) Type I Aortic Dissection, Ascending Aorta True Lumen (*TL*) (Superior), False Lumen (*FL*) (Inferior). (**b**) Type I Aortic Dissection, Ascending Aorta with color, Color flowing into false lumen True Lumen (*TL*) (Inferior), False Lumen (*FL*) (Superior)

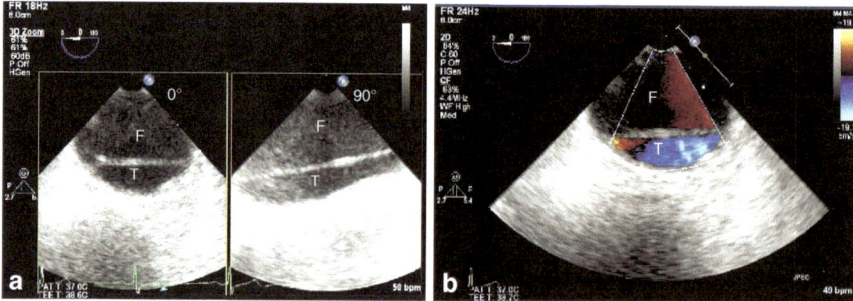

Fig. 8.35 (**a**) Type III Aortic dissection, Short Axis view with color, True lumen (*T*) (Inferior) False lumen (*F*) (Superior). (**b**) Type III Aortic dissection, Short Axis view with color, True lumen (*T*) (Inferior), False lumen (*F*) (Superior)

8.4
Pitfalls

TEE needs expertise for avoiding potential erroneous diagnosis resulting from misinterpretation of normal and abnormal anatomy.

- *Air* within the esophagus and stomach, or an air-filled trachea and bronchi intervening between probe and cardiac structures can consistently produce artifacts or interfere with certain tomographic views (Fig. 8.36).
- *Reverberation signals* or ghost shadows are common and result from impedance mismatch resulting in linear artifacts most commonly seen in the upper ascending and mid-descending aorta. Imaging of the upper ascending aorta with the horizontal plane is limited by a blind spot caused by interposed bronchus between the esophagus and upper ascending aorta.
- *Normal anatomy* may be interpreted abnormal. These include muscular trabeculations in the atrial appendage mistaken as mass or thrombus, the terminal portion of the partition between the left atrial appendage and left upper pulmonary vein appearing as a globular mass, fat-laden fossa ovalis or lipomatous hypertrophy of the atrial septum interpreted as a mass, and surgical sutures appearing filamentous or pedunculated and interpreted as mass or vegetations.
- *"Echo-free spaces"*: Certain normal structures generate echo-free spaces and may be incorrectly interpreted as cysts or abscesses. These include the transverse and the oblique sinus.
- *Other difficulties* that may be encountered during TEE include the adequate visualization and quantification of aortic valve regurgitation, aortic valve and pulmonary valve gradient estimation, and non-foreshortened visualization of the left ventricular apex.
- Finally, ultrasound transducers generate heat. During prolonged monitoring, the device may be required to be shut down periodically to allow cooling.

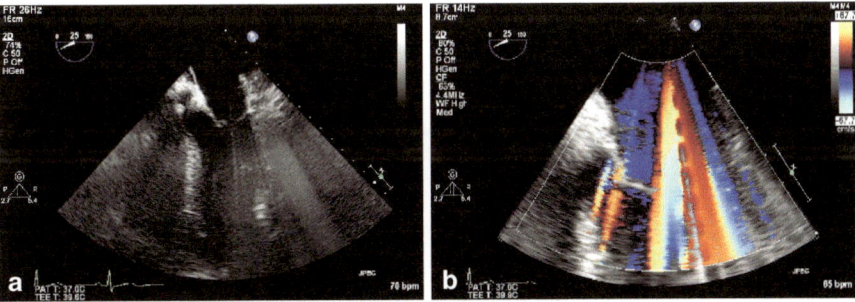

Fig. 8.36 (a) Example of artifact in the mid-esophageal view which interferes with image quality. Artifact can result from poor contact, presence of air in the esophagus, or from intracardiac structures of high density. (b) Example of color flow imaging artifact resulting from esophageal air interfering with probe contact

Intraoperative Transesophageal Echocardiography

9

Alina Nicoara and Madhav Swaminathan

A. Nicoara (✉)
Department of Anesthesiology, Yale University School of Medicine, West Haven, CT, USA
e-mail:alina.nicoara@yale.edu

T.P. Abraham (ed.), *Case Based Echocardiography*,
DOI: 10.1007/978-1-84996-151-6_9, © Springer-Verlag London Limited 2011

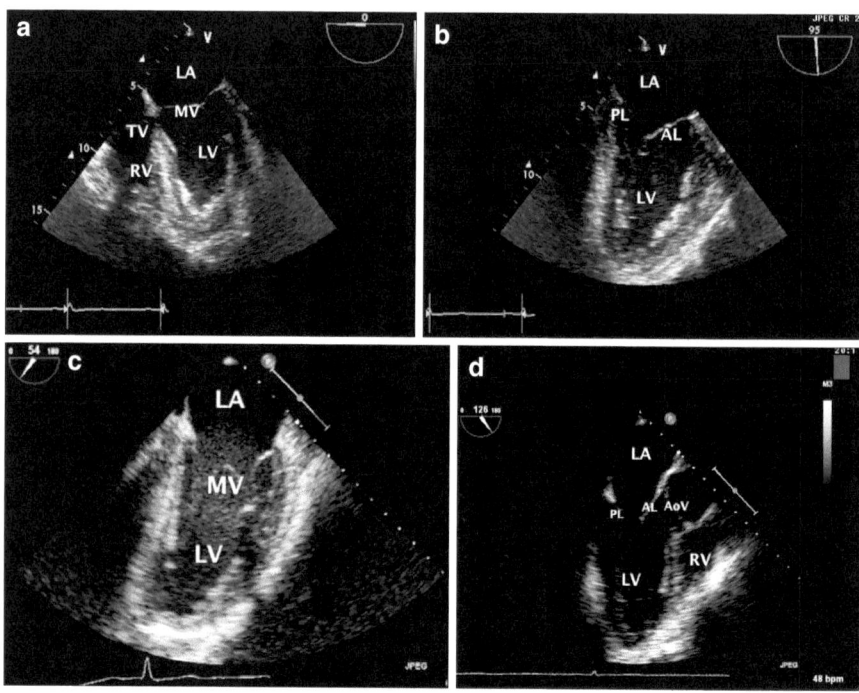

Fig. 9.1 At the mid-esophageal level, at an imaging depth of about 35 cm, several tomographic views can be obtained by adjusting the imaging angle. (**a**) Mid-esophageal four-chamber view (ME 4-Ch) is obtained at an imaging angle between 0° and 20° with slight retroflexion of the tip of the probe. This image shows the 4-Ch as well as the mitral and tricuspid valves and it is used to assess the size and function of the heart chambers and the structure and function of the valves. It is the usual starting point for most intraoperative imaging (*RA*, right atrium; *LA*, left atrium; *RV*, right ventricle; *LV*, left ventricle; *MV*, mitral valve; *TV*, tricuspid valve). (**b**) Mid-esophageal two chamber view (ME 2Ch) is obtained from the same position by advancing the multiplane angle to about 90°. It visualizes the mitral valve, the anterior and inferior walls of the LV as well as the apical cap, AL, anterior leaflet of the mitral valve; Pl, posterior leaflet of the mitral valve. (**c**) The mid-esophageal mitral commissural view is obtained at an imaging angle of about 60° and is used mainly to assess the structure and function of the mitral valve. The A2 segment of the anterior leaflet is seen in the middle of the image, while the P3 and P1 segments are seen on the left and right sides of the image, respectively. (**d**) The mid-esophageal long-axis view (ME LAX) at an imaging angle from 120° to 130° is mostly used to evaluate the motion of the anteroseptal (*right side of the image*) and inferolateral walls (*left side*) of the LV; presence of structural abnormalities of the MV such as prolapsed or flail leaflets and LV outflow tract pathology (*AoV*, aortic valve)

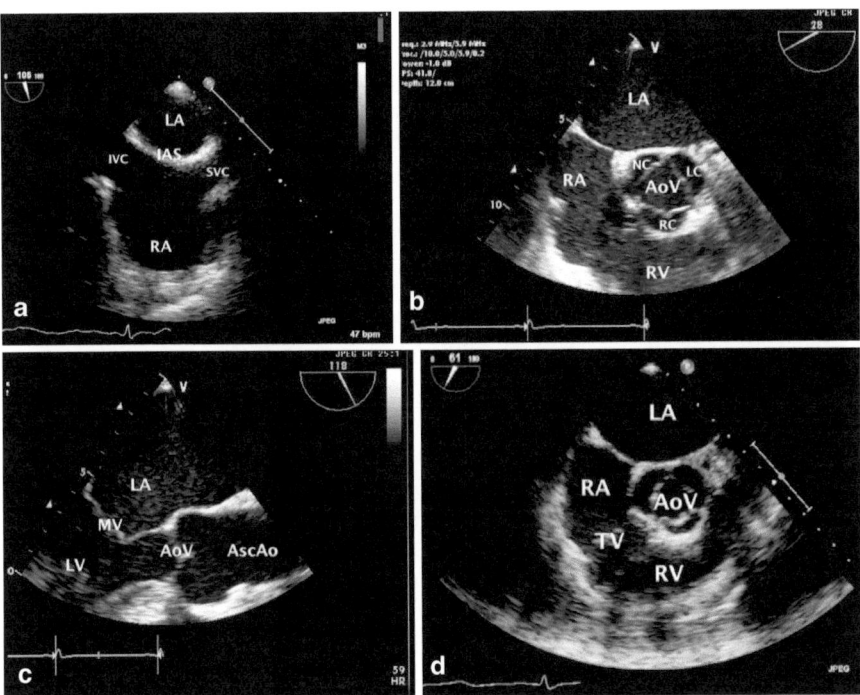

Fig. 9.2 (**a**) The mid-esophageal bicaval view is obtained at an imaging angle of about 90° by turning the probe slightly to the right. It is used mainly for the assessment of the integrity of the interatrial septum (IAS) and to guide placement of catheters and cannulae placed intraoperatively (*IVC*, inferior vena cava; *SVC*, superior vena cava; *LA*, left atrium; *RA*, right atrium). (**b**) The midesophageal aortic valve short-axis view (ME AV SAX) is obtained at the mid-esophageal level by rotating the angle to 30°–60°, placing the aortic valve in the center of the screen and decreasing the imaging depth to about 10 cm. This image is used to evaluate the aortic valve cusps, measure valve area by planimetry and visualize regurgitant jets using color flow Doppler (*AoV*, aortic valve; *RC*, right coronary cusp; *LC*, left coronary cusp; *NC*, non-coronary cusp; *RV*, right ventricle). (**c**) The mid-esophageal aortic valve long-axis view (ME AV LAX) visualizes the LV outflow tract, aortic valve, and ascending aorta. It is obtained at an imaging angle of about 120°–160°. Decreasing the imaging depth to about 10 cm also helps optimize the image. Similar to the SAX view, this view is used to evaluate the aortic valve cusps for the presence of vegetations or other masses and to assess the severity of aortic insufficiency with color flow Doppler (*Asc Ao*, ascending aorta; *MV*, mitral valve). (**d**) The mid-esophageal right ventricular inflow–outflow view is obtained from the ME 4Ch view by advancing the imaging angle to 60°–90° and placing the tricuspid valve in the center of the screen. This view is used to visualize the tricuspid valve (TV), the right ventricular outflow tract, the right ventricle free wall, and the pulmonary valve

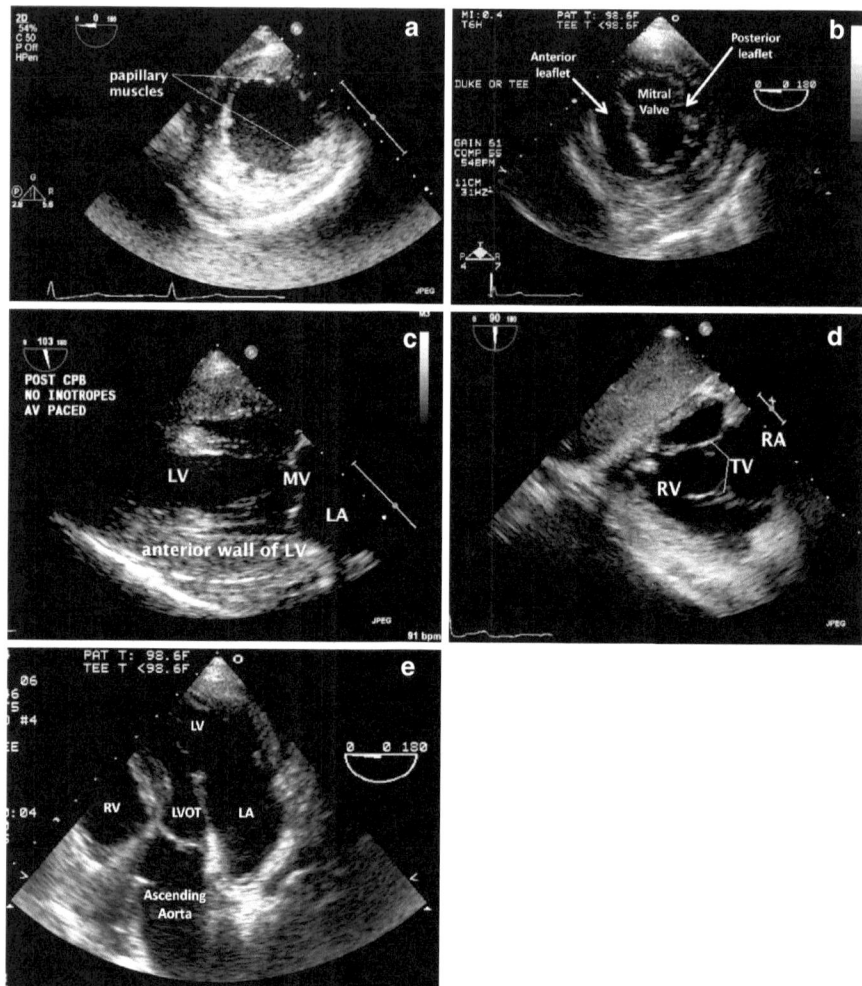

Fig. 9.3 From the mid-esophageal level, the probe can be further advanced into the stomach to the trans-gastric position. (**a**) Anteflexion of the probe until it makes contact with the gastric wall enables the transgastric mid-papillary short axis view (TG mid SAX). The left ventricle is seen in cross-section as a circular structure at the level of the papillary muscles. This view is mostly used to evaluate the function and size of the left ventricle as well as regional wall motion abnormalities. In addition, pericardial effu-sions can also be clearly seen. While evaluating wall motion abnormalities, it is important to note that the orientation of left ventricular walls is opposite to that of chest wall imaging. (**b**) The transgastric basal short-axis view (TG basal SAX) is obtained by further anteflexion and/or slight withdrawal of the probe. Similar to the TG mid SAX, the basal view is also used to assess the size and function of the LV. (**c**) The transgastric 2-Ch view is obtained by rotating the imaging angle to 90°. It visualizes the anterior and inferior left ventricular walls, the mitral valve and the subvalvular apparatus (*LV*, left ventricle; *LA*, left atrium; *MV*, mitral valve). (**d**) The transgastric right ventricular inflow view (TG RV inflow) is obtained from the TG mid SAX by rotating the imaging angle to about 100° and turning the probe slightly to the *right*. It visualizes the right ventricle in long axis (*RV*, right ventricle; *RA*, right atrium; *TV*, tricuspid valve). (**e**) The deep transgastric long axis view (deep TG LAX) is obtained by further advanc-ing the probe in the stomach and anteflexing in such a way that the probe is adjacent to the left ventricu-lar apex with the imaging angle at 0°. This view is used for measuring velocities across the aortic valve and left ventricular outflow tract using spectral Doppler (*LVOT*, left ventricular outflow tract)

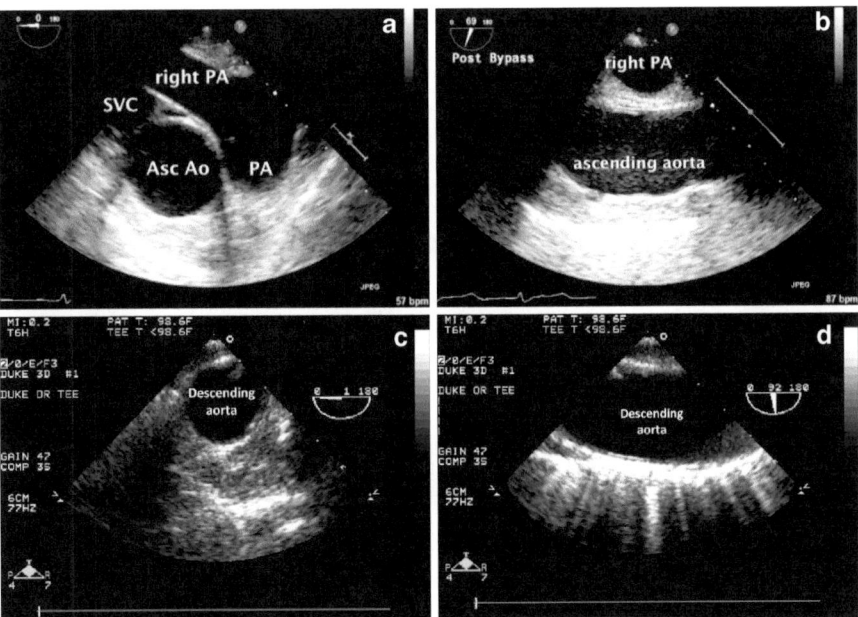

Fig. 9.4 TEE can be used to examine the proximal ascending aorta, the distal aortic arch, and the descending aorta. Because of the interposition of the trachea and the left main stem, the distal ascending aorta and the proximal aortic arch cannot always be examined (the echo "blind spot"). As these aortic segments are used most frequently for aortic cannulation and cross-clamping, the complete evaluation of these segments requires epiaortic scanning (**a**) Mid-esophageal ascending aorta short-axis view (ME asc aortic SAX) is obtained from the mid-esophageal level by slightly withdrawing and anteflexing the probe until the ascending aorta is seen in short axis (*Asc Ao*, ascending aorta; *PA*, pulmonary artery; *right PA*, right pulmonary artery; *SVC*, superior vena cava). (**b**) From this position, advancing the angle to about 90°–120° will generate the mid-esophageal ascending aorta long axis view (ME asc aortic LAX). Both views may be used to evaluate the ascending aorta for atheroma and dissection flaps, to evaluate the pulmonary artery for the presence of thrombus or for the position of the pulmonary artery catheter, and to assess the dimensions of the ascending aorta. (**c**) The descending aorta short-axis view is obtained by turning the probe to the left at an imaging angle of 0° until the descending aorta comes into view as a circle. The imaging depth should be decreased to about 6–8 cm and the aorta should also be examined distally as far as possible. (**d**) Forward rotation of the imaging angle to 90° generates the descending aorta long axis view. Both views of the descending aorta can be used to assess descending aorta for the presence of atheromatous plaque or dissection flaps. (**e**) By withdrawing the probe in the upper esophagus at an imaging angle of 0°, the circular shape of the descending aorta changes into a tubular shape of the aortic arch, thus enabling the upper esophageal aortic arch long-axis view (UE aortic arch LAX). (**f**) From this position, advancing the imaging angle to about 90° will generate the upper esophageal aortic arch short axis view (UE aortic arch SAX) (*PA*, pulmonary artery). Both views can be used to assess the aortic arch for the presence of atheromatous plaque, dissection flaps and other interventions like endovascular aortic stents. The UE aortic arch SAX can also be used to assess velocities across the pulmonary valve, which is oriented well to allow a spectral Doppler beam to be directed along transvalvular flow

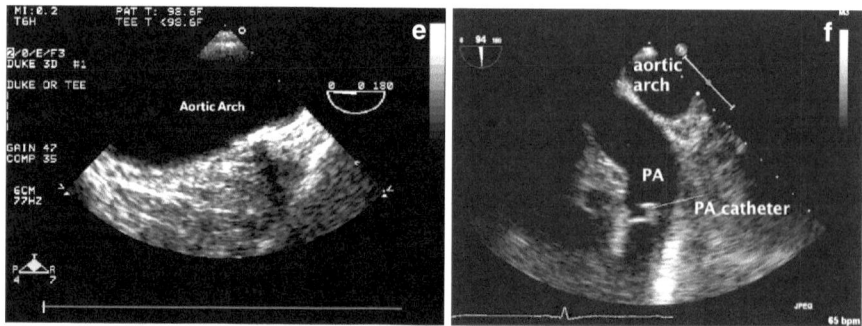

Fig. 9.4 (continued)

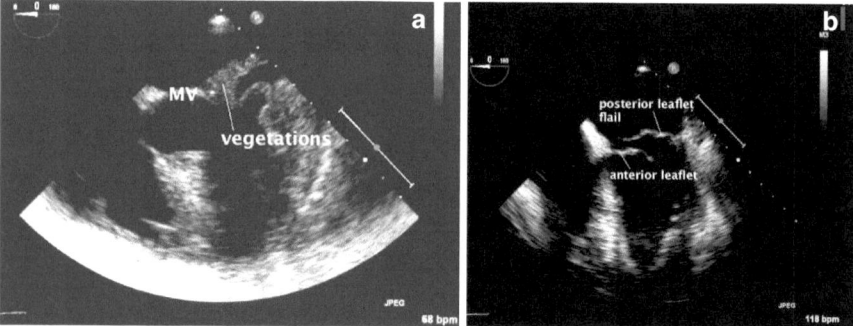

Fig. 9.5 Mitral valve pathology. (**a**) Mitral valve vegetations appear as irregular, heterogeneous masses originating most often from the atrial side. They are accompanied by valvular regurgitation and are prone to embolization, MV, mitral valve. (**b**) Posterior leaflet flail as seen in the ME 4-Ch view can be due to chordal elongation or rupture and usually leads to severe mitral regurgitation. (**c**) Mitral valve regurgitation can be due to degenerative disease of the mitral valve or subvalvular apparatus or due to changes in the geometry of the mitral valve annulus or the left ventricle. It is best assessed and quantified in the mid-esophageal views. (**d**) One of the methods of quantifying the mitral regurgitation is by measuring the vena contracta, which is the narrowest portion of the regurgitant jet. It is usually measured in the ME LAX view. (**e**) Measurement of the radius of the proximal isovelocity surface area (PISA) allows calculation of the effective regurgitant orifice area and of the regurgitant volume

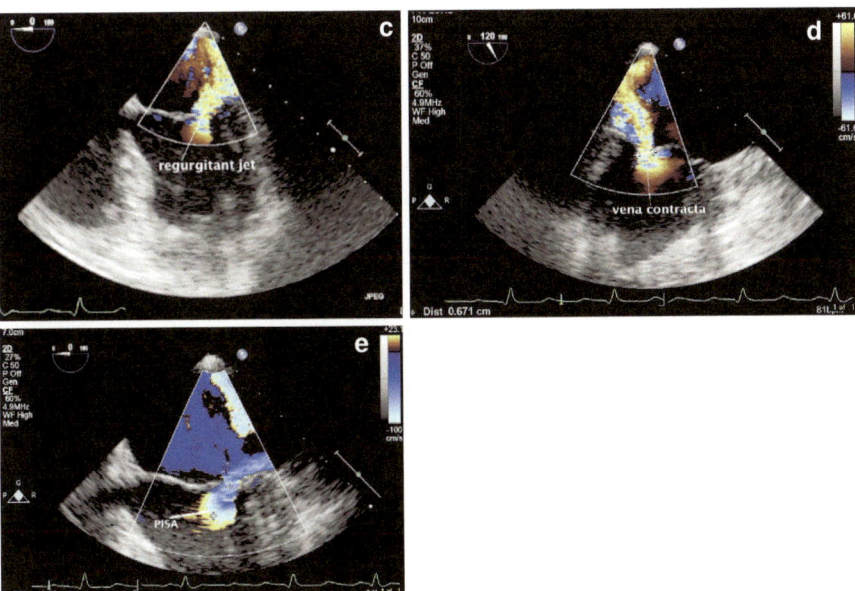

Fig. 9.5 (continued)

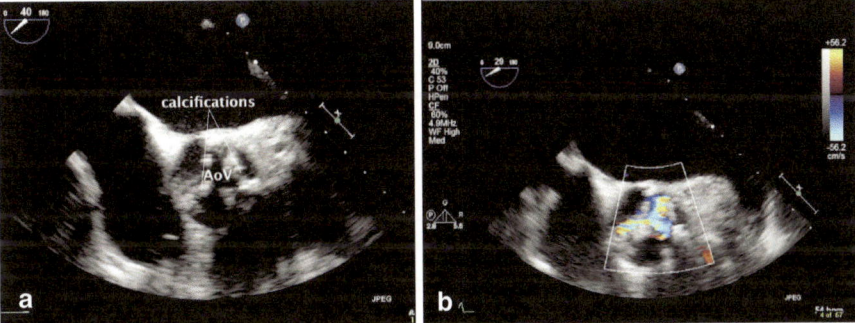

Fig. 9.6 Aortic valve pathology. (**a**) Aortic valve calcification, fibrosis, and thickening result in decrease in the flexibility of the cusps and fusion of the commissures with limitation of flow and aortic stenosis. The ME AV SAX view allows examination of the cusps for pathology. (**b**) Turbulent flow through a stenotic aortic valve can be observed with color flow Doppler in the ME AV SAX. (**c**) Bicuspid aortic valve, seen in ME AV SAX, is the most common congenital malformation of the aortic valve. (**d**) Aortic valve vegetations originate usually from the ventricular side of the valve are irregular and heterogeneous and lead to valvular regurgitation. TEE is the diagnostic modality of choice for endocarditis. Aortic valve vegetations are seen here in the ME AV LAX view. (**e**) The same lesions are also seen on the aortic valve cusps in the ME AV SAX view. (**f**) The ME AV LAX is the preferred view to quantify the severity of aortic valve regurgitation with color flow Doppler. (**g**) Aortic stenosis and aortic regurgitation can also be quantified using continuous wave Doppler in the deep TG LAX view and analyzing the velocities of the stenotic or the regurgitant lesions. This image depicts concomitant severe aortic stenosis and mild aortic regurgitation

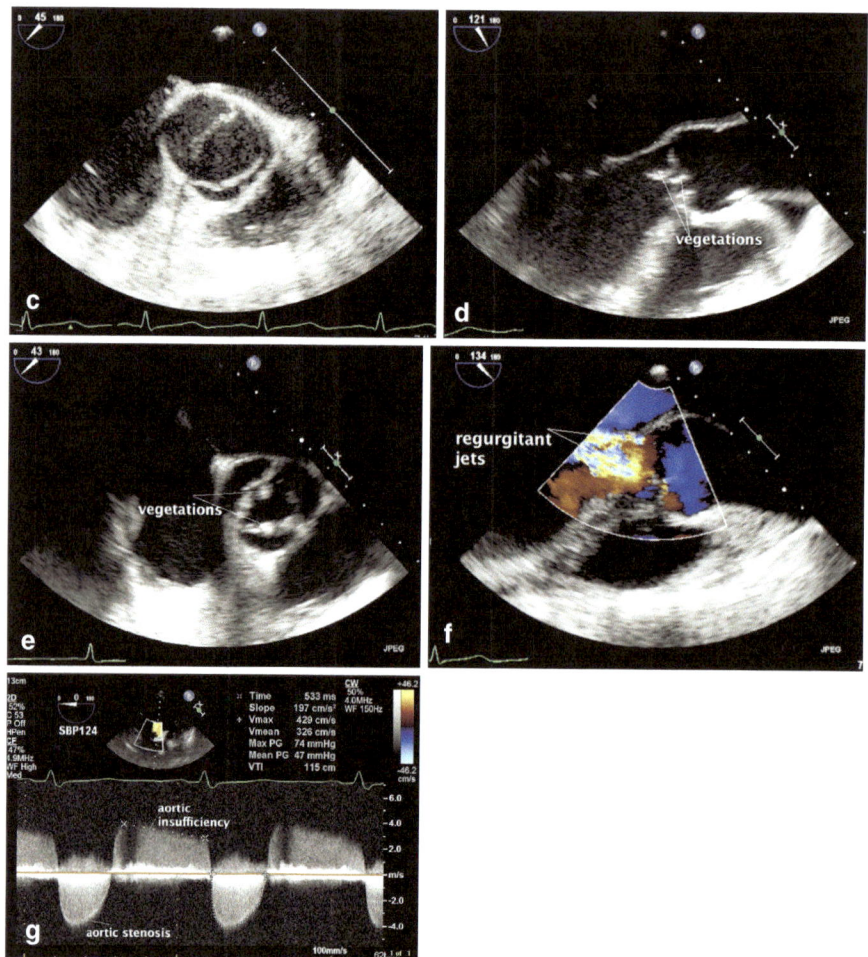

Fig. 9.6 (continued)

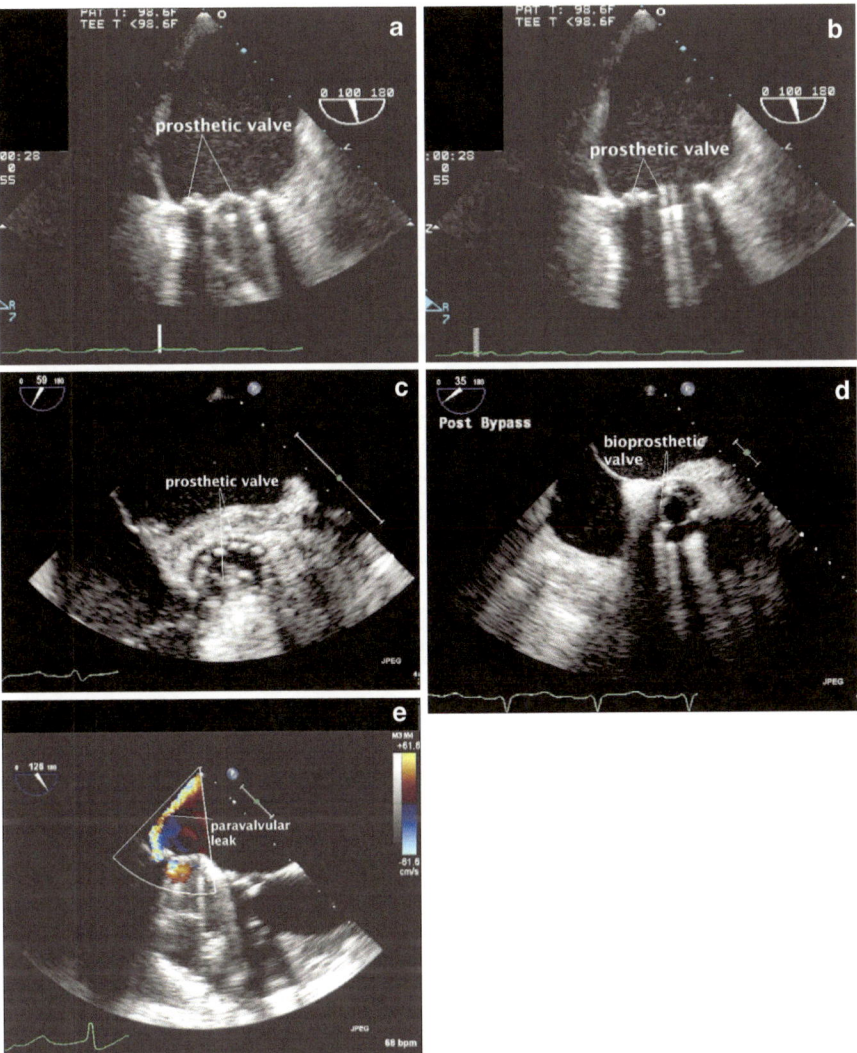

Fig. 9.7 Prosthetic valves. Transesophageal echocardiography can provide detailed information on prosthetic valves through high-quality two and three-dimensional echo images and Doppler examination. (**a**) Bileaflet mechanical valve in systole (*closed*) in the mitral position. (**b**) Bileaflet mechanical valve in diastole (*open*) in the mitral position. Prosthetic valves should be evaluated for the movement of the mechanical occluders according to specifications, stability, lack of rocking motion, and absence of attached fibrinous or thrombotic material. (**c**) An open bileaflet mechanical valve in the aortic position. (**d**) Bioprosthetic valve in the aortic position. The three supporting struts and the three leaflets are visible in open position. (**e**) In the ME LAX view, a significant regurgitant jet is visible originating from outside of the annulus of the bileaflet mechanical valve and representing a paravalvular leak

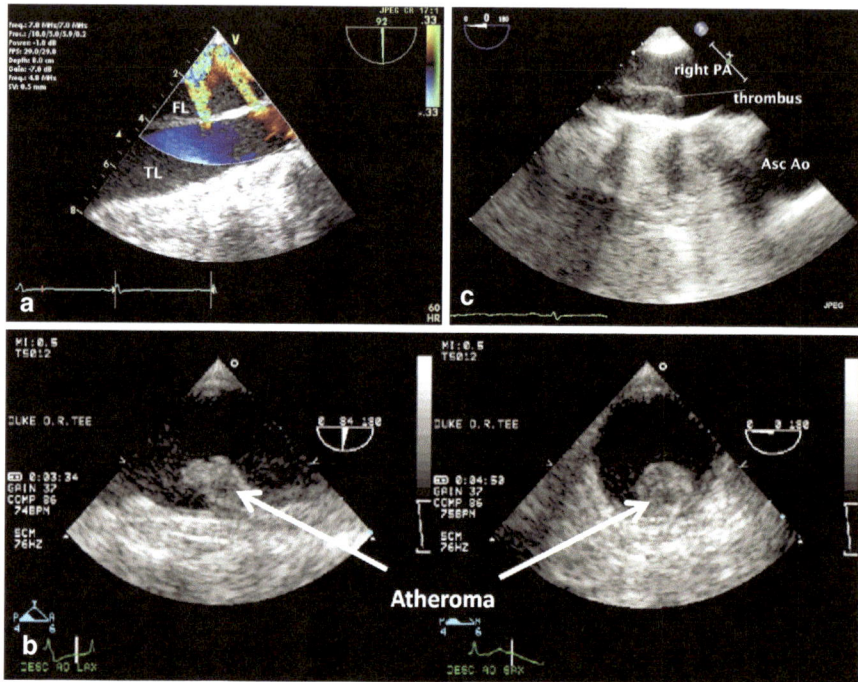

Fig. 9.8 Major vessels. (**a**) Dissection of the descending aorta with blood flow seen from the true lumen into the false lumen through multiple sites of entry in the descending aorta long axis view (*TL*, true lumen; *FL*, false lumen). (**b**) Large atheromatous plaque seen in the descending aorta in the long axis (*left*) and short axis (*right*) views. (**c**) Thrombus seen in the distal right pulmonary artery in the ME ascending aorta SAX view (*Asc Ao*, ascending aorta; *PA*, pulmonary artery)

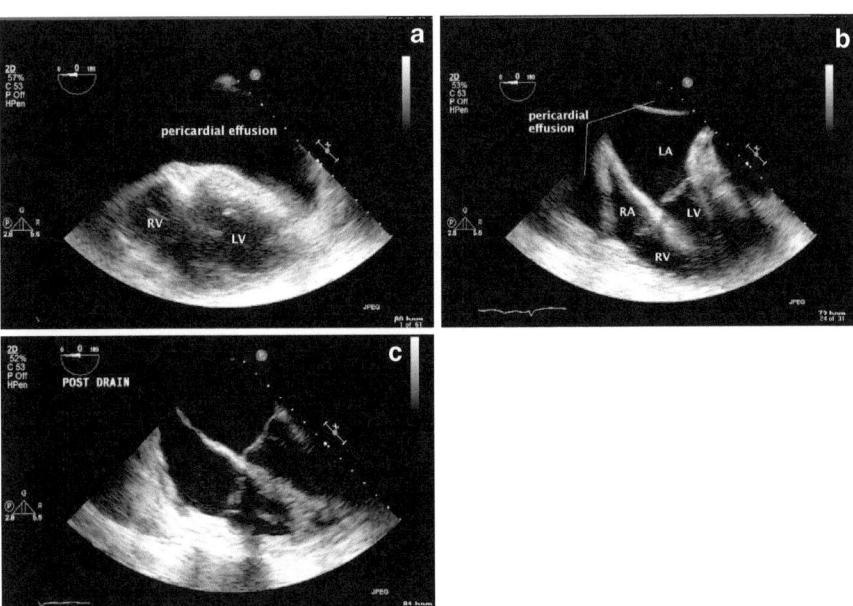

Fig. 9.9 TEE is a valuable tool in diagnosing pericardial effusions as a cause of hemodynamic instability. (**a**) In the TG mid SAX, the pericardial effusion is seen as an echolucent space posterior to the heart chambers (*RV*, right ventricle; *LV*, left ventricle). (**b**) In the ME 4-Ch view, the pericardial effusion is compressing on the right and left atria distorting the normal anatomy (*RA*, right atrium; *LA*, left atrium). (**c**) ME 4-Ch view in the same patient after drainage of the effusion

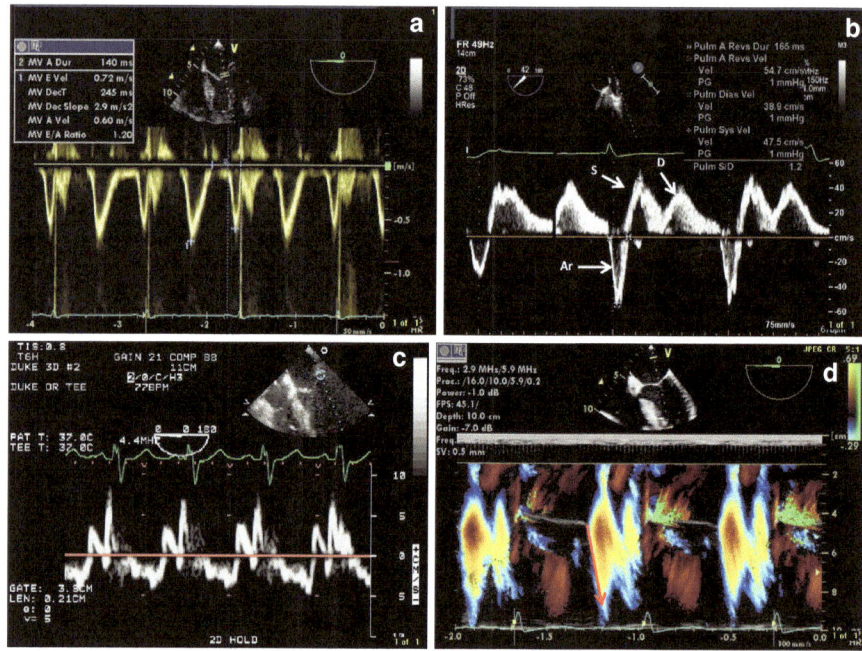

Fig. 9.10 Assessment of intraoperative diastolic function involves the comprehensive use of spectral Doppler. (**a**) Transmitral pulsed wave Doppler in the mid-esophageal 4-Ch view (Fig. 9.1a) demonstrating early (E) and late (A) diastolic flow velocities away from baseline. The direction of transmitral flow is in contrast to conventional chest wall imaging. (**b**) Pulsed wave Doppler of peak velocities in the left upper pulmonary vein. Forward flow in systole (S), diastole (D), and reversed flow (Ar) during atrial contraction can be seen. (**c**) Tissue velocity of the lateral mitral annulus is shown using tissue Doppler imaging. Two diastolic waves, early (E′) and late (A′) can be seen above baseline and a downward wave in systole (S′) as the base descends during this period. (**d**) Propagation velocity of early diastolic left ventricular filling assessed using color M-mode. The red arrow illustrates the slope that depicts propagation velocity

Fig. 9.11 Imaging of the descending aorta for dissections can sometimes be confounded. The bright echo-reflective posterior wall of the aorta can generate a mirror image distal to the actual image of the descending aorta. An intraaortic balloon pump A is seen in the lumen of the aorta, while its mirror image B can be seen in the aortic mirror image. This may be easily mistaken for a dissection

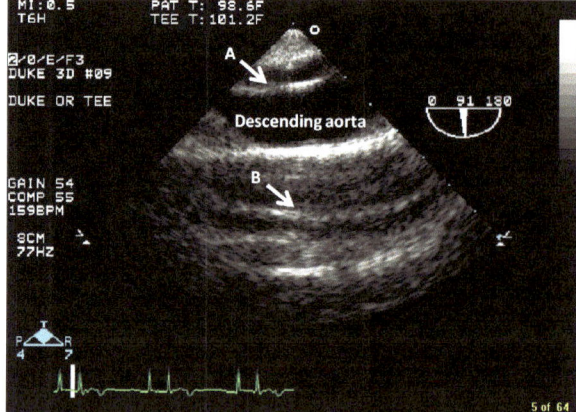

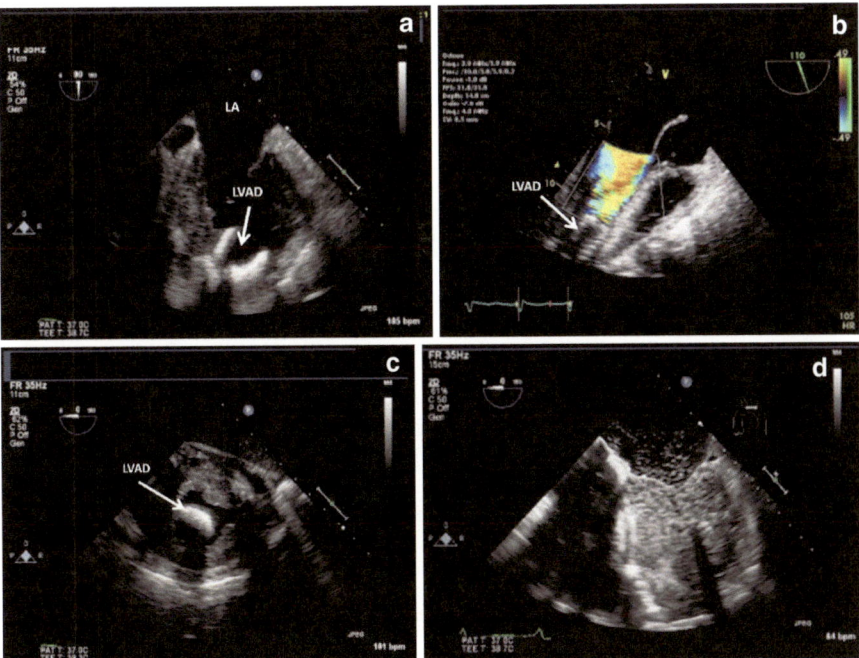

Fig. 9.12 TEE is particularly useful in the assessment of inflow and outflow cannulae of ventricular assist devices (VAD). (**a**) In this mid-esophageal 2-Ch view, a left-sided VAD inflow canula inserted in the left ventricular apex can be seen as an echo-dense object. (**b**) Color flow Doppler may be used to determine quality of flow across the device for assessment of obstruction. (**c**) The transgastric mid-short axis view shows the cannula in cross section. (**d**) While weaning from cardiopulmonary bypass, there may be a significant amount of air that can be seen on TEE as bright echo-reflective bubbles in the left ventricle. It is critical to perform de-airing procedures at this time

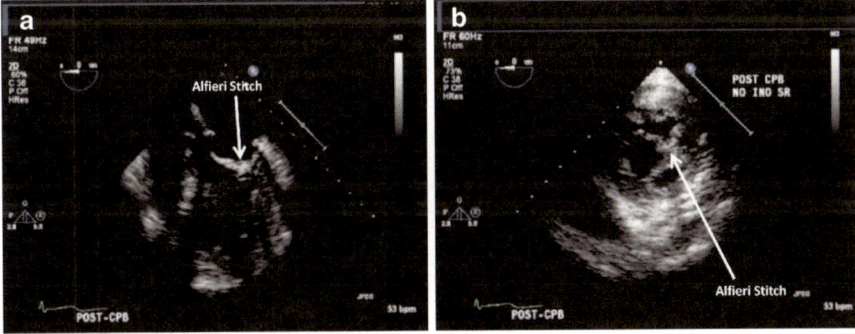

Fig. 9.13 A common adjuvant procedure during mitral valve surgery is an edge-to-edge repair (Alfieri technique) that is usually performed between the A2 and P2 scallops of the mitral valve for mitral regurgitation, or when there is excessive anterior leaflet tissue. On TEE imaging in the mid-esophageal 4-Ch (**a**) and transgastric basal short axis (**b**) views, the effects of the edge-to-edge stitch may be seen on the mitral valve. A double mitral opening can also be appreciated in the short axis views

Use of Echo Contrast in Routine Practice

10

Shizhen Liu and Mani A. Vannan

10.1
Introduction

Ultrasound contrast agents, used with contrast-specific imaging techniques, have an established role for diagnostic cardiovascular imaging in the echocardiography laboratory. It has approved indication of Left ventricular opacification (LVO) and enhancement of endocardial border delineation (EBD). Also, a number of investigative reports have confirmed the utility of the off-label use of contrast agents for assessment of myocardial perfusion (MCE).

10.2
What Are Ultrasound Contrast Agents?

- Microbubbles in contrast agent compose of gas and the shell.
- According to the different gas inside the microbubbles, contrast agents could be divided into two generations.
  - First generation: air
  - Second generation: perfluorocarbon or sulfur fluoride
- The Second generation agents have better stability and contrast effect and are in use now.

S. Liu (✉)
Department of Cardiovascular Medicine, The Ohio State University Medical Center,
Columbus, OH, USA
e-mail: shizhen.liu@osumc.edu

T.P. Abraham (ed.), *Case Based Echocardiography*,
DOI: 10.1007/978-1-84996-151-6_10, © Springer-Verlag London Limited 2011

10.3
Contrast Agents in Use

Agent	Size, mm (range)	Gas	Shell composition	Manufacture	Approved in
Levovist	2–3 (2–8)	Air	Lipid (palmitic acid)	Bayer Schering Pharma AG (Berlin, Germany)	Canada, Europe, Asia
Optison	4.7 (1–10)	Perfluoropropane	Human albumin	GE Healthcare (Princeton, NJ)	US, Canada
Definity	1.5 (1–10)	Perfluoropropane	Phospholipid	Lantheus Medical Imaging (North Billerica, MA)	US, Canada, Europe
SonoVue	2.5 (1–10)	Sulfur hexafluoride	Phospholipid	BRACCO Diagnostics (Milan, Italy)	Canada, Europe, Asia

10.4
Indication in Clinical Practice – 1 (Fig. 10.1)

LV volumes and LVEF	• Suboptimal image quality: Obesity; chronic obstructive pulmonary disease patients in intensive care settings; mechanically ventilated; chest deformities
	• Optimal image quality: need accurate, precise and repeatable measurements of absolute LV volumes, mass and global systolic performance

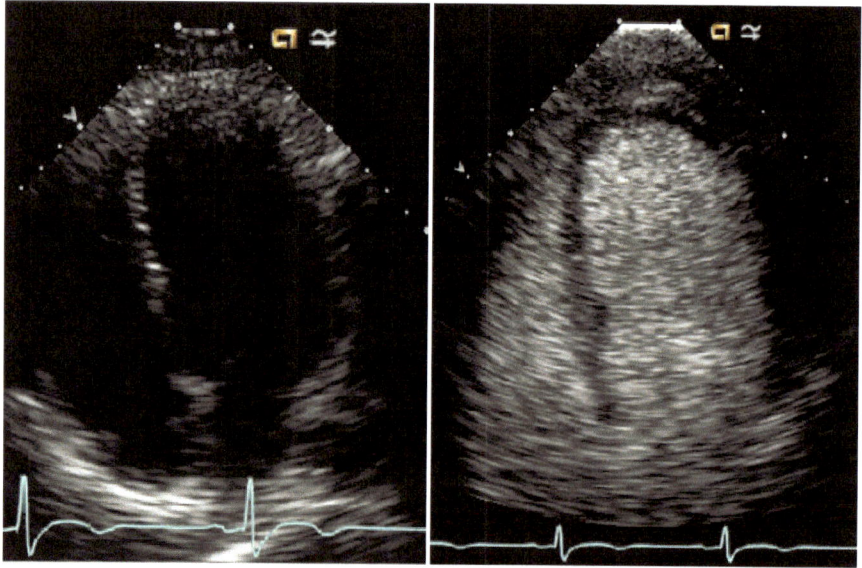

Fig. 10.1 Apical 4 chamber view before (*left*) and after (*right*) contrast

10.5
Indication in Clinical Practice – 2 (Fig. 10.2)

Confirm or exclude abnormalities in apex	• Apical aneurysm (Fig. 10.2, left)
	• Apical thrombus
	• Apical false tendons or trabeculations
	• Apical hypertrophic cardiomyopathy
	• Endocardial noncompaction

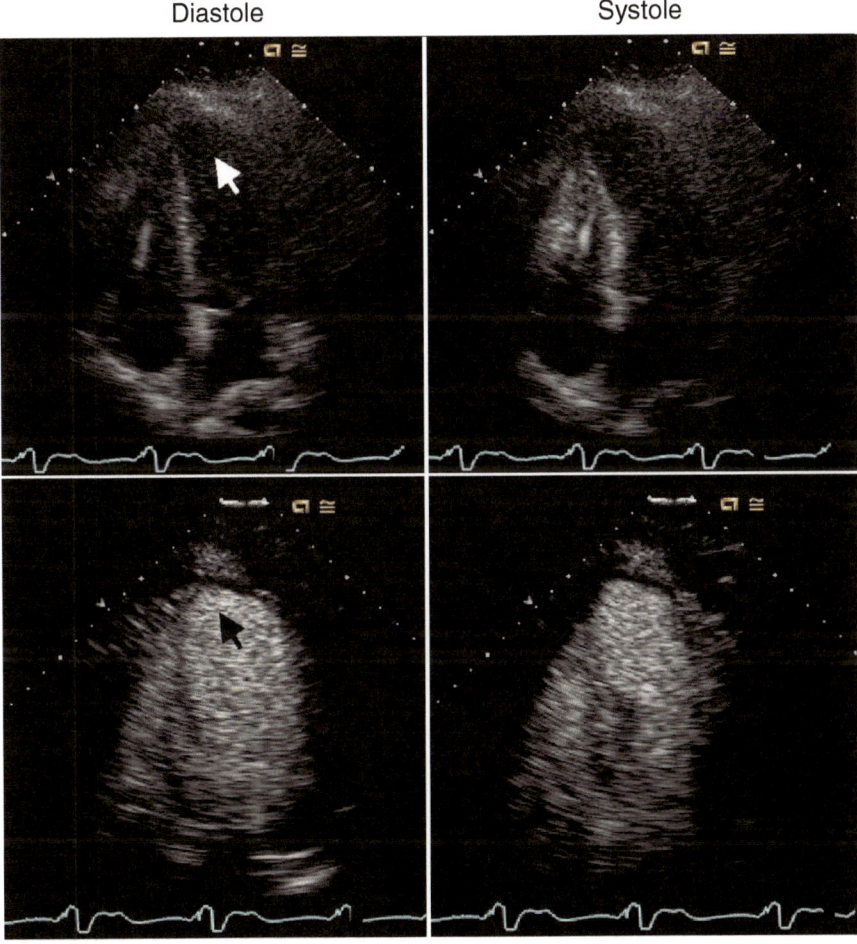

Fig. 10.2 LV aneurysm (*arrow*) is confirmed after contrast (*lower panel*)

10.6
Indication in Clinical Practice – 3

Cardiac chamber mass differentiation	• Stasis of blood: swirl within a region of blood stasis
	• Thrombus: complete contrast dropout
	• Tumor: reperfuse with contrast after several cardiac cycles
Cardiac structure differentiation	• Myocardial rupture
	• Pseudoaneurysm
	• Giant aortic sinus aneurysm differentiated with RA and/or cyst
Doppler enhancement	• Tricuspid regurgitation
	• Aortic stenosis
	• Pulmonary vein flow

10.7
Protocol for Routine Contrast Study – 1

- Laboratory setup
  - Team approach: physicians, sonographers, and nurses
  - Written document: indications; injecting and imaging protocols; personnel responsibilities
  - Reimbursement procedures establishment
  - Contrast agent storage

10.8
Protocol for Routine Contrast Study – 2

- Contrast procedure
  - Patient selection
  - Explain procedure to patient
  - Establish IV access
  - Determine optimal mode of administration (Table 10.1)
  - Optimize equipment settings (Table 10.2)

Table 10.1 Administration methods of contrast agent

CE administration	Characteristics
Bolus	• Quick and simple to perform with a high level of contrast enhancement.
	• Higher incidence of attenuation artifact. (Overcome by slowing the rate of bolus injection or using a dilute bolus.)
	• Need a slow flush with enough saline or 5% dextrose and water solution (D5W) to opacify the LV properly.
	• Flush is terminated as soon as contrast is seen in the RV and the contrast preset is activated.
Continuous infusion	• Control the injection of microbubbles more efficiently and are essential for quantitative perfusion studies.
	• IV setup is usually more complicated and time-consuming.

Table 10.2 Equipment settings for contrast echocardiography

Control	Adjustment
Mechanical Index (MI)	• 0.4–0.6. Select harmonic imaging
Overall gain	• Higher gain does not cause microbubble destruction
	• Lower MI requires higher gain
Time gain compensation (TGC)	• Greater TGC gain in greater depths
Compression (dynamic range)	• Medium dynamic range in LVO
Transducer frequency	• Lowest transmit frequency
Transmit focus	• Usually at distal location; move to apex as needed
Persistence	• Low or off
Depth	• Optimize depth to region of interest (e.g., LA is not needed during LVO)

10.9
Protocols for Stress Contrast Study

- Administration
  - In exercise stress echocardiography
    - Baseline and peak stages
  - In pharmacologic stress echocardiography
    - Baseline, low dose, and peak stages

- For peak images
  - Agent is given 15–20 s before termination of the test
  - Followed by a slower bolus of 2–3 mL of flush
  - Establish the optimal window in the non-contrast preset

10.10
Techniques, Problems, and How to Resolve

	Artifact	Causes	Solutions
LVO	Attenuation	• High concentration of microbubbles within the LV cavity • Rib or lung artifact	• Waiting for dissipating over time • Slowing the speed to inject the flush • Using a dilute bolus • Using infusion method • Repositioning transducer to minimize rib or lung artifact
	Swirling of the contrast	• MI setting is too high • Concentration of contrast is too low	• Lowering the MI • Increasing the amount of contrast injected • Moving the focus to the region of the swirling
MCE	False-positive perfusion	• High gain settings	• Using high MI impulse to differentiate: False-positive perfusion shows no reperfusion after high MI flash
	Blooming	• High gain settings	• Lowering the gain
	Motion artifact	• Always see when using power Doppler imaging methods	• Adjusting pulse repetition frequency (PRF) setting to minimize it

10.11
Safety

- Common adverse effects
  - Infrequent and mild: headache, weakness, fatigue, palpitations, nausea, dizziness, dry mouth, altered sense of smell or taste, dyspnea, urticaria, pruritus, back pain, chest pain, rash
  - Rarely: Allergic and potentially life threatening hypersensitivity reactions

10.12
FDA Recommendation for Definity and Optison

- Contraindication
  - Right-to-left, bidirectional, or transient right-to-left cardiac shunts
  - Hypersensitivity to perflutren
  - Hypersensitivity to blood, blood products, or albumin (applies to Optison only).
  - Intra-arterial injection
- Patients with pulmonary hypertension or unstable cardiopulmonary conditions
  - Monitoring of vital signs, electrocardiography, and cutaneous oxygen saturation during and for at least 30 min after

10.13
Summary

Contrast echocardiography is an important and a significant addition to a modern echocardiography laboratory. Successful implementation of contrast echo depends on a team effort, including appropriate dosing and administration of the agent, optimized system settings for contrast-enhanced study, and correct image acquisition and interpretation. Fully understanding the bubble physics and instrument setting, together with the indications, and contraindications for contrast-enhanced studies, will maximize the benefit to patients.

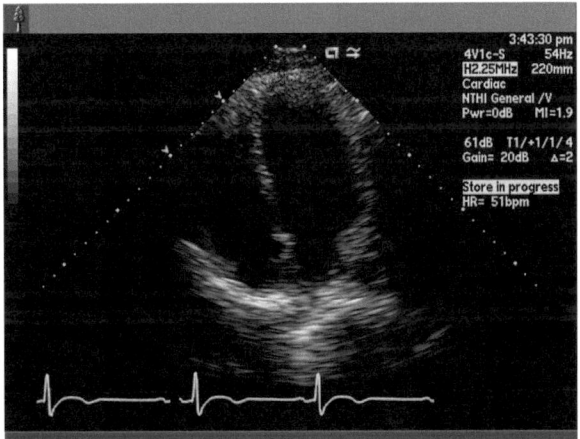

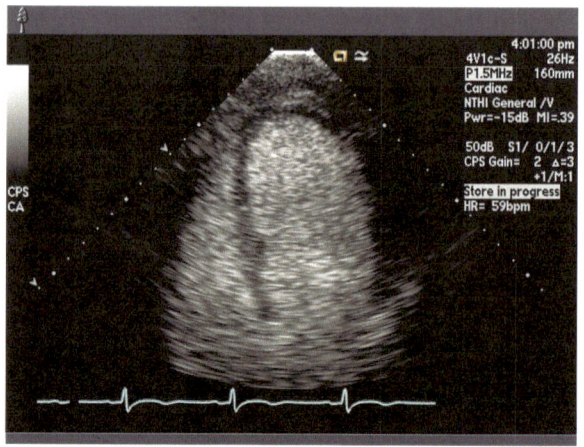

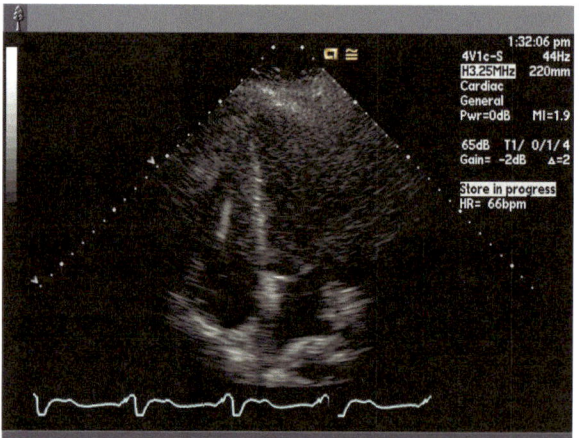

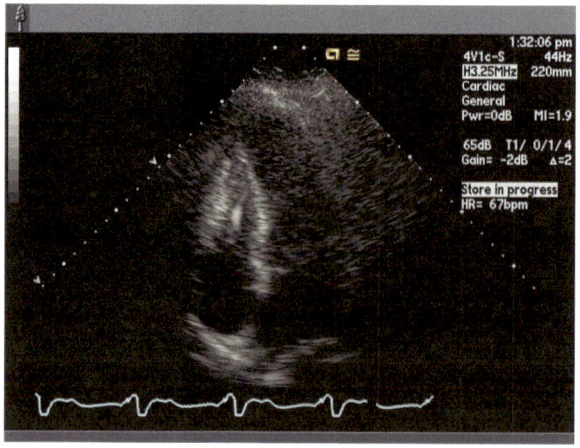

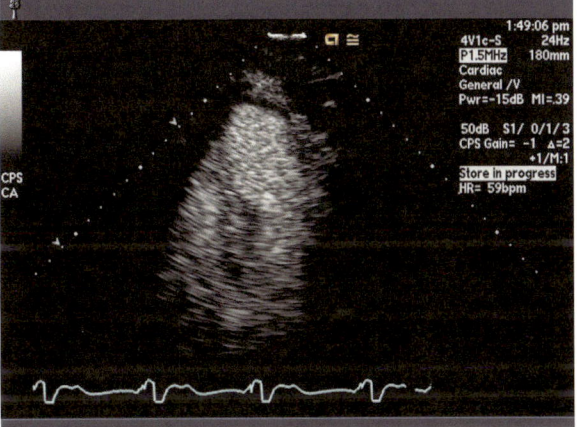

Three-Dimensional Echocardiography

11

Lissa Sugeng, Lynn Weinert, and Roberto M. Lang

11.1
Introduction

- Two-dimensional echocardiography (2DE) is one of the most widely used and well established noninvasive imaging tools in the cardiology.
- Within 50 years of its inception by Edler and Hertz, advancement in transducer and software technology has given birth to fully sampled matrix array transducers, which not only allows traditional two-dimensional echocardiography (2DE) but also has the capability of simultaneous biplane imaging and volumetric three-dimensional imaging.
- Real-time 3D echocardiography (RT3DE) is truly "real-time" when using narrow angled or zoom mode and near "real-time" with wide-angled scanning.
- RT3DE enhances the ability in diagnosis of valvular heart disease by allowing precise imaging planes which can be aligned perpendicular to the valve plane, placed at the tips of the valve leaflets and thus producing a perfect en-face view of the valve orifice.
  - In the assessment of mitral stenosis, three-dimensional echo results in accurate, reliable, and reproducible measurements of mitral valve area compared to conventional 2DE methods.[1-4]
  - Prolapsed or flail segments, valvular dehiscence, and perforation can be identified from a left atrial orientation simulating a "surgeon's view."
  - RT3DE imaging using matrix array probe in patients with good acoustic windows is feasible 83% of the time with adequate visualization of both anterior and posterior mitral leaflets.
  - The anterior mitral valve is best seen from a ventricular perspective regardless of acoustic window, the posterior leaflet from parasternal window, and both commissures well seen from a parasternal or apical window.[5]
  - RT3DE has also enhanced our understanding of ischemic mitral regurgitation, by imaging papillary muscle displacement.[6,7]

L. Sugeng (✉)
Section of Cardiology, Department of Medicine, Non-Invasive Cardiovascular Imaging Laboratory, University of Chicago Medical Center, Chicago, IL, USA
e-mail: lsugeng@medicine.bsd.uchicago.edu

T.P. Abraham (ed.), *Case Based Echocardiography*,
DOI: 10.1007/978-1-84996-151-6_11, © Springer-Verlag London Limited 2011

- RT3DE is accurate, reliable, and reproducible with less inter- and intra-observer variability in the assessment of left ventricular function and mass, using prior 3DE methods of acquisition and even more recent RT3DE technology.[7-19] In addition to global left ventricular function and volumes, regional volumes are obtained, which allow quantitation of left ventricular dyssynchrony.[20-23]
- The development of a fully sampled matrix RT3D transesophageal probe was made possible due to higher density electronics and micro-beam forming architecture within the probe.
- Instantaneous 3D imaging of the valves and ventricle readily provide information on valvular pathology for surgical planning, and can help assess the results of mitral valve repair.[23,24] RT3DE also plays a role in interventional procedures such as balloon mitral valvuloplasty, ASD and left atrial appendage device closure.[25-27]
- Three-dimensional echocardiography has evolved from a specialized research tool for a highly selected group of researchers that was obscure to the clinician due to cumbersome acquisition, lengthy processing, and off-line analysis. However, RT3DE now is a viable clinical tool mainly attributed to shorter acquisition time and ease of use, which is accommodated by a matrix array transducer and online visualization. It will certainly be a must have tool in most echo labs in the years to come.

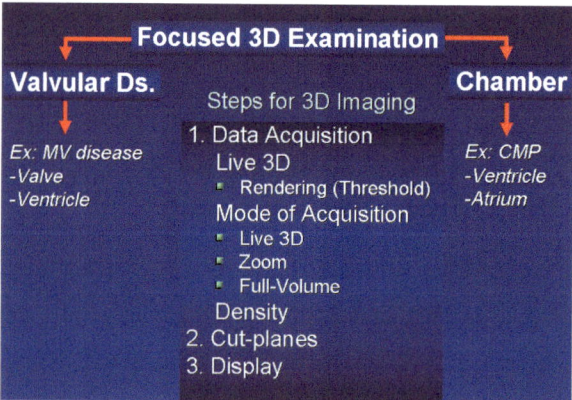

Fig. 11.1 RT3DE Examination Strategy. Incorporation of a three-dimensional echo examination in routine clinical echocardiographic study may pose challenges due to time constraints. Hence, performing a focused 3D examination is essential. Depending on the patient's pathology, a sonographer may focus on imaging the valve using a zoom mode of imaging to assess valve area or determine a prolapsing segment and acquire a full-volume of the left ventricle to quantitate left ventricular function. If the patient has a cardiomyopathy which requires a functional assessment, then a full-volume acquisition of the left ventricle should be obtained. There are essential steps for 3D imaging, which include: (1) data acquisition, (2) application of cut-planes, and (3) determination of the type of display

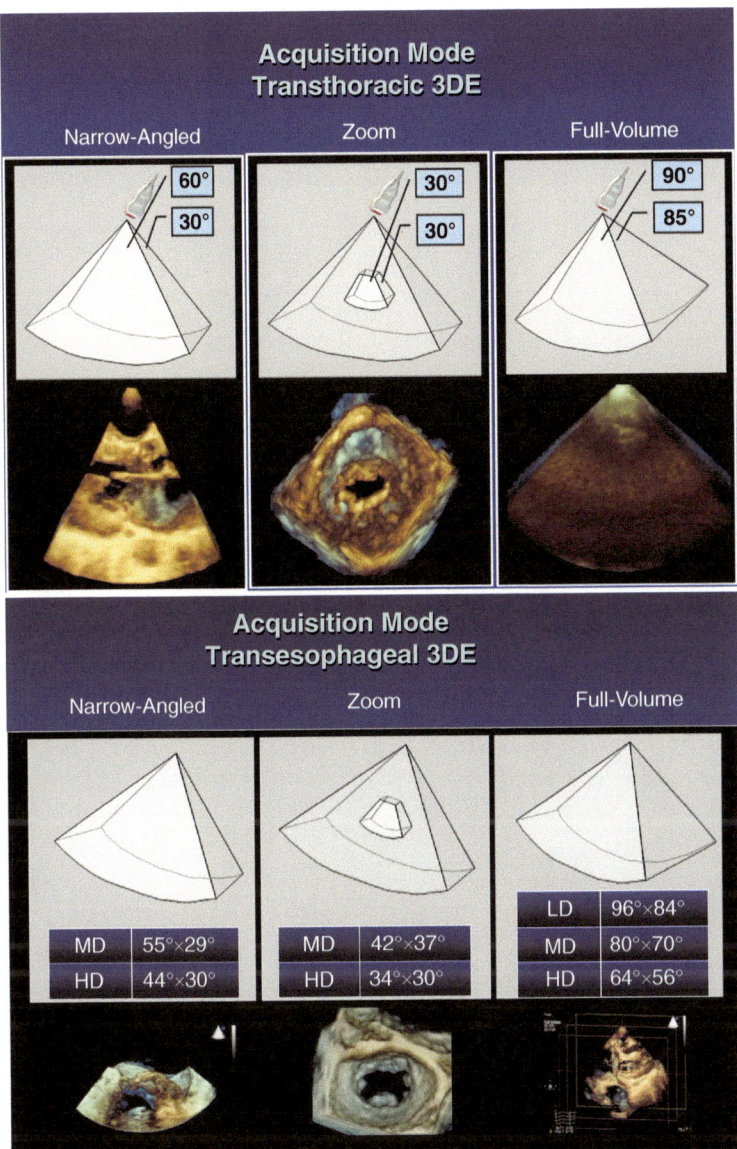

Fig. 11.2 There are three modes of acquisition for both transthoracic and transesophageal RT3DE: (1) narrow-angled, (2) zoom, and (3) full-volume. Narrow-angled and zoom mode of acquisition are both truly "real-time" since data is obtained in one beat. These two modes of acquisition are a small wedge volume of data and have the advantage of having less respiratory artifact. Adjustments of gain, TGC, compress or as generally referred as "thresholding" in 3D terms, are performed on a narrow-angled mode. A zoom mode of acquisition is preferably used for valvular or smaller structures. Ventricular function or atrial chambers need a larger volume scan, so a full-volume mode is chosen. This can be either a four beat acquisition or if higher frame rates are needed a seven beat acquisition which can encompass the entire ventricle

Density

Select Density

Mode of Acuisition		High Density	Medium Density	Low Density
	Live 3D	46° x 23°	58° x 29°	N/A
	3D Zoom	30° x 30°	38° x 38°	45° x 45°
	Full Volume	62° x 56°	78° x 70°	93° x 84°
	3D Color	28° x 28°	35° x 35°	42° x 42°

Fig. 11.3 Density settings for transthoracic RT3DE determine the volume resolution and size

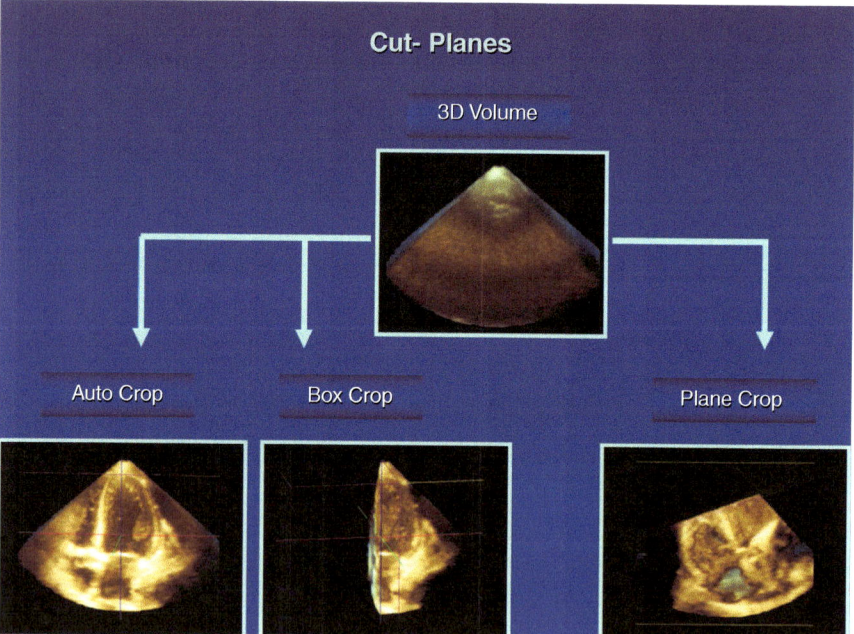

Fig. 11.4 Cut-planes. After 3D volume is acquired, cropping planes are applied to demonstrate certain pathology. There are three cropping tools: (1) auto crop, (2) box crop, and (3) plane crop. Auto crop is useful to automatically demonstrate 50% of a full-volume scan. This enables the operator to ensure that thresholding was sufficient during acquisition. The box crop tool allows six planes to be used to crop the volume acquired in a perpendicular fashion whereas, a plane crop aids the operator to demonstrate abnormalities from any direction

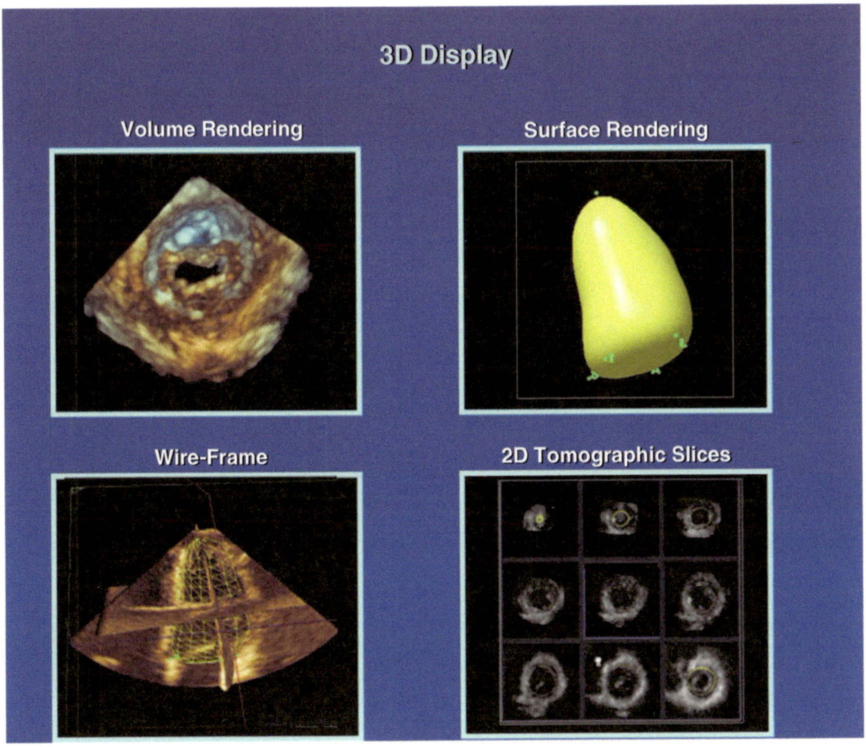

3D Display

Volume Rendering

Surface Rendering

Wire-Frame

2D Tomographic Slices

Fig. 11.5 3D Display. (1) Volume-rendering, (2) surface-rendering, (3) wire-frame, and (4) 2D tomographic slices

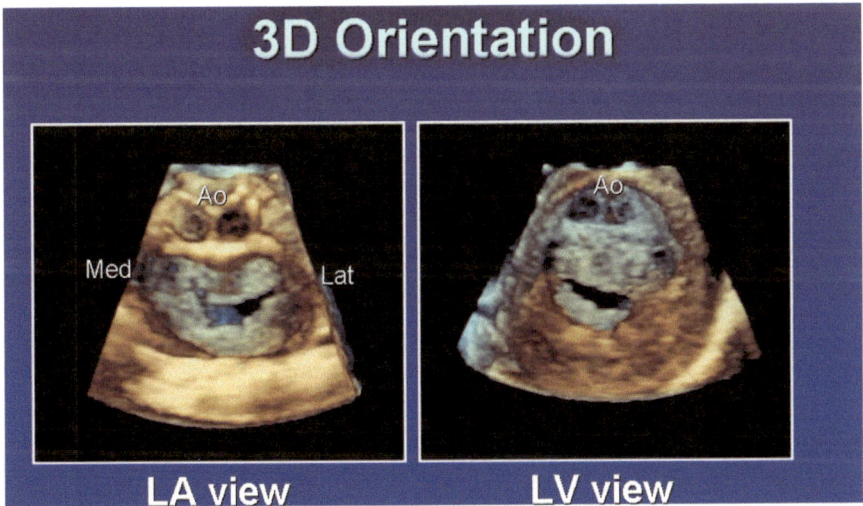

3D Orientation

Ao

Med   Lat

LA view

Ao

LV view

Fig. 11.6 3D Orientation is an important aspect of three-dimensional imaging. Imaging from a left atrial and left ventricular perspective, the mitral valve is displayed with the aortic valve at about 12 o'clock similar to a surgical view

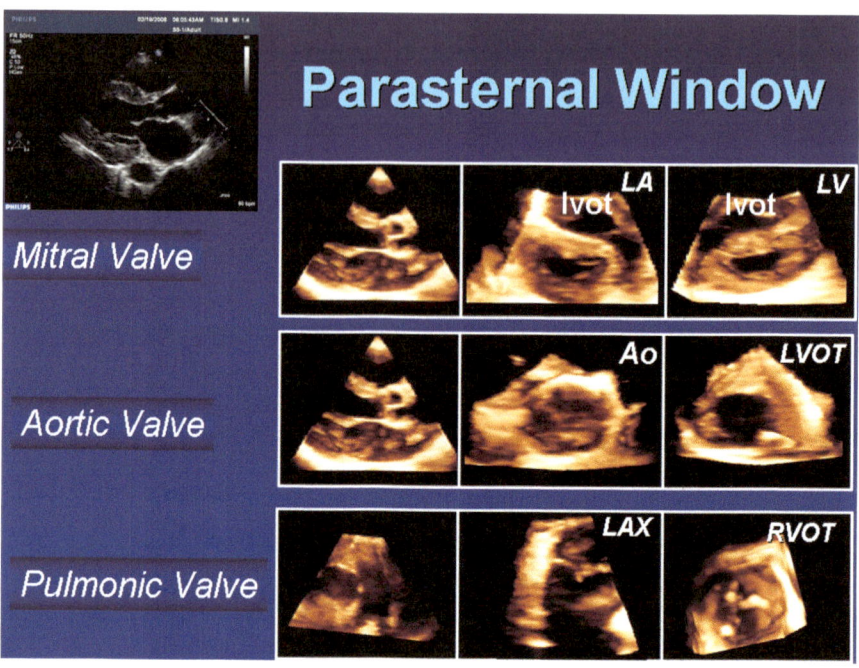

Fig. 11.7 These are examples of a normal mitral valve, aortic, and pulmonic valve obtained from a parasternal window. The first image on the left is all narrow-angled acquisitions. A zoom mode acquisition is displayed in the center and right panels

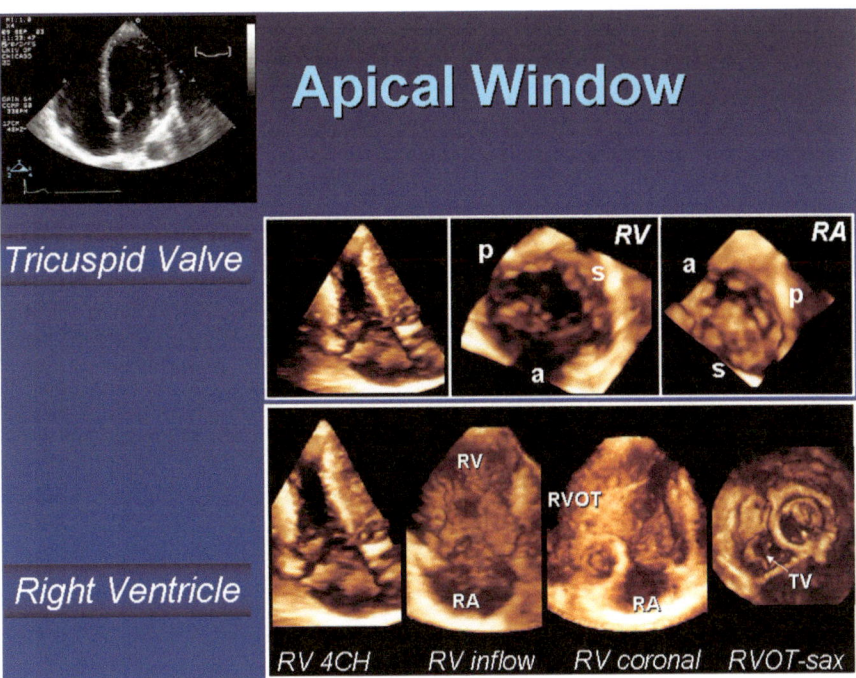

Fig. 11.8 Examples of a normal tricuspid valve on top. Imaging of the tricuspid valve is only partially viewed from a parasternal window, so the preferred window to obtain the entire tricuspid valve and annulus is from an apical approach. The first image is a narrow-angled acquisition of part of the right ventricle. A subsequent zoom mode acquisition was obtained to view the tricuspid valve from the right ventricle and the right atrium. The right ventricle is also only partially viewed from a parasternal window; hence similarly to the tricuspid valve the entire right ventricle is obtained from an apical approach. The first image (RV 4CH) is a narrow-angle acquisition of the right ventricle from an apical 4-chamber view. From a full-volume right ventricular data set, several cut planes can be applied to obtain: (1) RV inflow, (2) RV coronal, and (3) RVOT short-axis. *RV 4CH*, right ventricle 4-chamber; *RVOT*, right ventricular outflow; *a*, anterior leaflet; *p*, posterior leaflet; *s*, septal leaflet

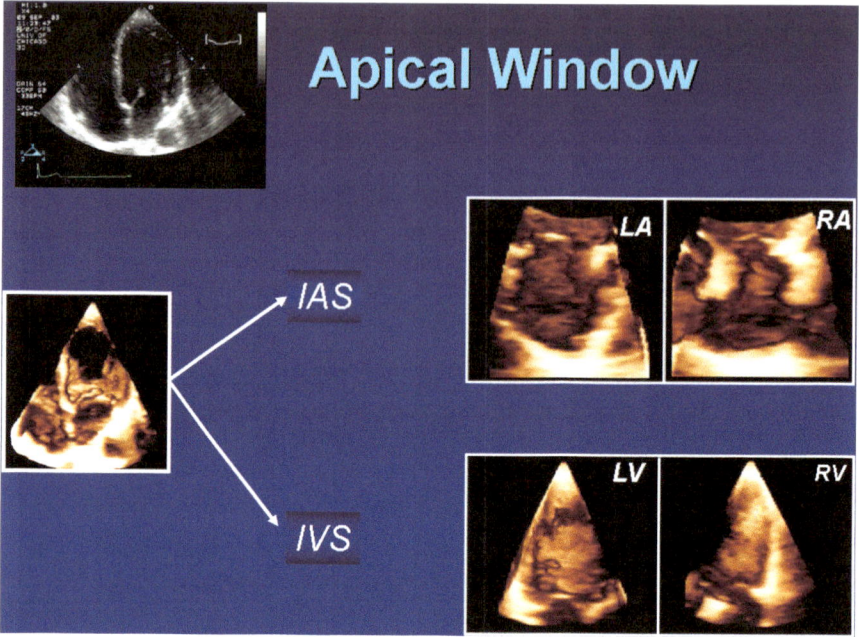

Fig. 11.9 The interatrial septum (IAS) and interventricular septum (IVS) are both acquired from an apical window. On the left is a narrow-angle acquisition of a left ventricular 4-chamber view. A zoom mode of acquisition is chosen to obtain the IAS and IVS. Both structures can be viewed from the left or right sided chambers

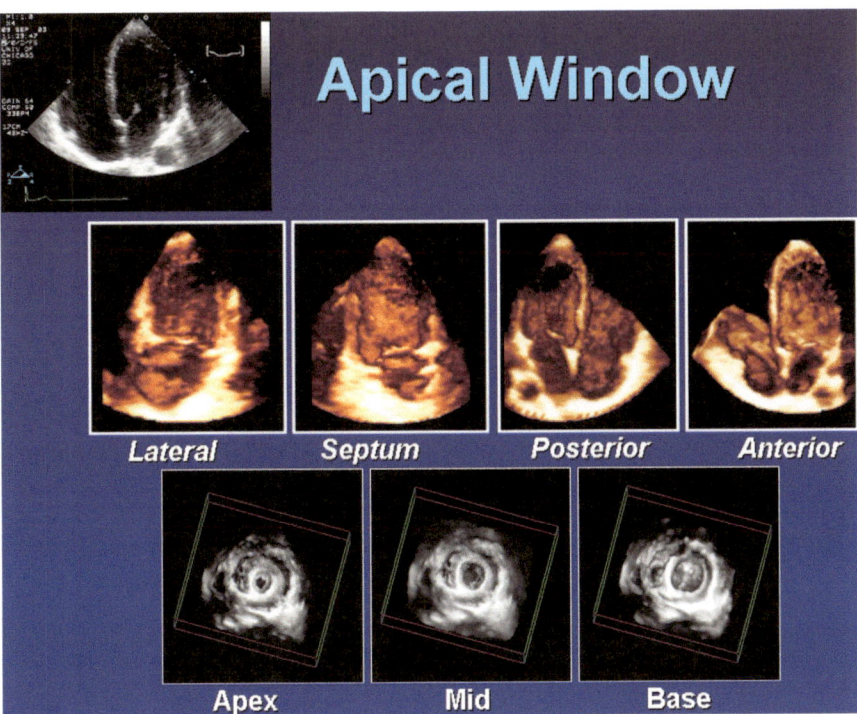

Fig. 11.10 The left ventricle is acquired using a full-volume mode of acquisition. From this pyramidal volume, many cut-planes can be applied to view different walls of the ventricle (*top row*). Using a box crop, the operator can view the lateral, septal, posterior, and anterior walls. Using the same method, a short-axis plane can be utilized to obtain multiple views of the left ventricle as seen on the bottom panel

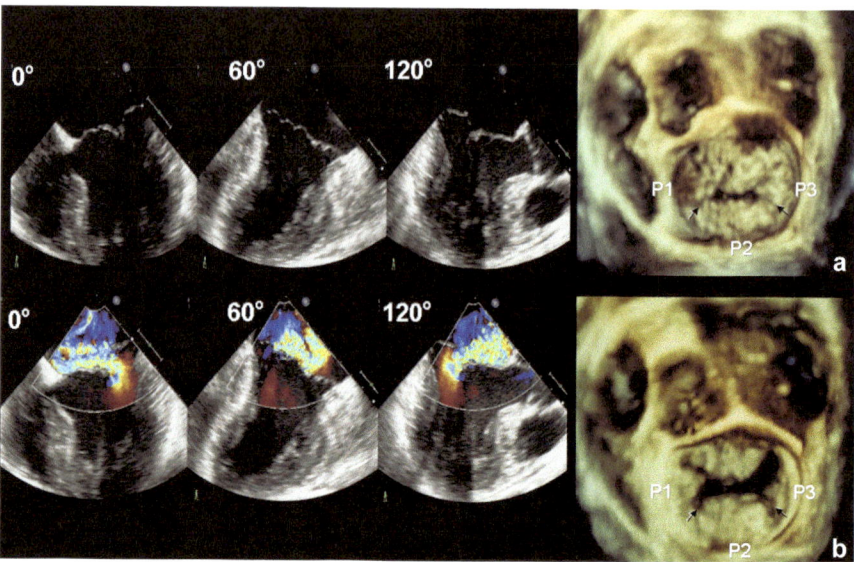

Fig. 11.11 A fully sampled 3D matrix transesophageal echo (3DMTEE). The image shows routine two-dimensional echo in the top and bottom panels performed on a patient with bileaflet mitral valve prolapse and severe eccentric mitral regurgitation (*bottom panel*) at 0°, 60°, and 120°. Using a zoom mode, the mitral valve is displayed from a *left* atrial view in systole (*Panel A*) and diastole (*Panel B*). In systole, all three segments of the posterior and corresponding anterior segments are prolapsing. The *arrows* designate the location of the posterior leaflet indentations demarcating the separation of P1, P2, and P3 which are better seen in diastole

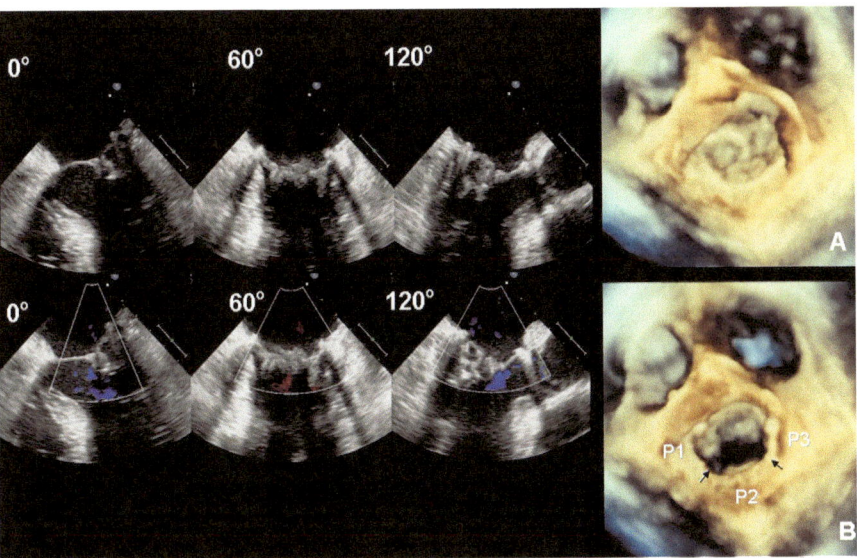

Fig. 11.12 Intraoperative evaluation of this same patient in Fig. 11.11 was performed post-repair. Routine 2D imaging was performed at 0°, 60°, and 120° with and without color. Post-repair there was not any residual mitral regurgitation. Using a zoom mode, the mitral valve is displayed from a left atrial view in systole (*Panel A*) and diastole (*Panel B*). In systole, all three segments of the posterior and corresponding anterior segments appear well opposed with a flexible mitral ring. Gore-Tex chords were placed to repair this valve without any resection performed. These chords are not readily seen and in diastole the demarcation of the posterior leaflet indentations can still be appreciated

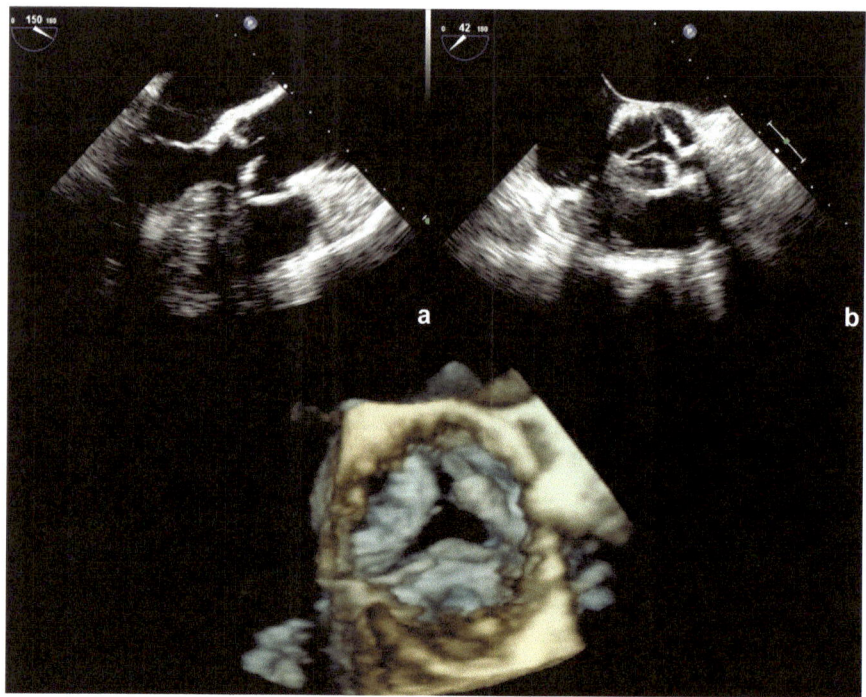

Fig. 11.13 In the two top panels a long-axis and short-axis of the aortic valve are demonstrated (**a** and **b**). There is moderate aortic sclerosis seen on the aortic leaflets as also viewed on a three-dimensional image of the valve from an aortic perspective (*bottom panel*)

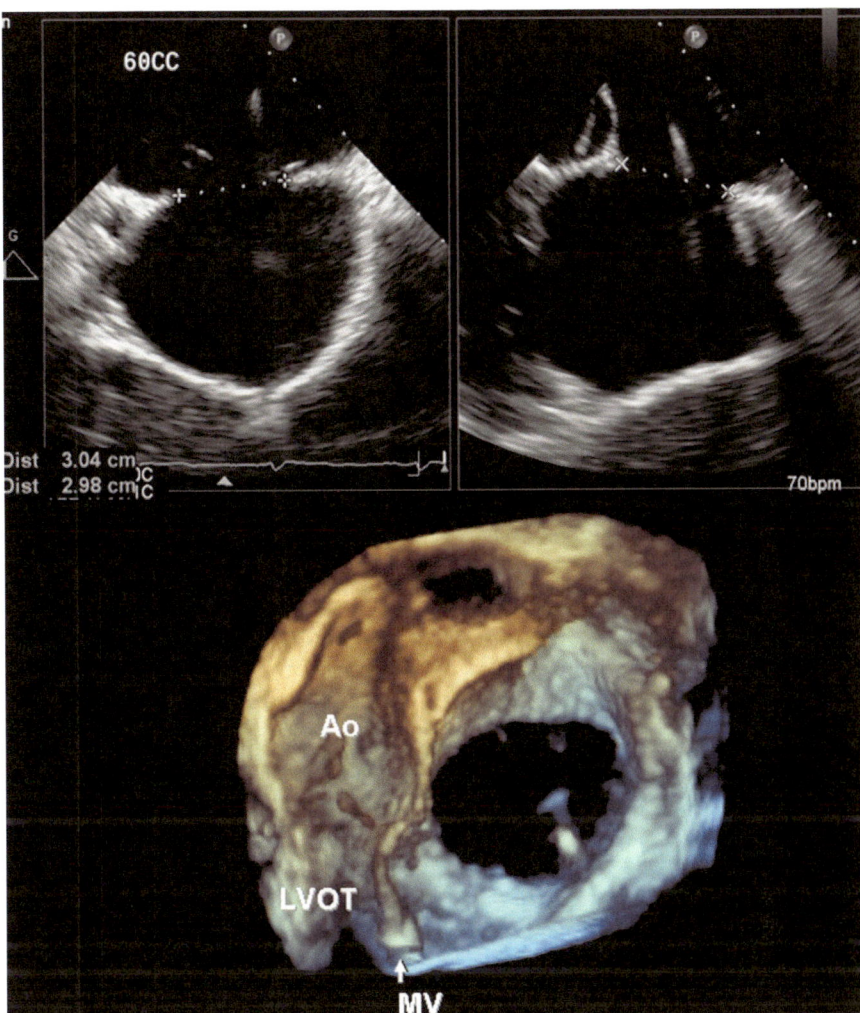

Fig. 11.14 Example of a patient with a secundum atrial septal defect demonstrated using simultaneous biplane 2D imaging, which was performed during closure of this defect. The diameter of the ASD measured in 2D was 3.04 and 2.93 cm with sufficient rim to place a device. Three-dimensional echo imaging allows en-face visual assessment of this ASD from a left atrial perspective (*bottom*). A wire is seen crossing the ASD in 2D as well as 3D

References

1. Zamorano J, Perez d I, Sugeng L, et al. Non-invasive assessment of mitral valve area during percutaneous balloon mitral valvuloplasty: role of real-time 3D echocardiography. *Eur Heart J.* 2004;25(23):2086-2091.

2. Zamorano J, Cordeiro P, Sugeng L, et al. Real-time three-dimensional echocardiography for rheumatic mitral valve stenosis evaluation: an accurate and novel approach. *J Am Coll Cardiol.* 2004;43(11):2091-2096.

3. Sugeng L, Weinert L, Lammertin G, et al. Accuracy of mitral valve area measurements using transthoracic rapid freehand 3-dimensional scanning: comparison with noninvasive and invasive methods. *J Am Soc Echocardiogr.* 2003;16(12):1292-1300.

4. Binder TM, Rosenhek R, Porenta G, Maurer G, Baumgartner H. Improved assessment of mitral valve stenosis by volumetric real-time three-dimensional echocardiography. *J Am Coll Cardiol.* 2000;36(4):1355-1361.

5. Sugeng L, Coon P, Weinert L, et al. Use of real-time 3-dimensional transthoracic echocardiography in the evaluation of mitral valve disease. *J Am Soc Echocardiogr.* 2006;19(4):413-421.

6. Kwan J, Shiota T, Agler DA, et al. Geometric differences of the mitral apparatus between ischemic and dilated cardiomyopathy with significant mitral regurgitation: real-time three-dimensional echocardiography study. *Circulation.* 2003;107(8):1135-1140.

7. Watanabe N, Ogasawara Y, Yamaura Y, et al. Geometric differences of the mitral valve tenting between anterior and inferior myocardial infarction with significant ischemic mitral regurgitation: quantitation by novel software system with transthoracic real-time three-dimensional echocardiography. *J Am Soc Echocardiogr.* 2006;19(1):71-75.

8. Gopal AS, Keller AM, Rigling R, King DL Jr, King DL. Left ventricular volume and endocardial surface area by three-dimensional echocardiography: comparison with two-dimensional echocardiography and nuclear magnetic resonance imaging in normal subjects. *J Am Coll Cardiol.* 1993;22(1):258-270.

9. Gopal AS, Keller AM, Shen Z, et al. Three-dimensional echocardiography: in vitro and in vivo validation of left ventricular mass and comparison with conventional echocardiographic methods. *J Am Coll Cardiol.* 1994;24(2):504-513.

10. Gopal AS, Schnellbaecher MJ, Shen Z, Boxt LM, Katz J, King DL. Freehand three-dimensional echocardiography for determination of left ventricular volume and mass in patients with abnormal ventricles: comparison with magnetic resonance imaging. *J Am Soc Echocardiogr.* 1997;10(8):853-861.

11. Jacobs LD, Salgo IS, Goonewardena S, et al. Rapid online quantification of left ventricular volume from real-time three-dimensional echocardiographic data. *Eur Heart J.* 2006;27(4):460-468.

12. Jenkins C, Bricknell K, Hanekom L, Marwick TH. Reproducibility and accuracy of echocardiographic measurements of left ventricular parameters using real-time three-dimensional echocardiography. *J Am Coll Cardiol.* 2004;44(4):878-886.

13. King DL, Harrison MR, King DL Jr, Gopal AS, Martin RP, DeMaria AN. Improved reproducibility of left atrial and left ventricular measurements by guided three-dimensional echocardiography. *J Am Coll Cardiol.* 1992;20(5):1238-1245.

14. King DL, Gapal AS. Three-dimensional echocardiography: use of additional spatial data for measuring left ventricular mass. *Mayo Clin Proc.* 1994;69(3):293-295.

15. Kuhl HP, Franke A, Merx M, Hoffmann R, Puschmann D, Hanrath P. Rapid quantification of left ventricular function and mass using transoesophageal three-dimensional echocardiography: validation of a method that uses long-axis cutplanes. *Eur J Echocardiogr.* 2000;1(3):213-221.

16. Kuhl HP, Schreckenberg M, Rulands D, et al. High-resolution transthoracic real-time three-dimensional echocardiography: quantitation of cardiac volumes and function using semi-automatic border detection and comparison with cardiac magnetic resonance imaging. *J Am Coll Cardiol.* 2004;43(11):2083-2090.

17. Maehle J, Bjoernstad K, Aakhus S, Torp HG, Angelsen BA. Three-dimensional echocardiography for quantitative left ventricular wall motion analysis: a method for reconstruction of endocardial surface and evaluation of regional dysfunction. *Echocardiography.* 1994;11(4):397-408.

18. Mor-Avi V, Sugeng L, Weinert L, et al. Fast measurement of left ventricular mass with real-time three-dimensional echocardiography: comparison with magnetic resonance imaging. *Circulation.* 2004;110(13):1814-1818.

19. Sapin PM, Schroder KM, Gopal AS, Smith MD, DeMaria AN, King DL. Comparison of two- and three-dimensional echocardiography with cineventriculography for measurement of left ventricular volume in patients. *J Am Coll Cardiol.* 1994;24(4):1054-1063.

20. Bacha EA, Zimmerman FJ, Mor-Avi V, et al. Ventricular resynchronization by multisite pacing improves myocardial performance in the postoperative single-ventricle patient. *Ann Thorac Surg.* 2004;78(5):1678-1683.

21. Kapetanakis S, Cooklin M, Monaghan MJ. Mechanical resynchronisation in biventricular pacing illustrated by real time transthoracic three dimensional echocardiography. *Heart.* 2004;90(5):482.

22. Kapetanakis S, Kearney MT, Siva A, Gall N, Cooklin M, Monaghan MJ. Real-time three-dimensional echocardiography: a novel technique to quantify global left ventricular mechanical dyssynchrony. *Circulation.* 2005;112(7):992-1000.

23. Sugeng L, Shernan SK, Salgo IS, et al. Live 3-dimensional transesophageal echocardiography initial experience using the fully-sampled matrix array probe. *J Am Coll Cardiol.* 2008;52(6):446-449.

24. Sugeng L, Shernan SK, Weinert L, et al. Real-time three-dimensional transesophageal echocardiography in valve disease: comparison with surgical findings and evaluation of prosthetic valves. *J Am Soc Echocardiogr.* 2008;21(12):1347-1354.

25. Lodato JA, Cao QL, Weinert L, et al. Feasibility of real-time three-dimensional transesophageal echocardiography for guidance of percutaneous atrial septal defect closure. *Eur J Echocardiogr.* 2009;10(4):543-548.

26. Shah SJ, Bardo DM, Sugeng L, et al. Real-time three-dimensional transesophageal echocardiography of the left atrial appendage: initial experience in the clinical setting. *J Am Soc Echocardiogr.* 2008;21(12):1362-1368.

27. Messika-Zeitoun D, Brochet E, Holmin C, et al. Three-dimensional evaluation of the mitral valve area and commissural opening before and after percutaneous mitral commissurotomy in patients with mitral stenosis. *Eur Heart J.* 2007;28(1):72-79.

Stress Echocardiography

12

Sebastian Kelle

12.1
Purpose

- Detection of myocardial ischemia and viability
- Baseline echo to identify regional LV function
- Wall motion abnormalities (WMA) are one of the earliest signs of myocardial ischemia during stress
- Exercise or pharmacologic stress
- Dobutamine is the preferred pharmacological stress agent for the detection of inducible WMA

12.2
Indications

- Inconclusive exercise test or inability to exercise
- Suspected coronary artery disease
- Assessment of ischemia in patients with known CAD
- Patients post revascularization and atypical chest pain
- Assessing extent of ischemia
- Guidance for intervention (PCI or CABG)
- Assessment of viability
- Preoperative risk assessment
- Documenting exercise capacity
- Risk stratification and prognosis
- Assessment of response to treatment
- Assessment of low gradient aortic stenosis or mitral valve stenosis
- Dyspnea of possible cardiac origin

S. Kelle
Department of Cardiology, German Heart Institute Berlin, Berlin, Germany
e-mail: kelle@dhzb.de

T.P. Abraham (ed.), *Case Based Echocardiography*,
DOI: 10.1007/978-1-84996-151-6_12, © Springer-Verlag London Limited 2011

12.3
Contraindications

- Unstable angina pectoris
- Acute myocardial infarction (within 2 days)
- Uncontrolled arrhythmias causing symptoms of hemodynamic compromise
- Symptomatic severe aortic stenosis
- Uncontrolled symptomatic heart failure
- Active endocarditis or acute myocarditis or pericarditis
- Acute aortic dissection or aortic aneurysm
- Acute pulmonary or systemic embolism
- Acute noncardiac disorders that may affect exercise performance or may be aggravated by exercise
- Severe hypertension
- Hemodynamically significant left ventricular outflow tract obstruction
- Known HOCM
- Hypokalemia

12.4
Dobutamine

- Given in incremental doses starting with 5–10 µg/kg/min and increasing at 10, 20, 30 and 40 µg/kg/min to simulate exercise
- Low-dose stages (up to 20 µg/kg/min) viability and ischemia assessment in segments with WMA at rest
- Half life 2 min/steady state 10 min
- Positive inotropy
  - Stimulates LV myocardial function
  - Recruits hibernating myocardium
- Positive chronotropy
  - Increases heart rate
  - Increases oxygen consumption
  - Induces ischemia

12.5
Contraindications for Dobutamine/Atropine

1. Severe arterial hypertension (>220/120 mmHg)
2. BP<90 mmHg systolic
3. Unstable angina pectoris
4. Acute myocardial infarction
5. Second or third degree AV Block or sick-sinus-syndrome (no pacemaker)

6. Severe aortic stenosis (AVA < 1 cm^2)
7. HOCM
8. Acute Perimyocarditis or Endocarditis
9. Glaucoma

12.6
Side Effects

- Palpitations, nausea, headache, chills, urinary urgency, anxiety
- Angina, hypotension, cardiac arrhythmias
- Premature atrial or ventricular contractions – 4%
- Ventricular fibrillation or myocardial infarction: 1/2,000

12.7
Monitoring Requirements

1. Heart rate and rhythm: continuously
2. Blood pressure: every 3 min
3. Symptoms: continuously
4. Wall-motion-abnormalities: every dose increment
5. Imaging < 3 min
6. Cover all segments
7. ST-Segment changes

12.8
Visual Assessment of Left Ventricular WMA, the Standard Scoring System is Applied Per Myocardial Segment

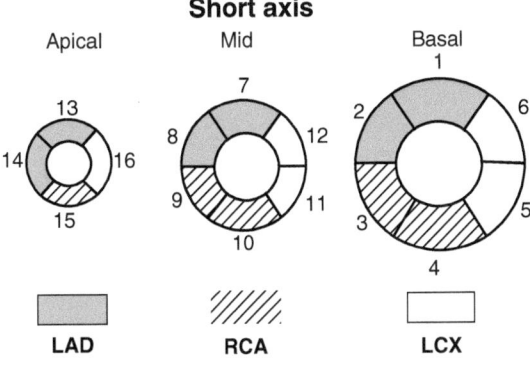

Scoring system
1, normokinesis
2, hypokinesis
3, akinesis
4, dyskinesis
5, aneurysmal

12.9
Performance

Patient instructions:
No β-blockers and nitrates 24 h prior to the examination

- Optimal ECG
- Select optimal windows (whole window for left ventricle)
- Use tissue harmonic imaging
- Highest frame rate
- Continuous monitoring
- Cine-loops at baseline, low- and high-dose
- Record several cycles
- Use intravenous contrast agents when two or more segments are not well visualized

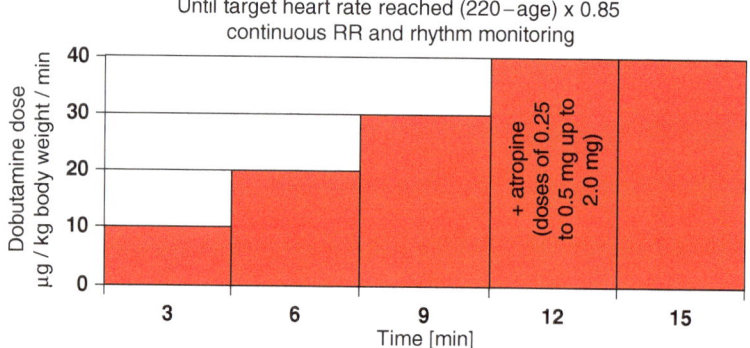

Baseline	Low dose 10-20 µg/kg/min	High-dose 40 µg/kg/min	Test result

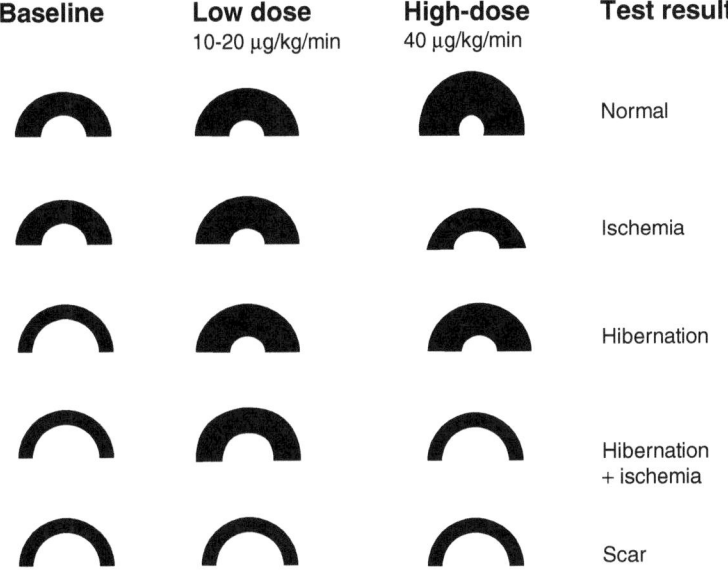

Normal

Ischemia

Hibernation

Hibernation
+ ischemia

Scar

12.10
Termination Criteria

- Submaximal heart rate reached ($[220 - \text{age}] \times 0.85$)
- Maximum dose reached (40 µg/kg/min dobutamine + 2 mg atropine)
- Systolic RR decrease > 20 mmHg below the baseline level or decrease > 40 mmHg from a previous level
- RR increase > 240/120 mmHg
- Intolerable symptoms (chest pain, nausea)
- New or worsening WMA in $N \geq 2$ adjacent LV segments
- ST depression > 3 mm
- Symptomatic or complex cardiac tachycardia

Ischemia is defined as a new WMA or a biphasic response.

12.11
Myocardial Viability

1. Myocardial stunning: result of *acute* ischemic insult leading to contractile dysfunction despite adequate reperfusion
2. Hibernating myocardium: reversible left ventricular dysfunction due to *chronic* coronary artery disease that improves after revascularization

12.12
Interpretation

- Report – description of
  - Hemodynamics
  - ECG changes
  - Clinical symptoms
  - Reached maximum heart rate
  - Stress level
  - Wall motion score at rest and stress
- Baseline
  - Left ventricular cardiac chamber volumes, ejection fraction, mass and regional wall motion, valves, aortic root
- Stress
  - New wall motion abnormalities during stress in segments with normal wall motion at rest or worsening or biphasic response in segments with wall motion abnormality at rest
  - Extent of ischemia
  - Assessment of ischemic mitral valve regurgitation
  - Assessment of aortic gradient

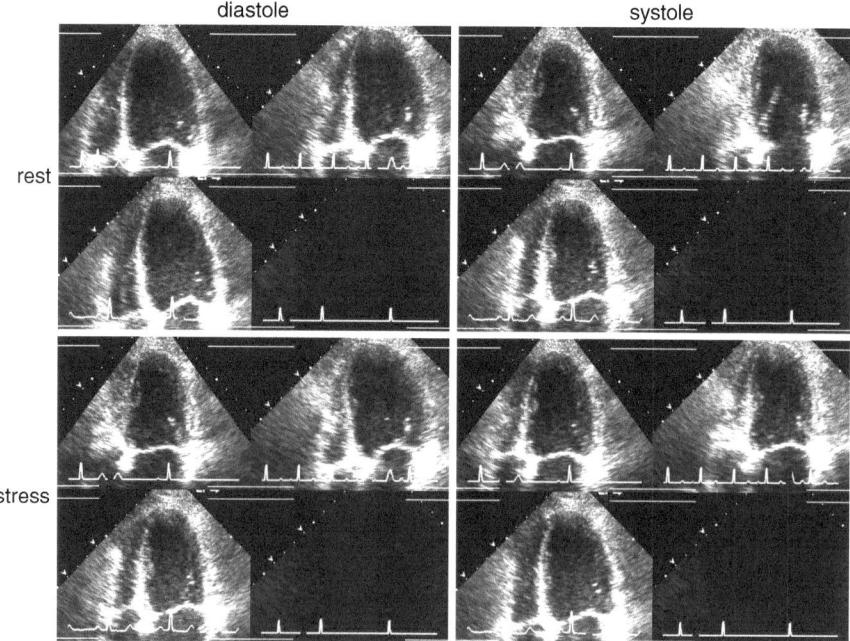

Fig. 12.1 Exercise stress echocardiogram images. Apical four-chamber view showing rest images (top row) and normal left ventricular wall motion. During stress imaging (bottom row) there is an anteroapical wall motion abnormality indicating exercise-induced ischemia in the distribution of the left anterior descending coronary artery.

Mechanical Dyssynchrony Assessment

Gabe B. Bleeker, Nico R. Van de Veire, Theodore P. Abraham, Eduard R. Holman, and Jeroen J. Bax

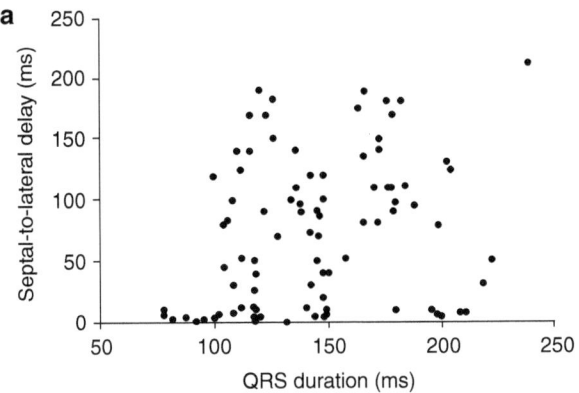

Fig. 13.1 Currently, the resynchronization of left ventricular (LV) dyssynchrony (present before pacemaker implantation) is considered to be the key mechanism of response following cardiac resynchronization therapy (CRT). Identification of LV dyssynchrony is, therefore, needed to select patients with high likelihood of response to CRT. In the current guidelines, a widened QRS complex (>120 ms) is used as a marker of LV dyssynchrony. Recent data, however, have indicated that QRS duration is a poor marker of LV dyssynchrony, with poor predictive value for response to CRT. Since this observation, several echocardiographic techniques, such as color-coded tissue Doppler imaging (TDI), have been evaluated for the ability to directly quantify LV dyssynchrony. (a) Results of a recent study illustrating the lack of correlation between LV dyssynchrony (expressed as the septal-to-lateral delay) and QRS duration in 90 heart failure patients with LV ejection fraction <35% and NYHA class III-IV heart failure ($r=0.26$, $P=NS$) (Reprinted with permission from Ref.[1]). (b) Example of a heart failure patient with a narrow QRS complex (110 ms) and a delay of 85 ms between the peak systolic velocity (PSV) of the septum and lateral wall, indicating the presence of LV dyssynchrony (*arrows* indicate peak systolic velocities, *AVO* aortic valve opening, *AVC* aortic valve closure). (c) Example of a patient with a wide QRS complex (160 ms) without a delay in peak systolic velocity between the septum and the lateral wall, indicating the absence of LV dyssynchrony (*arrows* indicate peak systolic velocities, *AVO* aortic valve opening, *AVC* aortic valve closure)

G.B. Bleeker (✉)
Department of Cardiology, Leiden University Medical Center, Leiden, The Netherlands
e-mail: g.b.bleeker@lumc.nl

T.P. Abraham (ed.), *Case Based Echocardiography*,
DOI: 10.1007/978-1-84996-151-6_13, © Springer-Verlag London Limited 2011

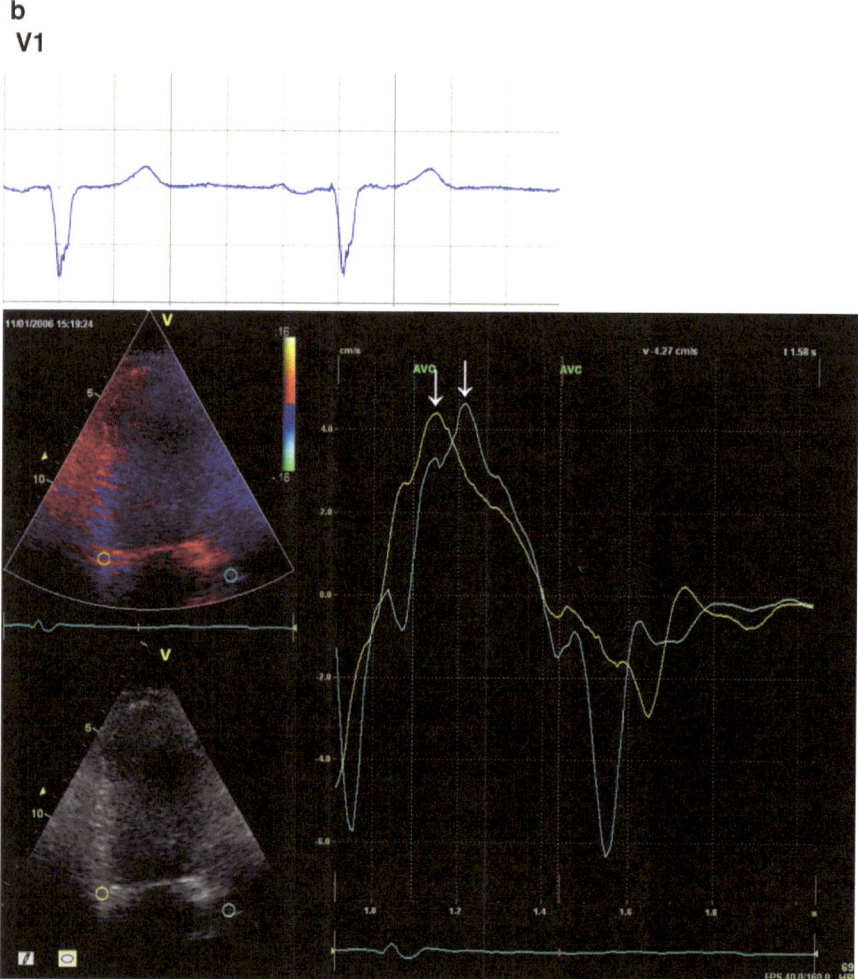

Fig. 13.1 (continued)

c

V1

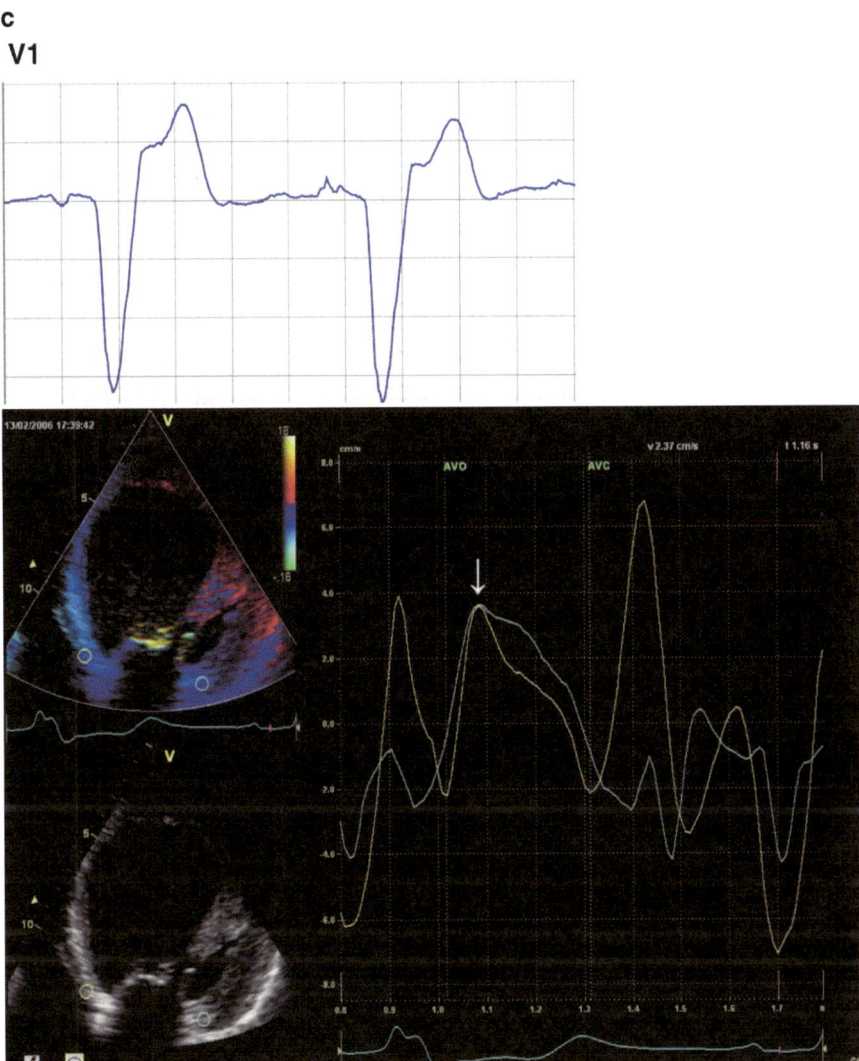

Fig. 13.1 (continued)

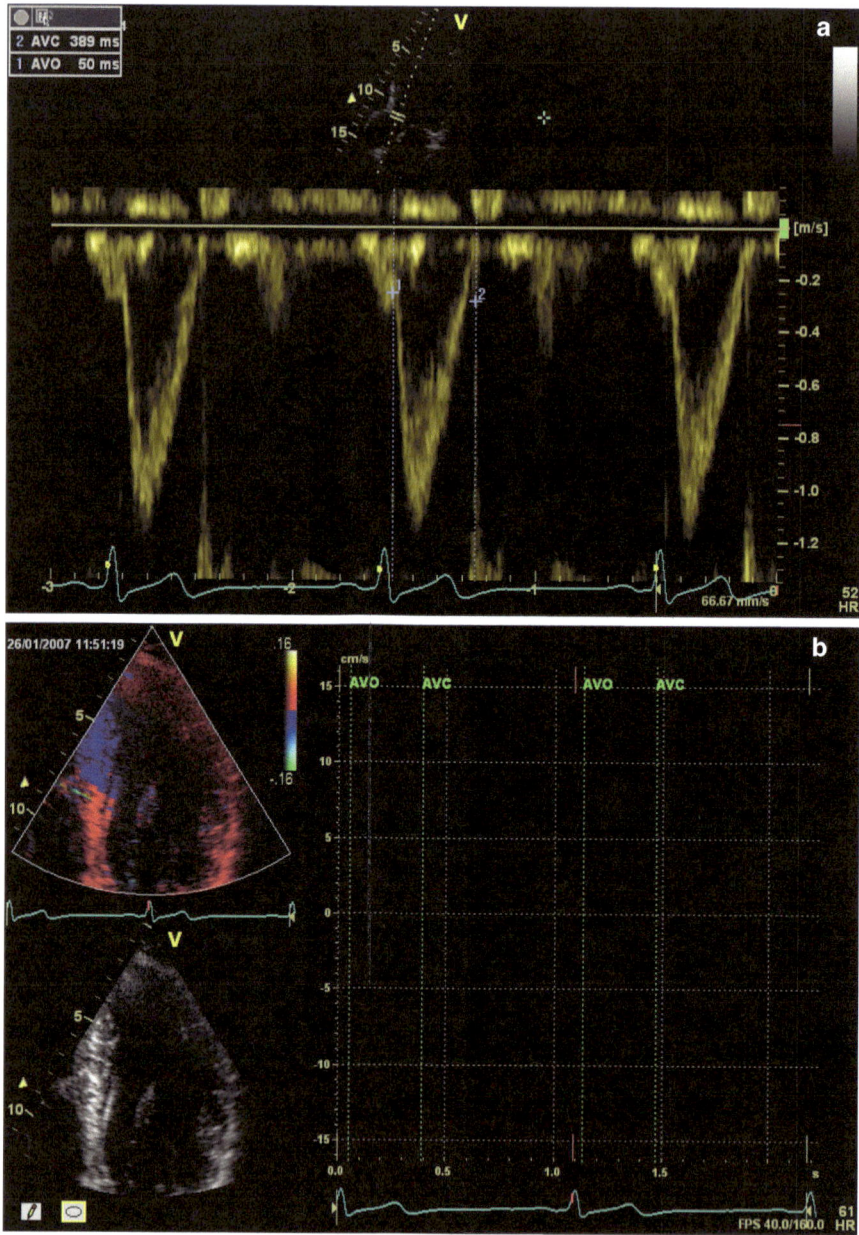

Fig. 13.2 The first step in LV dyssynchrony measurement from TDI is to define the ejection period. Using the "event timing function," the timing of aortic valve opening (AVO) and closure (AVC) can be defined from the pulsed-wave Doppler recording in the LV outflow tract (**a**). After marking the AVO and AVC in the pulsed-wave Doppler recording, the timing of the ejection phase is automatically displayed in the TDI-analysis window (**b**)

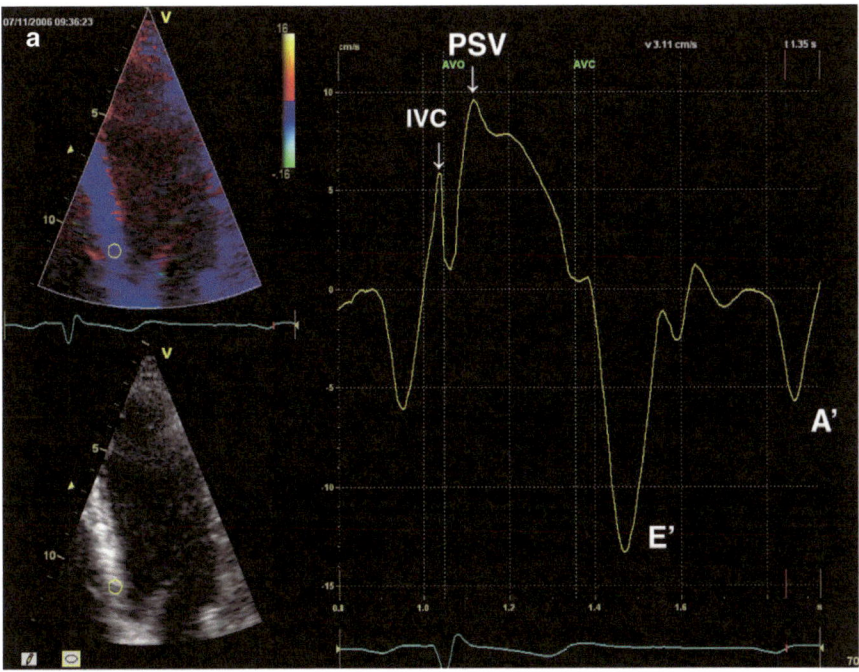

Fig. 13.3 (**a**) Example of a TDI curve derived from the basal septum in a normal individual in the 4-chamber view. The sample volume is placed in the region of interest (here the basal septum), and a TDI curve will be automatically derived indicating the peak systolic velocity (PSV), which is within the ejection phase between aortic valve opening (AVO) and closure, (AVC), and diastolic parameters (E′ and A′). Do not confuse the peak of isovolumic contraction (IVC) with the peak systolic velocity (PSV). (**b**) Example of a TDI curve derived from the basal lateral wall in a normal individual (4-chamber view, for explanation see Fig. 13.3a). (**c**) Example of a TDI curve derived from the basal inferior wall in a normal individual (2-chamber view, for explanation see Fig. 13.3a). (**d**) Example of a TDI curve derived from the basal anterior wall in a normal individual (2-chamber view, for explanation see Fig. 13.3a). (**e**) LV dyssynchrony can be calculated as the delay in time-to-peak systolic velocity between the basal septum and the lateral wall (referred to as septal-to-lateral delay (*2-segmental model*, cutoff value 60 ms[6]). Example of a normal individual without a delay in peak systolic velocity, indicating absence of LV dyssynchrony. (**e, f**) Another described method to quantify LV dyssynchrony by measuring the time-to-maximum delay between the peak systolic velocities among the four basal LV walls (septum, lateral, inferior, and anterior walls (*4-segmental model*, derived from Fig. 13.3a–d) (most frequently dyssynchrony is observed between the septum and lateral wall, cutoff value 65 ms[7]). When the time-to-peak systolic velocity is measured in multiple views, the beginning of the QRS complex can be used as a reference point

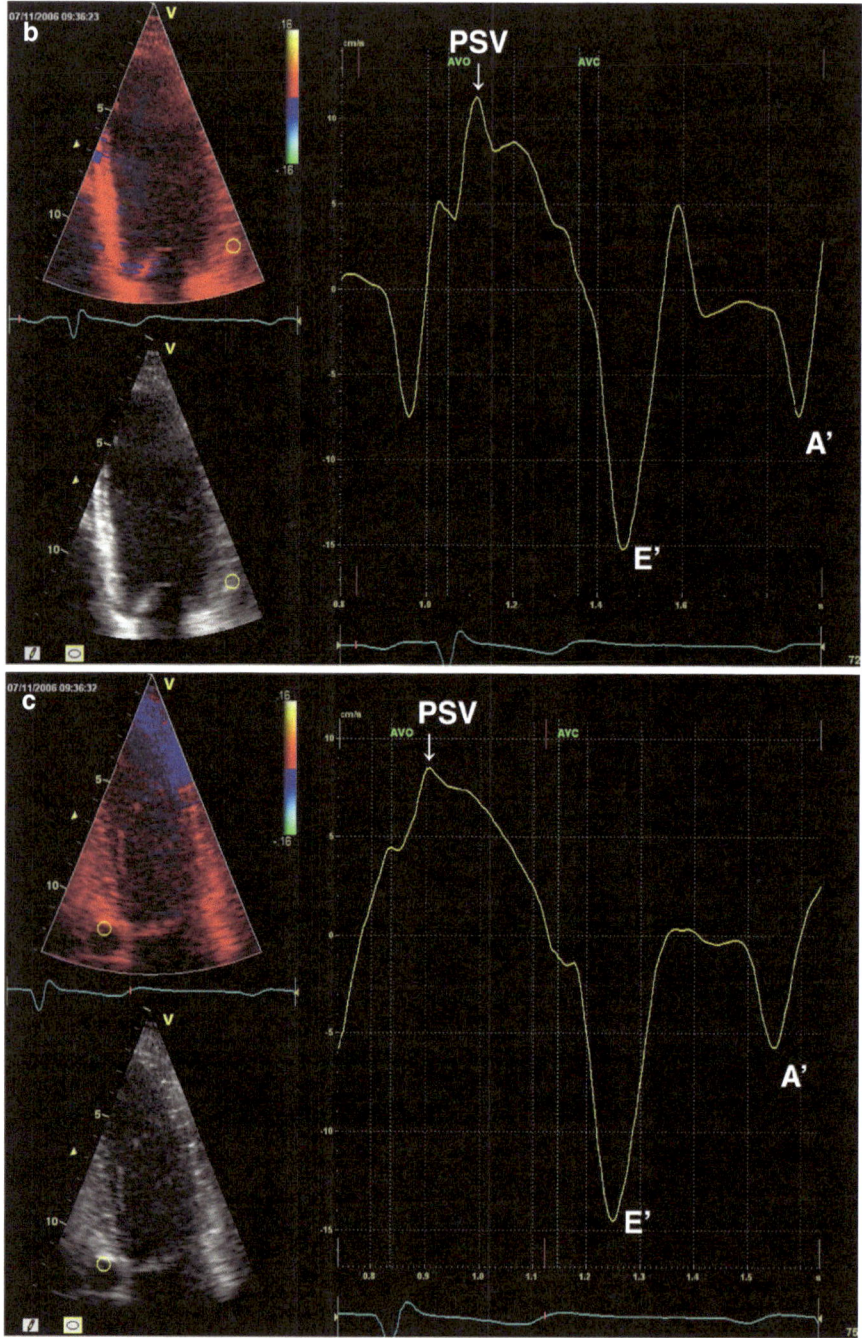

Fig. 13.3 (continued)

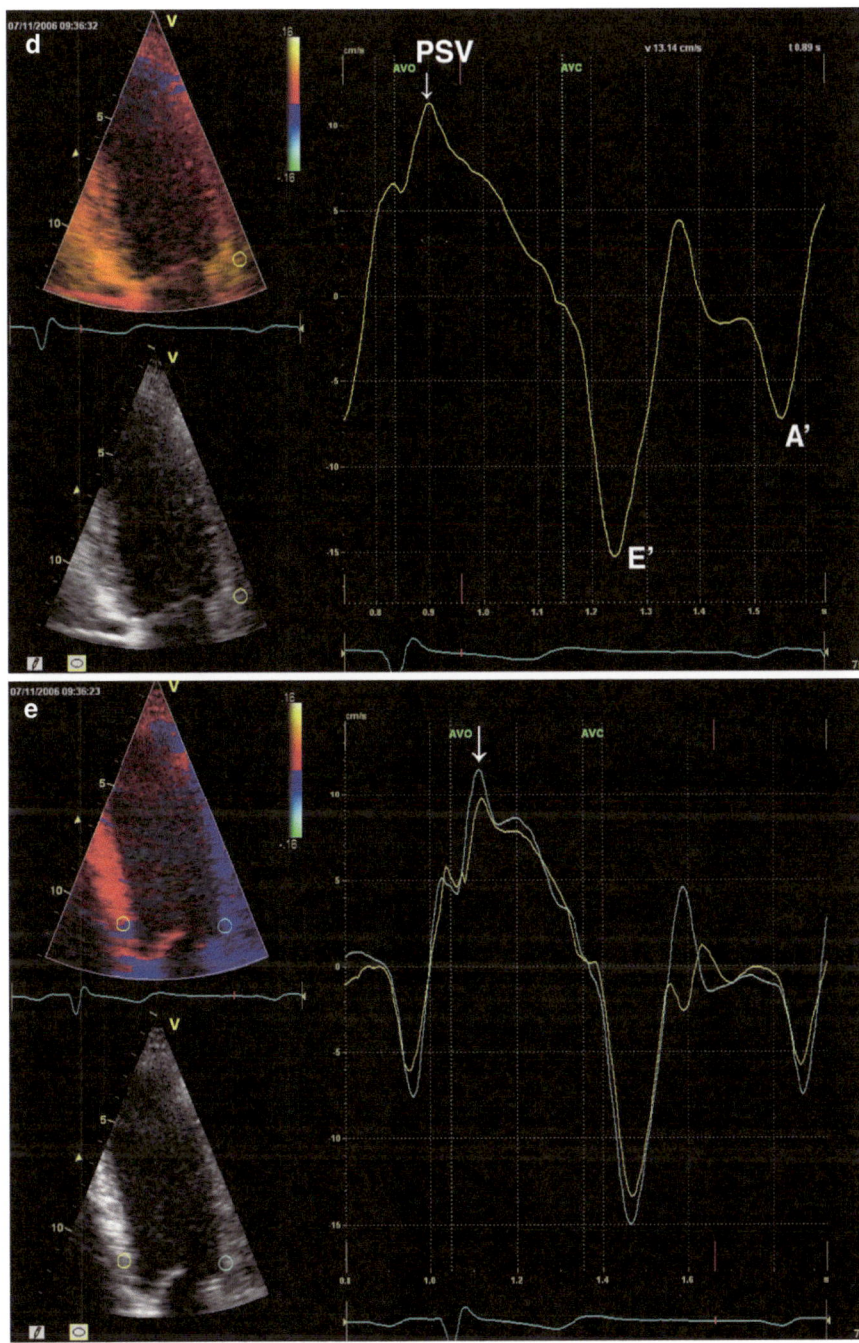

Fig. 13.3 (continued)

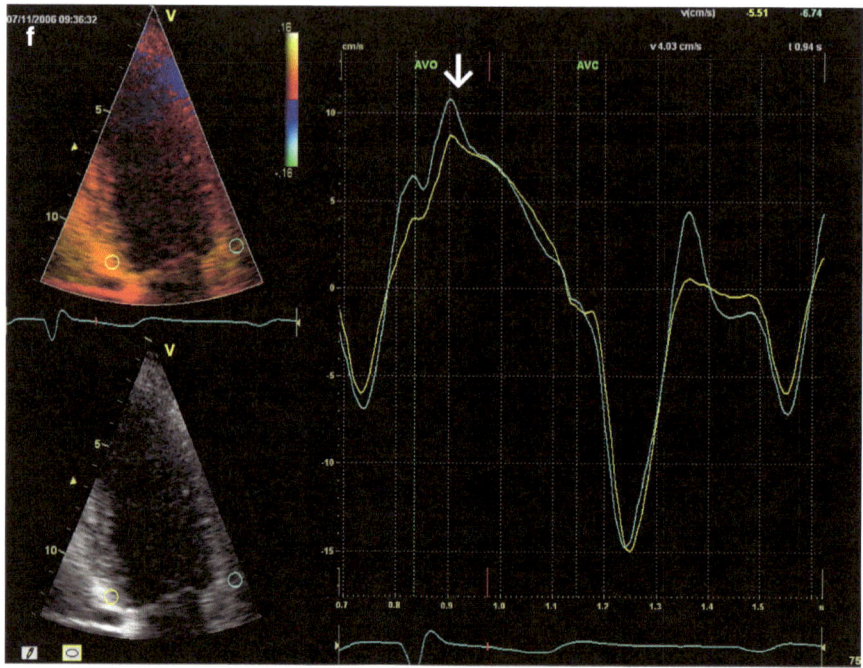

Fig. 13.3 (continued)

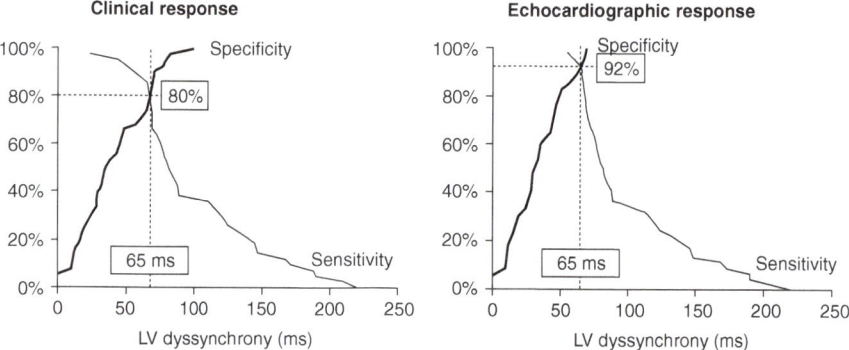

Fig. 13.4 ROC curve analysis to determine the predictive value for response following CRT using the 4-segmental LV dyssynchrony model (maximum delay among four basal segments), demonstrating a sensitivity and specificity of 80% to predict clinical response (defined as improvement in NYHA class≥1 score and improvement≥25% in 6-min walking distance) at a cutoff level of 65 ms for LV dyssynchrony. In addition, this approach yielded a sensitivity and specificity of 92% to predict reverse LV remodeling after CRT (defined as improvement in LV end-systolic volume≥15%) at a cutoff level of 65 ms for LV dyssynchrony. Reprinted with permission from reference[8]

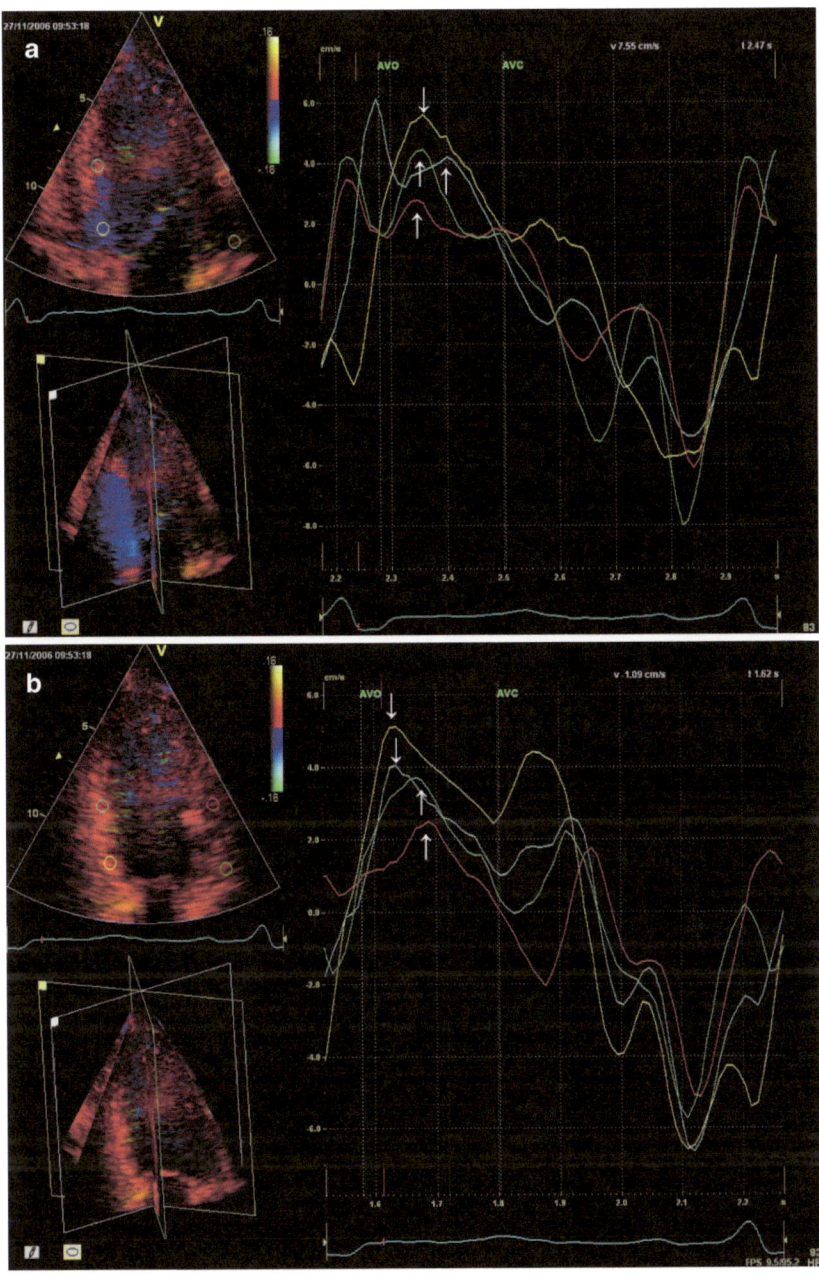

Fig. 13.5 Illustration of the *12-segmental model* for LV dyssynchrony measurement (Yu-index[8]). The time-to-peak systolic velocities during the ejection phase in each view are measured (by using the beginning of the QRS complex as a reference point). The myocardial velocity curves are derived from the basal and mid parts of the following LV segments: septum and lateral wall (4-chamber view, **a**), inferior and anterior wall (2-chamber view, **b**) and antero-septal and posterior wall (3-chamber view, **c**). LV dyssynchrony is defined as the standard deviation of the time-to-peak systolic velocity for all 12 segments (cutoff value 32 ms[8])

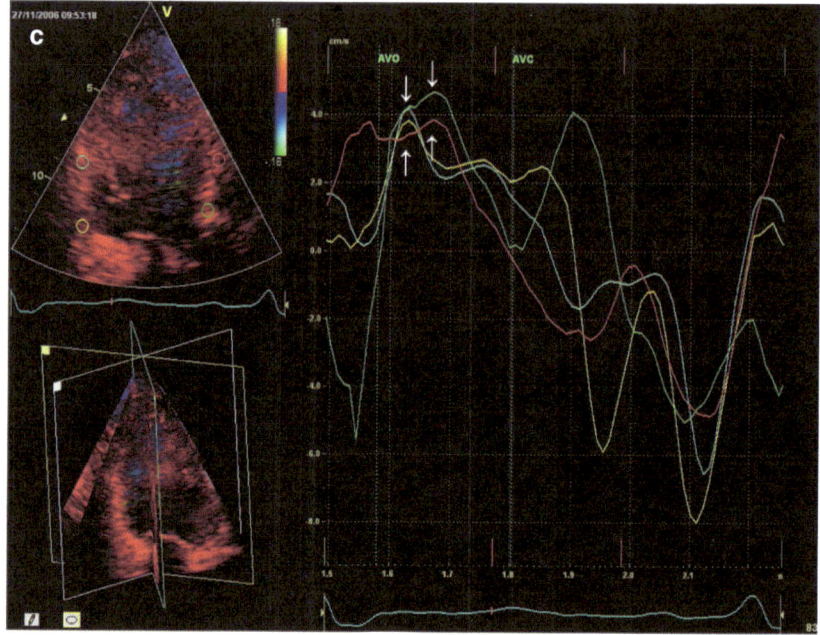

Fig. 13.5 (continued)

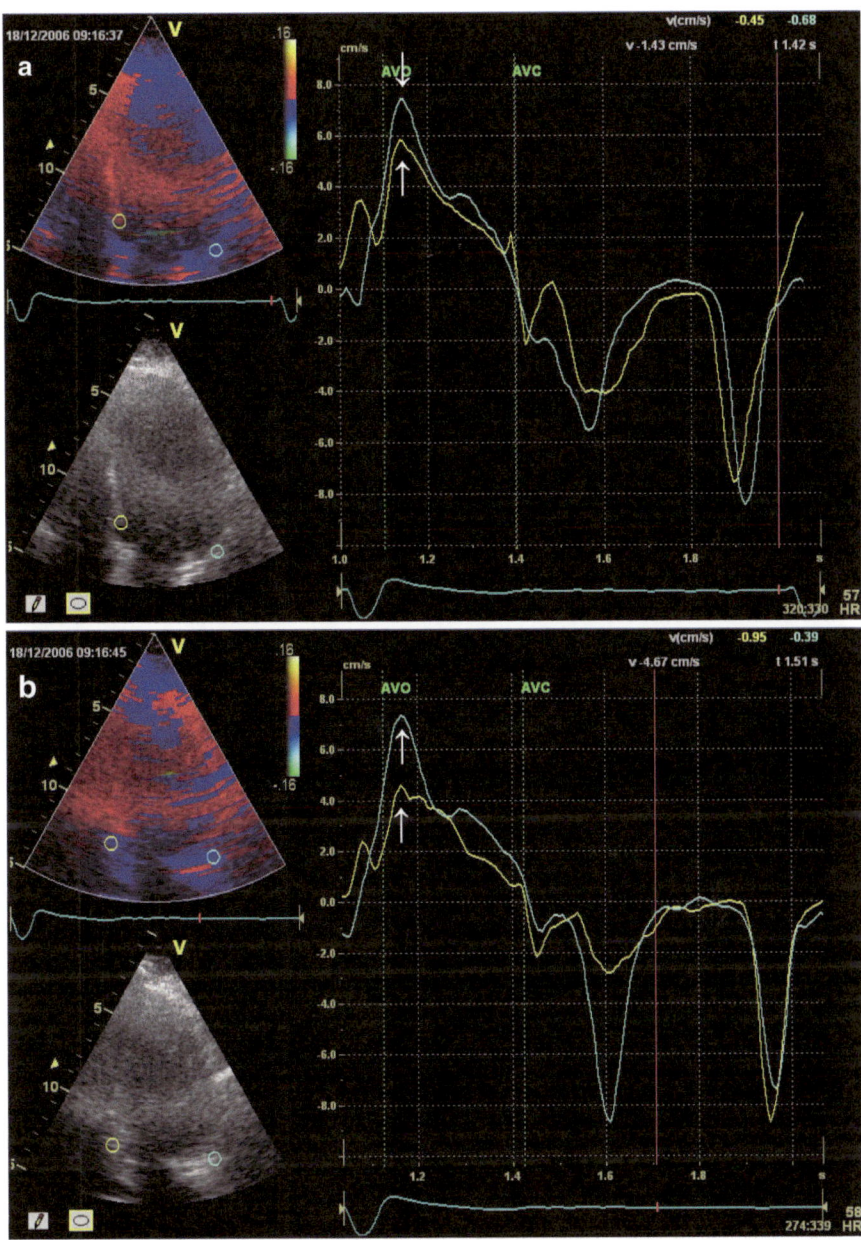

Fig. 13.6 Measurement of LV dyssynchrony using the 4-segmental model. Example of a patient without a delay in time-to-peak systolic velocity between the septum and the lateral wall (4-chamber view, **a**) and the inferior and anterior wall (2-chamber view, **b**), indicating the absence of LV dyssynchrony (*Arrows* indicate peak systolic velocities, *AVO* aortic valve opening, *AVC* aortic valve closure)

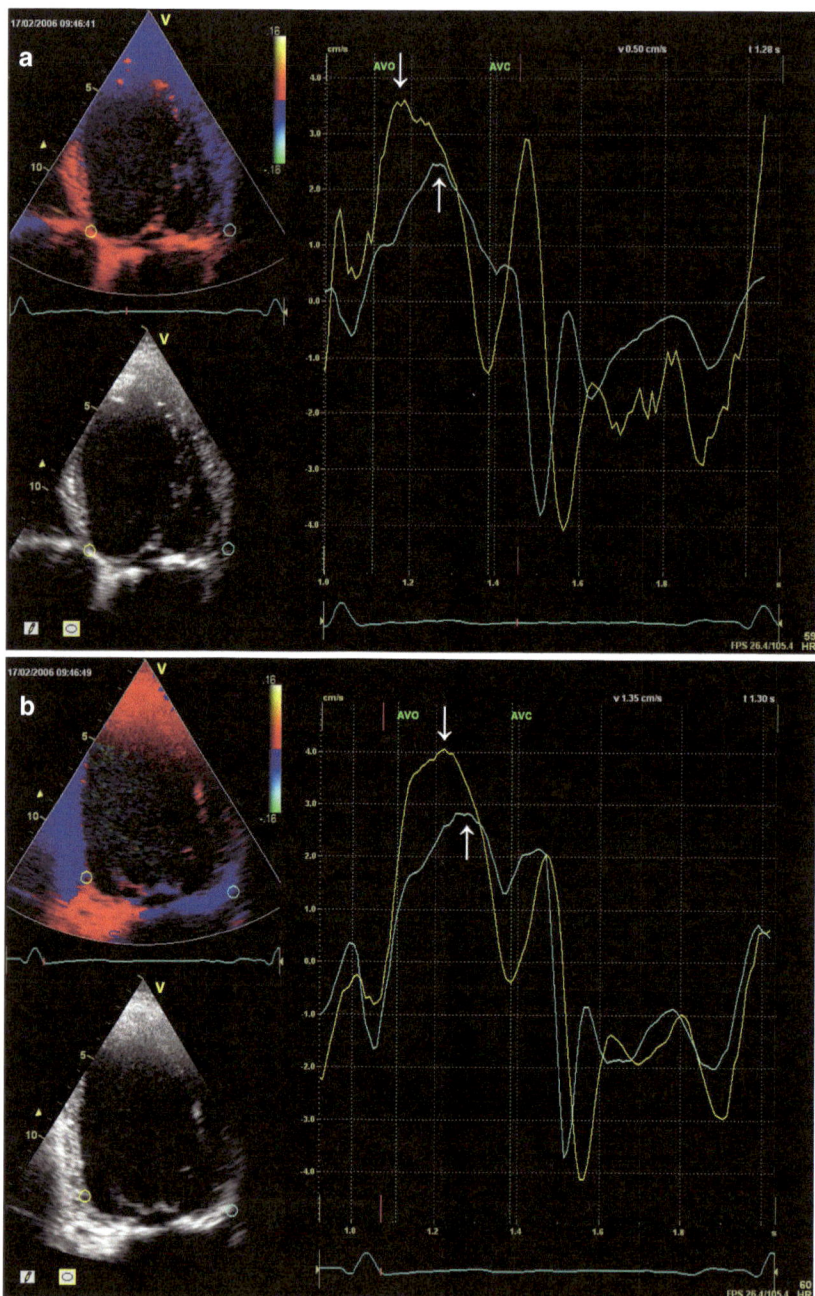

Fig. 13.7 Measurement of LV dyssynchrony using the 4-segmental model. Example of a patient with substantial LV dyssynchrony. In the 4-chamber view, a delay in time-to-peak systolic velocity of 120 ms is observed between the septum and the lateral wall (**a**) and a delay of 60 ms is present between the inferior and anterior walls (**b**). The maximum delay among the four segments is well above the cutoff value of 65 ms, indicating the presence of LV dyssynchrony (*Arrows* indicate peak systolic velocities, *AVO* aortic valve opening, *AVC* aortic valve closure)

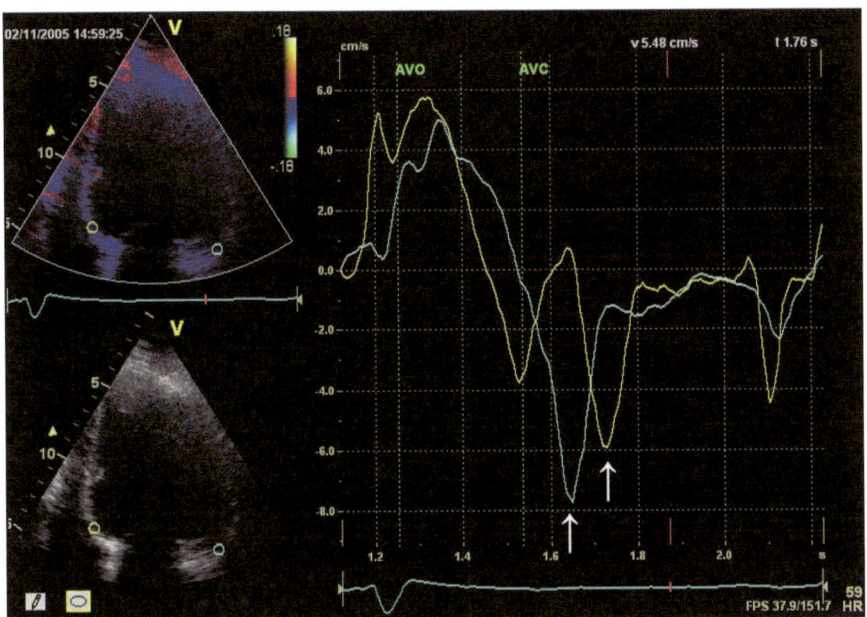

Fig. 13.8 Measurement of diastolic dyssynchrony within the left ventricle. Example of a patient with a delay of 90 ms between the time to peak E′-wave of the septum and lateral wall. At present, the role of diastolic dyssynchrony in CRT remains to be defined. No cutoff value for diastolic dyssynchrony has been proposed in the literature (*Arrows* indicate peak E′-wave)

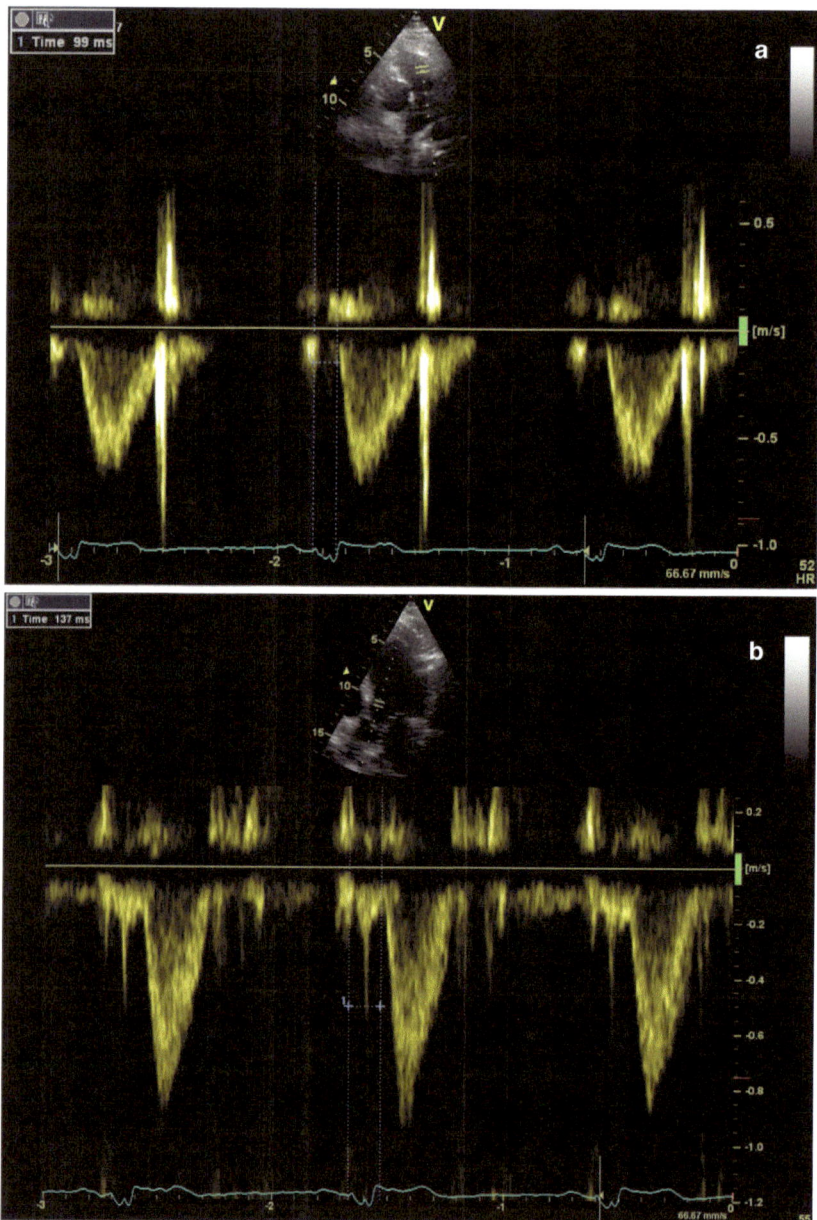

Fig. 13.9 Measurement of interventricular dyssynchrony (dyssynchrony between the left and right ventricles). The first method measures the difference in the pre-ejection times between the pulmonary flow (**a**, 99 ms) and the aortic flow (**b**, 137 ms). The difference between both pre-ejection times represents the interventricular dyssynchrony (38 ms in this example, proposed cutoff values range between 40 and 50 ms). Recent studies, however, have now clearly demonstrated that interventricular dyssynchrony is a poor predictor of response after CRT implantation. Another described method for interventricular dyssynchrony calculation is to measure the delay in peak systolic velocity between the LV lateral wall and the right ventricular free wall (**c**, *arrows* indicate peak systolic velocities)

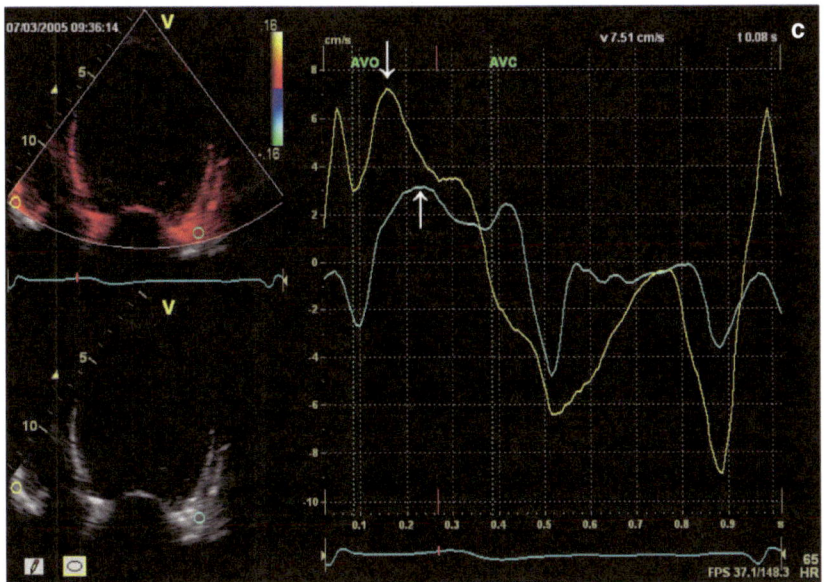

Fig. 13.9 (continued)

Table 13.1 Most commonly used echocardiographic techniques for LV dyssynchrony quantification. All clinically proven parameters of dyssynchrony – from JACC review

Echocardiographic technique	Parameter	Author
M-mode echocardiography	Difference in systolic inward motion between septum and posterior wall.	Pitzalis et al.[2,3]
Pulsed-wave TDI	Difference in time-to-onset of systolic velocity between septum and lateral wall.	Garrigue et al.[4]
	– Maximum difference in time-to-onset/peak systolic velocity among 12 basal and mid-LV segments.	Bordachar et al.[5]
	– Standard deviation in time-to-onset/peak systolic velocity among 12 basal and mid-LV segments.	
Color-coded TDI	Difference in time-to-peak systolic velocity between basal septum and lateral wall (septal-to-lateral delay).	Bax et al.[6] (Fig. 13.3)
	Maximum delay in time-to-peak systolic velocity among four basal segments.	Bax et al.[7] (Figs. 13.3 and 13.4)
	Standard deviation of the time-to-peak systolic velocity among 12 basal and mid-LV segments (Yu-index).	Yu et al.[8] (Fig. 13.5)
Tissue synchronization imaging	– Qualitative assessment of LV dyssynchrony based on color maps.	Yu et al.[9]
	– Standard deviation of the time-to-peak systolic velocity among 12 basal and mid-LV segments.	
Strain (rate) imaging (derived from TDI)	Difference in time-to-peak radial strain between septum and posterior wall.	Dohi et al.[10]
	Difference in time-to-peak strain between septum and lateral wall.	Popovic et al.[11]
2D strain (speckle tracking)	Difference in time-to-peak radial strain between septum and posterior wall.	Suffoletto et al.[12]
Real-time 3D echocardiography	Standard deviation of time-to-minimal regional volume among 16 segments (systolic dyssynchrony index).	Kapetanakis et al.[13]

TDI tissue Doppler imaging, *LV* left ventricular

Table based on Ref.[14]

Table 13.2 Algorithm for LV dyssynchrony measurement using color-coded TDI. Focus on the criteria you use clinically – may be 2–3 major ones for example, septal to lateral wall delay; maximum delay and Yu index

Step1:

Define the ejection phase by measuring the timing of the aortic valve opening and closure from the pulsed-wave Doppler signal in the LV outflow tract (Fig. 13.2).

Step 2:

Use the TDI curves to measure the time difference between the beginning of the QRS complex and the peak systolic velocity

In the following LV segments (Fig. 13.3):

  – Basal septum and basal lateral wall (apical 4-chamber view)

  – Basal anterior and basal inferior wall (apical 2-chamber view)

Additional measurements for the 12-segmental model (Yu-index, Fig. 13.5)

  – Mid-septal and mid-lateral wall (apical 4-chamber view)

  – Mid-anterior and mid-inferior wall (apical 2-chamber view)

  – Basal and mid-antero-septum and basal and mid-posterior LV wall (apical 3-chamber view)

Step 3:

The measurements from step 2 can be used to calculate the following parameters for LV dyssynchrony:

  – Time-delay between the peak systolic velocity of the basal septum and lateral wall (septal-to-lateral delay, cutoff value 60 ms[6]).

  – Maximum time delay among four basal segments (septum, lateral, inferior and anterior LV segments, cutoff value 65 ms[7]).

  – Standard deviation of the time-to-peak systolic velocity among 12 LV segments (Yu-index, cutoff value 32 ms[8]).

TDI tissue Doppler imaging, *LV* left ventricular

Table 13.3 Pitfalls in LV dyssynchrony measurement using color-coded TDI. Common pitfalls with dyssynchrony analysis and how to overcome them Suggested references: up to five general references where they can go for more details

Pitfalls	Solution
Which peak should be measured?	The measurement of the peaks should be limited to the ejection phase. Use the event timing function, which marks the opening and closure of the aortic valve (Fig. 13.2).
	In the event of multiple positive peaks in the ejection phase, take the peak with the highest systolic velocity.
	Do not confuse the peak systolic velocity with the peak of isovolumetric contraction.
Arrhythmias	Record the TDI-images during at least three consecutive beats in normal sinus rhythm. Avoid measurement of LV dyssynchrony during atrial and ventricular extrasystoles.
	During persistent atrial arrhythmias, LV dyssynchrony should be calculated within the same heartbeat. In addition, the measurements should be repeated/confirmed within other heartbeats.
Noisy signals	Ensure a frame rate of at least 100 frames per second (the higher the better). A high frame rate can be achieved by narrowing the apical 4-, 2- and 3-chamber TDI recordings down to the left ventricle (i.e., excluding the right ventricle and the atria).

TDI tissue Doppler imaging, *LV* left ventricular

References

1. Bleeker GB, Schalij MJ, Molhoek SG, et al. Relationship between QRS duration and left ventricular dyssynchrony in patients with end-stage heart failure. *J Cardiovasc Electrophysiol.* 2004;15:544-549.
2. Pitzalis MV, Iacoviello, Romito R, et al. Cardiac resynchronization therapy tailored by echocardiographic evaluation of ventricular asynchrony. *J Am Coll Cardiol.* 2002;40:1615-1622.
3. Pitzalis MV, Iacoviello, Romito R, et al. Ventricular asynchrony predicts a better outcome in patients with chronic heart failure receiving cardiac resynchronization therapy. *J Am Coll Cardiol.* 2005;45:65-69.
4. Garrigue S, Reuter S, Labeque JN, et al. Usefullness of biventricular pacing in patients with congestive heart failure and right bundle branch block. *Am J Cardiol.* 2001;88:1436-1441.
5. Bordachar P, Lafitte S, Reuter S, et al. Echocardiographic parameters of ventricular dyssynchrony validation in patients with heart failure using sequential biventricular pacing. *J Am Coll Cardiol.* 2004;44:2154-2165.
6. Bax JJ, Marwick TH, Molhoek SG, et al. Left ventricular dyssynchrony predicts benefit of cardiac resynchronization therapy in patients with end-stage heart failure before pacemaker implantation. *Am J Cardiol.* 2003;92:1238-1240.
7. Bax JJ, Bleeker GB, Marwick TH, et al. Left ventricular dyssynchrony predicts response and prognosis after cardiac resynchronization therapy. *J Am Coll Cardiol.* 2004;44:1834-1840.

8. Yu CM, Chau E, Sanderson JE, et al. Tissue Doppler echocardiographic evidence of reverse remodeling and improved synchronicity by simultaneously delaying regional contraction after biventricular pacing therapy in heart failure. *Circulation*. 2002;105:438-445.

9. Yu CM, Zhang Q, Fung JW, et al. A novel tool to assess systolic asynchrony and identify responders of cardiac resynchronization therapy by tissue synchronization imaging. *J Am Coll Cardiol*. 2005;45:677-684.

10. Dohi K, Suffoletto MS, Schwartzman D, et al. Utility of Echocardiographic radial strain imaging to quantify left ventricular dyssynchrony and predict acute response to cardiac resynchronization therapy. *Am J Cardiol*. 2005;96:112-116.

11. Popovic ZB, Grimm RA, Perlic G, et al. Noninvasive assessment of cardiac resynchronization therapy for congestive heart failure using myocardial strain and left ventricular peak power as parameters of myocardial synchrony and function. *J Cardiovasc Electrophysiol*. 2002;13:1203-1208.

12. Suffoletto MS, Dohi K, Cannesson M, et al. Novel speckle-tracking radial strain from routine black-and-white echocardiographic images to quantify dyssynchrony and predict response to cardiac resynchronization therapy. *Circulation*. 2006;113:960-968.

13. Kapetanakis S, Kearney MT, Siva A, et al. Real-time Three-dimensional echocardiography. *Circulation*. 2005;112:992-1000.

14. Bax JJ, Abraham T, Barold SS, et al. Cardiac resynchronization therapy. Part 1-Issues before device implantation. *J Am Coll Cardiol*. 2005;46:2153-2167.

Post Cardiac Resynchronization Therapy (CRT) Optimization Protocol

14

Hsin-Yueh Liang

14.1
Cardiac Optimization Protocol

14.1.1
Scheduling Requirements

1. 2-h slot
2. Sonographer
3. Programmer and pacemaker specialist
4. A physician who is familiar with echo and pacemaker

14.1.2
Protocol

1. Interrogate pacemaker and print out baseline settings, read low rate, hysteresis rate, max tracking rate, AV/PV delay, and VV offset
2. Determine percentage of A sense V sense (ASVS), A sense V pace (ASVP), A pace V sense (APVS), and A pace V pace (APVP) from histogram
3. Set VV offset as zero (simultaneous bi-ventricular pacing)

H.-Y. Liang
Division of Cardiology, Department of Medicine, China Medical University Hospital, Taichung, Taiwan
e-mail: liangsy2@gmail.com

T.P. Abraham (ed.), *Case Based Echocardiography*,
DOI: 10.1007/978-1-84996-151-6_14, © Springer-Verlag London Limited 2011

14.1.2.1
PV Optimization

Set pacer to the intrinsic rhythm (ASVS), make sure wide QRS from surface ECG on the echo machine and intracardiac electrogram (IEG) on the pacer programmer, usually the intrinsic PV delay is longer than 200 ms

A. Wait for at least 30 s at each setting before start of echo record
B. PW Doppler on MV at mitral annulus, measure VTI of A wave, and total mitral inflow (Fig. 14.1).
C. PW Doppler at LVOT, measure VTI of LVOT (Fig. 14.2)
D. Decrease PV delay until A sense V pace (ASVP), make sure narrow QRS from the surface ECG and IEG
E. Repeat this sequence of imagines (point A to C)
F. Decrease PV delay by 30 ms intervals and repeat this sequence of imagines (point A to C)
G. Repeat point F until there is mitral A wave truncation (Fig. 14.3).
H. The optimal PV delay is the setting, which yields maximal LVOT VTI with narrow QRS complex
I. Determine the optimal PV delay by VTI of mitral inflow in case maximal LVOT VTI is present at two different settings

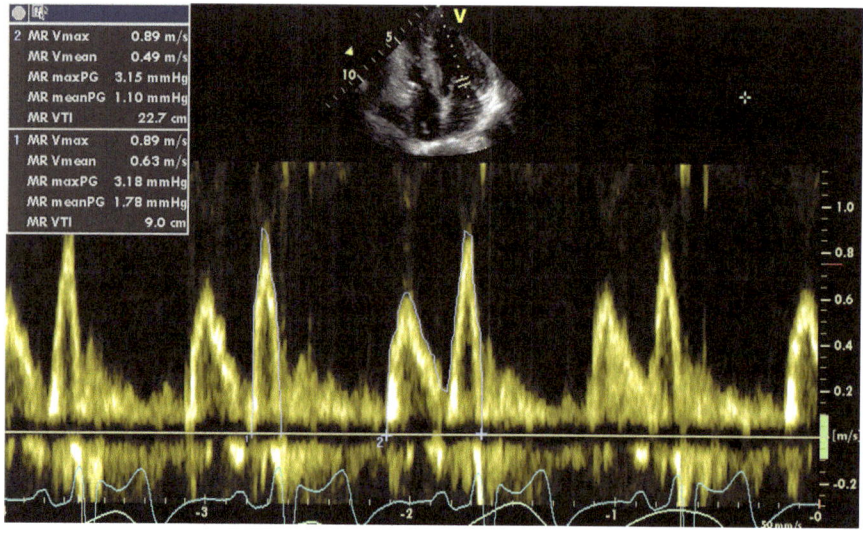

Fig. 14.1 VTI of A wave (*left*) and mitral inflow (*right*)

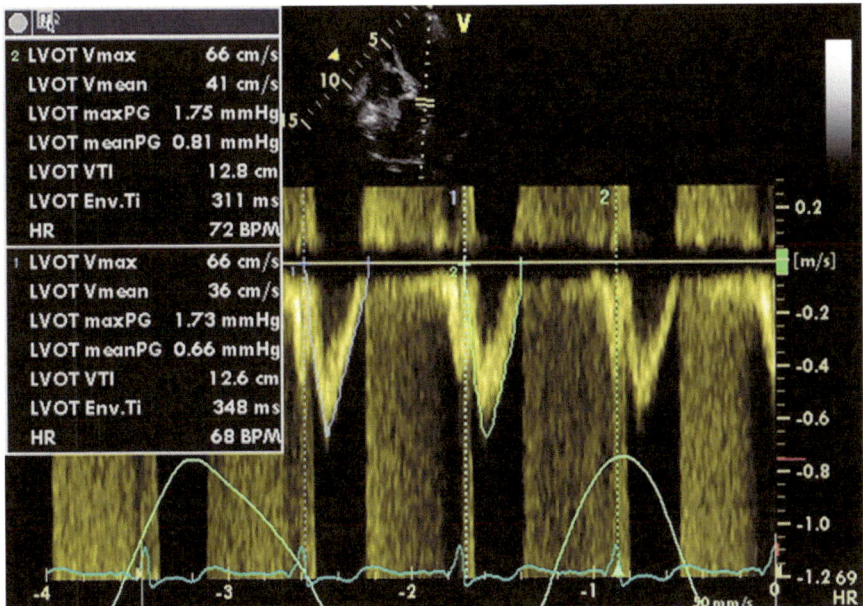

Fig. 14.2 VTI of LVOT

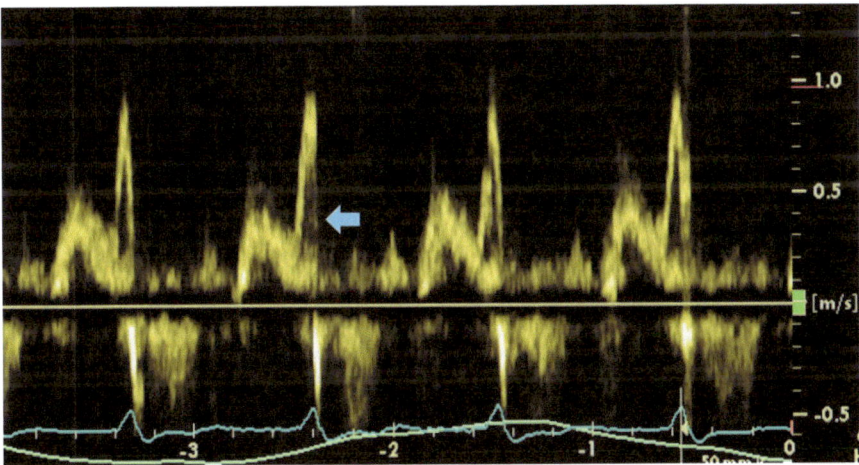

Fig. 14.3 A wave truncation (*arrow*)

14.1.2.2
AV Optimization

Set pacer from APVS (pace at a rate higher than the intrinsic cardiac beats, about 10 beat/min), make sure wide QRS from the surface ECG and IEG

A. Wait for at least 30 s at each setting before start of echo record
B. PW Doppler on MV at mitral annulus, measure VTI of A wave and total mitral inflow
C. PW Doppler at LVOT, measure VTI of LVOT
D. Decrease AV delay until A pace V pace (APVP), make sure narrow QRS from the surface ECG and IEG
E. Repeat this sequence of imagines (point A to C)
F. Decrease AV delay by 30 ms intervals and repeat this sequence of imagines (point A to C)
G. Repeat point F until there is mitral A wave truncation
H. The optimal AV delay is the setting, which yields maximal LVOT VTI with narrow QRS complex
I. Determine the optimal AV delay by VTI of mitral inflow in case maximal LVOT VTI is present at two different settings

14.1.2.3
VV Optimization

A. Set PV delay as the optimal one obtained from the procedure above
B. Change VV settings as follows and obtain images (point A to C) at each setting
    i. RV pre-excitation by 30 ms
    ii. RV pre-excitation by 60 ms
    iii. LV pre-excitation by 30 ms
    iv. LV pre-excitation by 60 ms
C. Set AV delay as the optimal one obtained from the procedure above
D. Change VV settings as follows and obtain images (point A to C) at each setting
    i. RV pre-excitation by 30 ms
    ii. RV pre-excitation by 60 ms
    iii. LV pre-excitation by 30 ms
    iv. LV pre-excitation by 60 ms
E. The optimal VV offset (including simultaneous offset) is the setting, which yields maximal LVOT VTI with narrow QRS complex
F. If the optimal VV offset at PV delay is different from the one at AV delay, determine the clinically optimal VV offset based on the percentage of ASVP and APVP from the initial interrogation

Echocardiographic Assessment of the Right Ventricle

15

Hisham Dokainish

15.1
Introduction

1. Echocardiography is a commonly used noninvasive modality to assess right ventricular (RV) morphology and function.
2. Two-dimensional echocardiographic variables include RV size, interventricular septal morphology and motion, and RV function using fractional area change, ejection fraction, and tricuspid annular plane systolic excursion (TAPSE).
3. Conventional Doppler variables include RV stroke volume and cardiac output and pulmonary artery systolic and diastolic pressure using the pulmonic and tricuspid regurgitation signals, respectively.
4. Emerging echocardiographic techniques to assess RV function include tissue Doppler imaging, speckle-based strain and strain rate imaging, and three-dimensional echocardiography.
5. A comprehensive echo-Doppler approach to the RV, incorporating many of these variables in concert, can result in an accurate assessment of RV size, function, and hemodynamics.

H. Dokainish
Department of Cardiology, Baylor College of Medicine, 6620 Main Street-11A.08, 77030, Houston, TX, USA
e-mail: hishamd@bcm.tmc.edu

T.P. Abraham (ed.), *Case Based Echocardiography*,
DOI: 10.1007/978-1-84996-151-6_15, © Springer-Verlag London Limited 2011

1. 2D echocardiographic variables in assessing of right ventricular size (Fig. 15.1).
   - Most but not all patients with abnormal RV function or significantly elevated pulmonary artery pressures have an enlarged RV.
   - Normal RV diastolic diameter in the apical 4-chamber view is <3.8 cm.

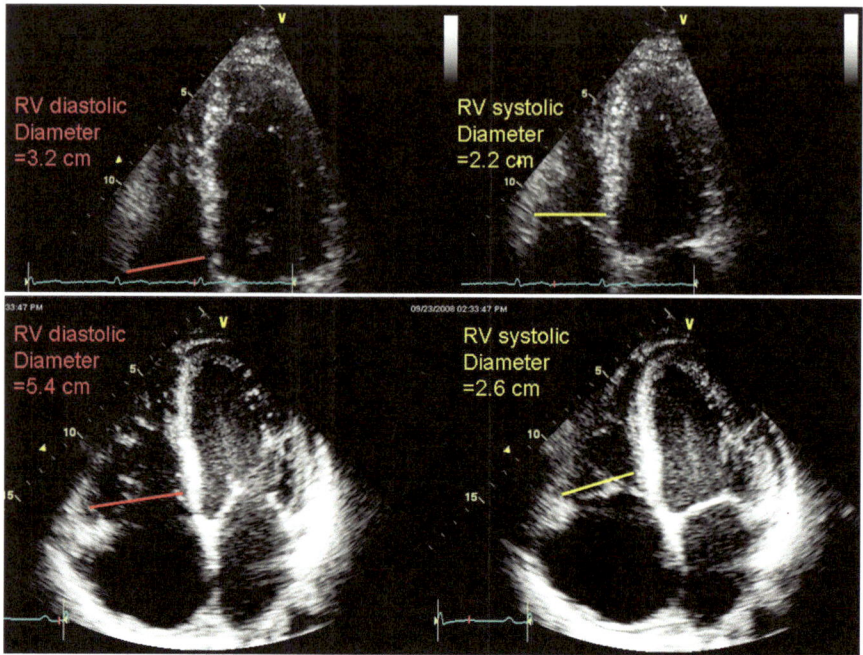

Fig. 15.1 In the *top panel*, RV diastolic diameter is 3.2 cm and RV systolic diameter is 2.2 cm, consistent with normal RV size In the *bottom panel*, RV diastolic dimension=5.4 cm and systolic dimension=2.6 cm, consistent with moderate to severe RV dilation

2. Right ventricular (RV) fractional area change for the assessment of RV function (Fig. 15.2).
   - Normal values are <32 cm² for RV diastolic area, <20 cm² for RV systolic area, and >35% for RV FAC.

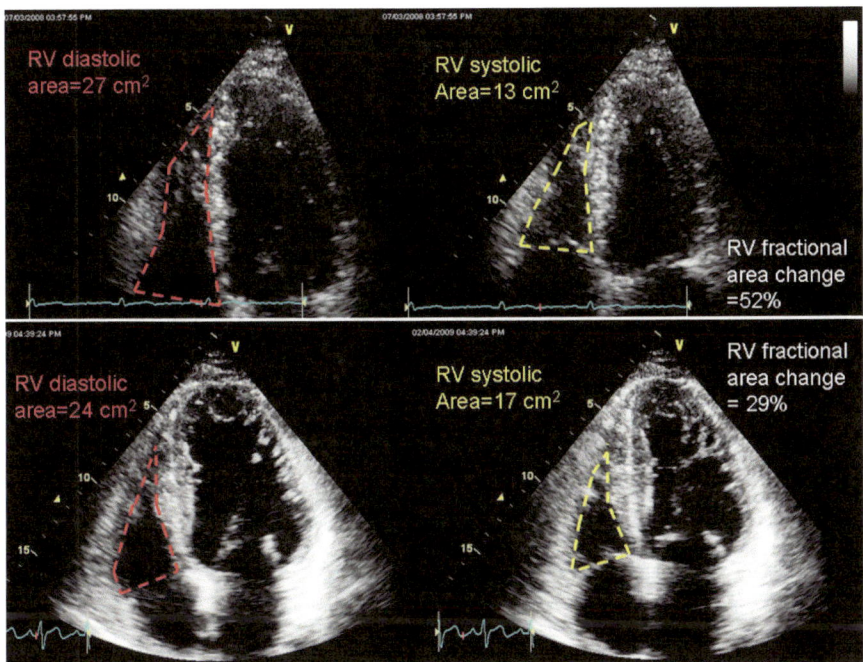

Fig. 15.2 In the *top panel*, RV diastolic area = 27 cm², RV systolic area = 13 cm², and FAC = (27–13)/27 = 52%. In the *bottom panel*, RV diastolic area = 24 cm², RV systolic area = 17 cm², and FAC = (24–17)/24 = 29%, consistent with mild-to-moderate RV dysfunction. Note should be made that the RV is not dilated in the *bottom panel*, despite the depressed systolic function

3. Right ventricular (RV) volumes and ejection fraction (EF) (Fig. 15.3).
   • In patients with severe pulmonary hypertension, echocardiography shows a severely
     enlarged RV and a small left ventricle (LV) compressed by RV enlargement.
   • The right atrium can be severely enlarged, with the interatrial septum bulging to the
     left, indicating elevation of RA pressure.

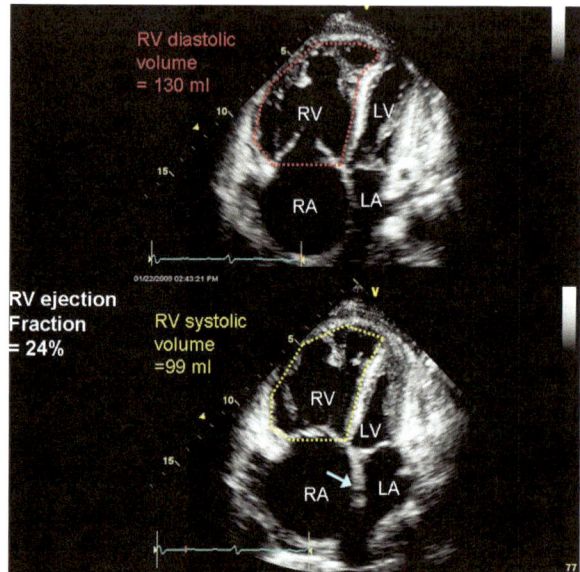

Fig. 15.3 In the *top panel*, RV
diastolic volume = 130 mL
and in the *bottom panel*, RV
systolic volume = 99 mL,
giving an RVEF = (130–
99)/130 = 24%, consistent
with severe RV dysfunction.
RVEF >45% is consistent
with normal RV systolic
function

4. Right ventricular (RV) tricuspid annular plane systolic excursion (TAPSE) (Fig. 15.4).
   - The image can be viewed by placing an M-mode cursor through the tricuspid annular plane that gives a longitudinal excursion in centimeter – referred to as TAPSE – a measure of longitudinal RV systolic function.
   - Normal TAPSE is >1.5 cm, while ≤1.5 is associated with RV dysfunction and adverse prognosis since RV disease results in decreased longitudinal RV excursion.
   - The sole use of TAPSE – or any measure of RV function in isolation – can result in errors.
   - Many variables of RV performance by echocardiography and Doppler should be used for accurate assessment of RV function.

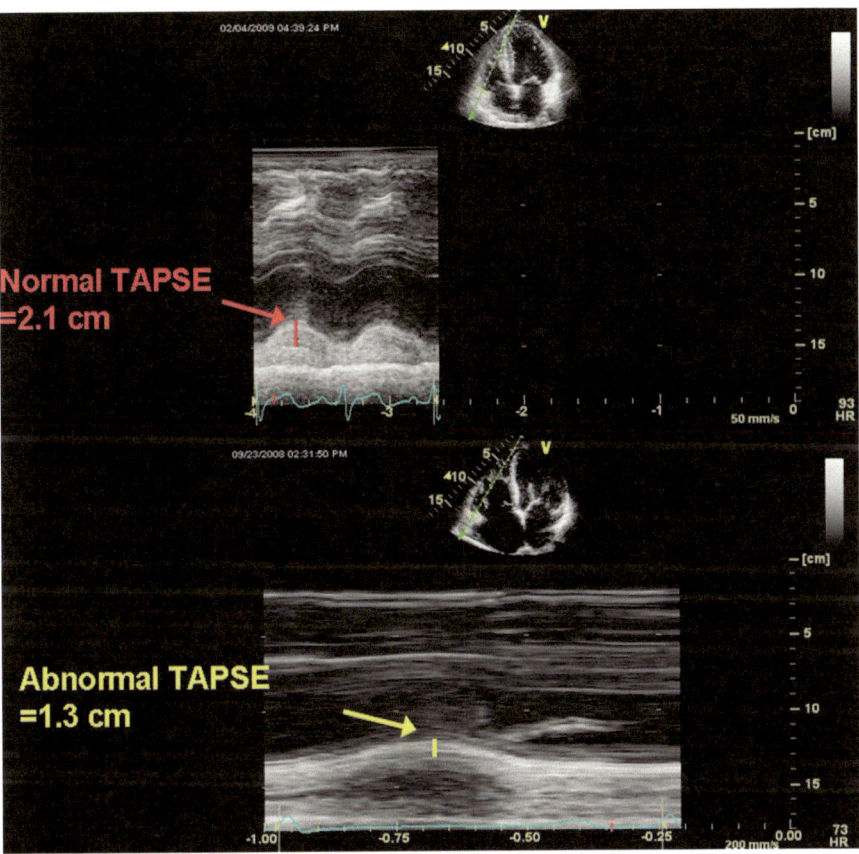

Fig. 15.4 The top image shows a TAPSE of 2.1 cm in a patient with diabetes but normal RV systolic function. The *bottom image* shows an abnormal TAPSE of 1.3 cm, consistent with moderate RV dysfunction

5. Right ventricular (RV) eccentricity index (RVEI) (Fig. 15.5).
   - RV dilates in response to volume overload and pushes the interventricular septum (IVS) toward the left ventricle (LV), compressing the LV.
   - In RV volume overload, the IVS flattens in diastole, and normalizes in systole, as the increase in systolic LV pressure pushes the IVS back toward the RV.
   - The dilation, which is primarily due to RV pressure overload flattens the IVS in both systole and diastole quantified using RVEI, which is the ratio of the LV orthogonal diameters in both diastole and systole.
   - RVEI that remains >1 in both diastole and systole is consistent with pressure overload.
   - High RVEI only confined to diastole, normalizing to ~1 in systole, is consistent with RV volume overload.

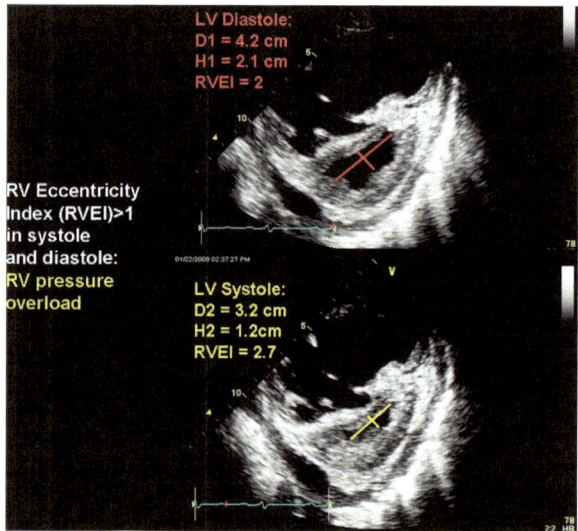

Fig. 15.5 In the *top panel*, the longitudinal LV diastolic diameter (D1)=4.1, while diastolic height=2.1 cm, and RVEI = 4.1/2.1 = 1.95. In the *bottom panel*, longitudinal systolic diameter (D2) = 3.2 cm, systolic height=1.2 cm, and RVEI =3.2/1.2 =2.7

6. Comprehensive Doppler assessment of right ventricular function (Fig. 15.6).

- The parameters assessed include Right ventricle (RV) stroke volume (SV), cardiac output (CO), cardiac index (CI), tricuspid regurgitation (TR) velocity, and right atrial pressure (RAP).
- Normal RV CO is >4.0 L/min (though this measure is very heart rate-dependent), and normal RV CI is >2.5 L/min/m^2.

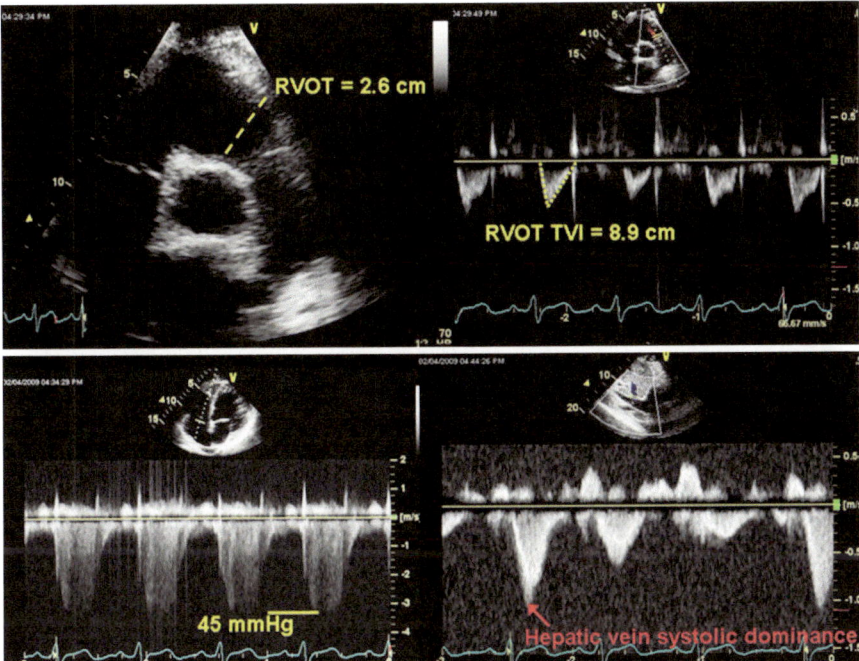

Fig. 15.6 Echocardiography showed a left ventricular ejection fraction=34%, and a mildly dilated RV (4.3 cm) which was moderately depressed in function. To calculate RV CO using the RV outflow tract (RVOT) diameter and time velocity integral (TVI), RV cross-sectional area=(2.6/2)^2 * 3.14=5.3 cm^2, and RVOT TVI=8.9 cm, resulting in RV SV=(5.3 cm^2 * 8.9 cm)=47 mL. Therefore, CO=47 mL * 95 bpm=4.47 L/min, and RV CI = 2.2 L/min/m^2, indicative of significantly depressed RV function

7. Comprehensive Doppler assessment of right ventricular (RV) hemodynamics in a patient with cor pulmonale (Fig. 15.7).

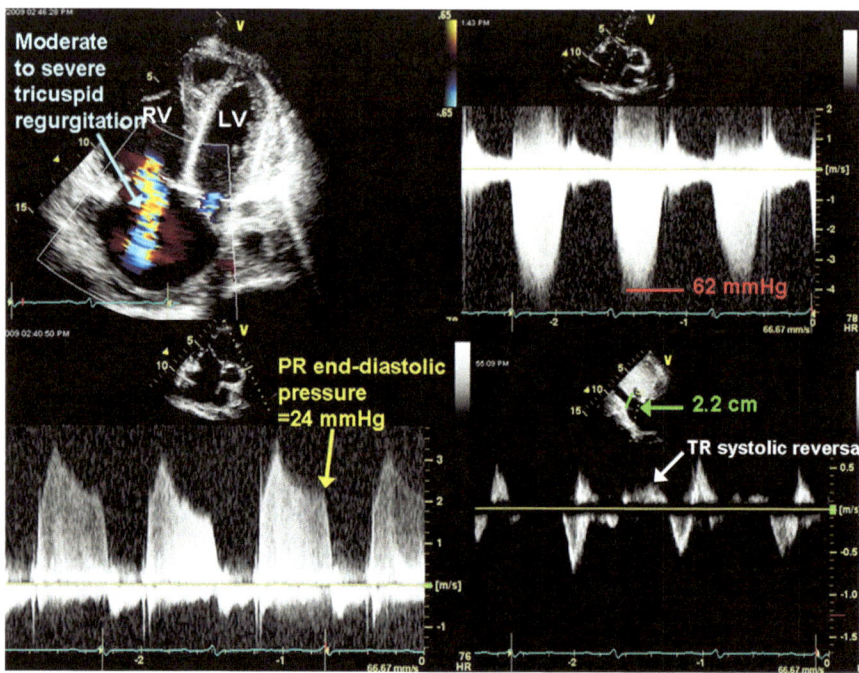

Fig. 15.7 Comprehensive Doppler assessment of right ventricular (RV) hemodynamics in a patient with cor pulmonale. This 36-year-old woman with primary pulmonary hypertension presented for routine follow-up. On echocardiography, she had a severely enlarged right ventricle (RV) with severely depressed function; the left ventricle (LV) is compressed by the RV. *Top left panel* shows moderate-to-severe tricuspid regurgitation (TR) due to incomplete leaflet coaptation from RV dilatation. Continuous wave Doppler (*top right*) shows a dense TR signal with a peak gradient of 62 mmHg. *Bottom right panel* shows that right atrial pressure is significantly elevated due to a dilated inferior vena cava (>2.0 cm, *green arrow*), with significant TR causing some reflux into the hepatic veins (*white arrow*), giving an RAP estimate of 20 mmHg. Therefore, estimated pulmonary artery systolic pressure (PASP) = 62 + 20 = 82 mmHg. *Bottom left panel* shows use of the pulmonic regurgitation (PR) signal for estimation of RV end-diastolic pressure (EDP), equivalent to PAEDP in patients without pulmonary outflow tract obstruction. Therefore, estimated PAEDP =24 + 20 mmHg (RA pressure estimate)=44 mmHg. Overall, PA pressure can be estimated at 82/44 mmHg, consistent with severe pulmonary hypertension

8. Demonstration of right ventricular (RV) systolic dysfunction by tissue Doppler (TD) imaging (Fig. 15.8).

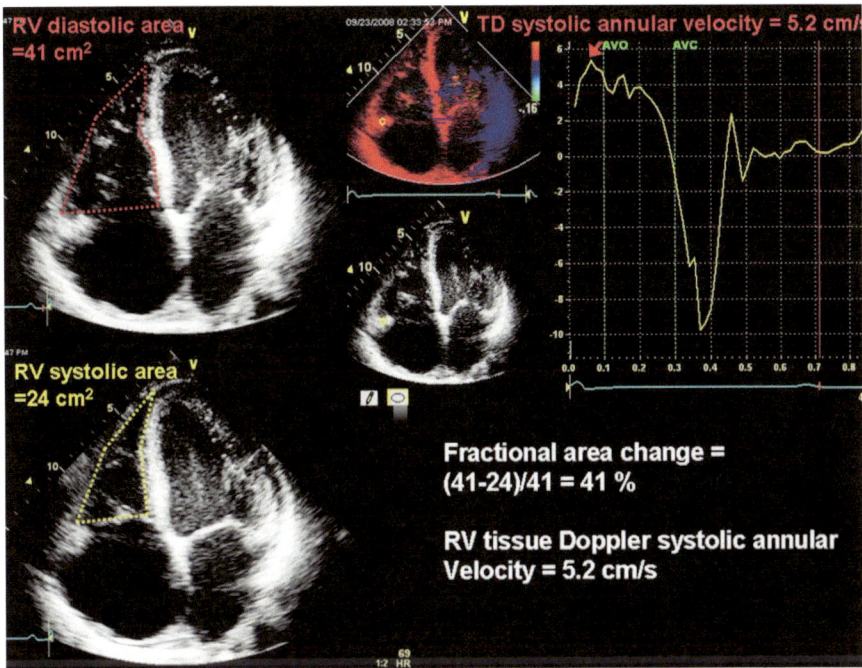

Fig. 15.8 Demonstration of right ventricular (RV) systolic dysfunction by tissue Doppler (TD) imaging. This 53-year-old man with atrial fibrillation presented with increasing dyspnea. Echocardiography revealed a severely dilated RV with a diastolic area (*top left*) of 41 cm², a systolic area (*bottom left*) = 24 cm² and fractional area change = 41%, suggesting normal RV systolic function. However, tissue Doppler (TD) imaging (*top right*) reveals a systolic annular velocity at the lateral tricuspid annulus = 5.2 cm/s, consistent with significant RV contractile impairment (Normal TD RV systolic annular velocity is >8 cm/s using color Doppler-derived TD imaging). Therefore, in the setting of severe TR, although RV FAC is within normal, TD imaging demonstrates evidence of RV systolic dysfunction (see Fig. 15.10)

9. Advanced echocardiographic variables in a patient with a normal heart (Fig. 15.9).
   - Tissue Doppler (TD) imaging can be applied to measure the longitudinal velocity of the RV free wall to assess function.
   - In normal subjects, the normal TD systolic annular velocity >8 cm/s using color-derived TD imaging.
   - Using non-Doppler based speckle tracking, strain imaging can be applied to assess deformation of the RV myocardium.
   - The peak strain in normal subject is <−16%, while the rate of deformation, strain rate, is < −0.9 s−1.
   - These advanced tissue Doppler and speckle-derived strain indices can help identify RV myocardial disease in patients with relatively normal "conventional" echocardiographic indices, such as RV fractional area change

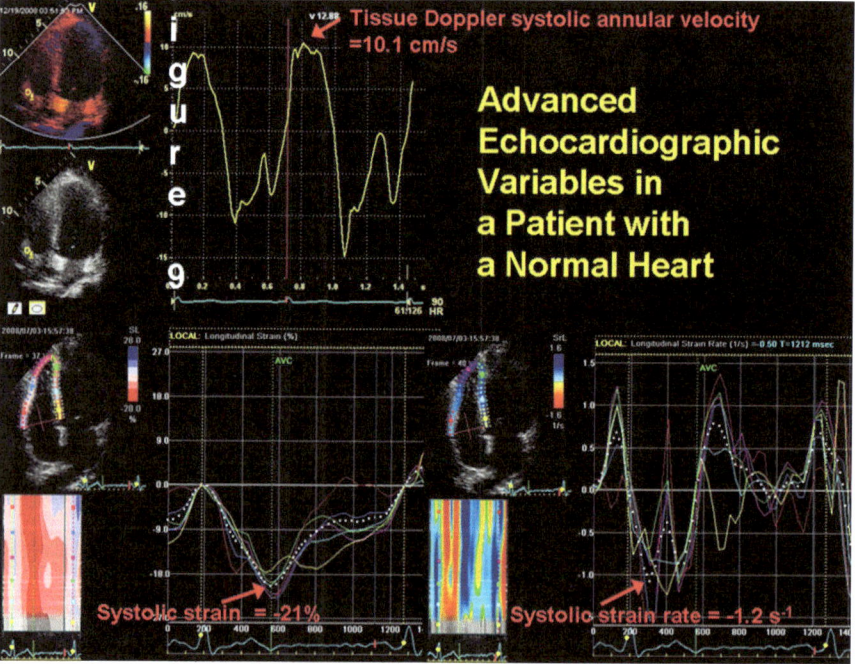

Fig. 15.9 Advanced echocardiographic variables in a patient with a normal heart. Tissue Doppler (TD) imaging can be applied to measure the longitudinal velocity of the RV free wall (see Fig. 15.8) to assess function. In this normal subject, the TD systolic annular velocity was 10.1 cm/s, (normal >8 cm/s using color-derived TD imaging). Using non-Doppler-based speckle tracking, strain imaging is applied to assess deformation of the RV myocardium. The peak strain in this subject was −21% (normal <−16%), while the rate of deformation, strain rate, was −1.2 s−1 (normal <−0.9 s−1). These advanced tissue Doppler and speckle-derived strain indices can help identify RV myocardial disease in patients with relatively normal "conventional" echocardiographic indices, such as RV fractional area change (see Figs. 15.8 and 15.10)

10. Advanced right ventricular (RV) echocardiographic variables in a patient with severe tricuspid regurgitation and atrial fibrillation (Fig. 15.10).
    - Tissue Doppler and speckle-based strain variables can point to depressed systolic function patients with severe tricuspid regurgitation, despite normal "conventional" echocardiographic variables such as FAC.

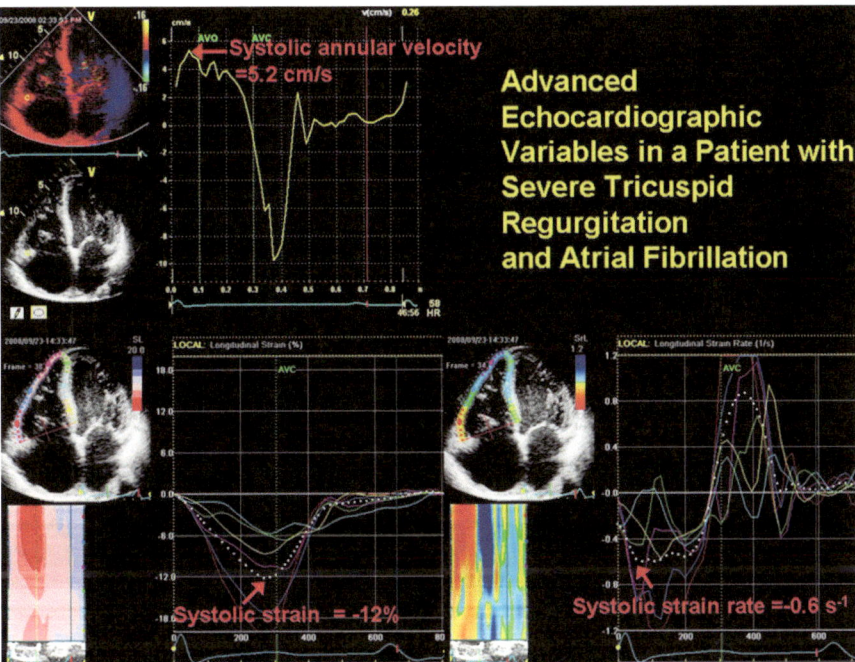

Fig. 15.10 Advanced right ventricular (RV) echocardiographic variables in a patient with severe tricuspid regurgitation and atrial fibrillation. This 53-year-old patient (same patient as in Fig. 15.8) underwent further advanced RV quantification. The right ventricle (RV) was moderately to severely dilated (5.3 cm) with RV fractional area change (FAC) = 41% (normal >35%). Tissue Doppler (TD) imaging revealed a systolic annular velocity = 5.2 cm/s (normal >8 cm/s using color Doppler-derived TD imaging), indicating depressed systolic longitudinal velocity. Speckle-based strain imaging revealed a peak strain of –12% in the RV free wall (normal < –16%), and peak systolic strain rate of = –0.6 s^{-1} (normal < –0.9%), indicating depressed systolic RV myocardial deformation. Therefore, these TD and speckle-based strain variables point to depressed systolic function in this patient with severe tricuspid regurgitation, despite normal "conventional" echocardiographic variables such as FAC

11. Three-dimensional echocardiography for the assessment of right ventricular (RV) function in a patient with severe primary pulmonary hypertension (Fig. 15.11).
    • Full volume acquisition of the heart over six or seven cardiac cycles can produce large volume images of the heart, which can readily be cropped, and rotating in multiple dimensions allows superior morphological and functional diagnosis.

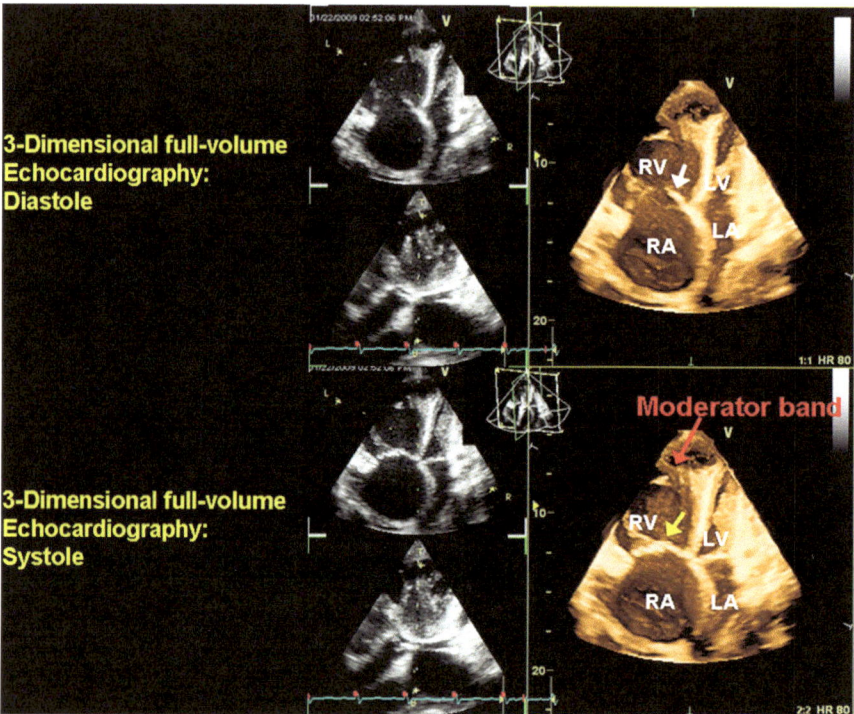

Fig. 15.11 Three-dimensional echocardiography for the assessment of right ventricular (RV) function in a patient with severe primary pulmonary hypertension. Full volume acquisition of the heart over six or seven cardiac cycles can produce large volume images of the heart – which can readily be cropped and rotating in multiple dimensions – allowing superior morphological and functional diagnosis. The *top image* depicts the severely dilated RV during diastole, with the tricuspid valve (TV) open (*white arrow*). The *bottom image* shows the RV during systole, with the TV closed (*yellow arrow*), and little change in RV volume compared to diastole, indicative of poor RV systolic function. Note the severely dilated RV and RA compressing the small left ventricle (LV) and left atrium (LA), respectively. The moderator band is also well seen (*red arrow*)

Aortic Valve Stenosis and Regurgitation

16

Vuyisile T. Nkomo

V.T. Nkomo
Division of Cardiovascular Diseases and Internal Medicine, Mayo Clinic, Rochester, MN, USA
e-mail: nkomo.vuyisile@mayo.edu

T.P. Abraham (ed.), *Case Based Echocardiography*,
DOI: 10.1007/978-1-84996-151-6_16, © Springer-Verlag London Limited 2011

185

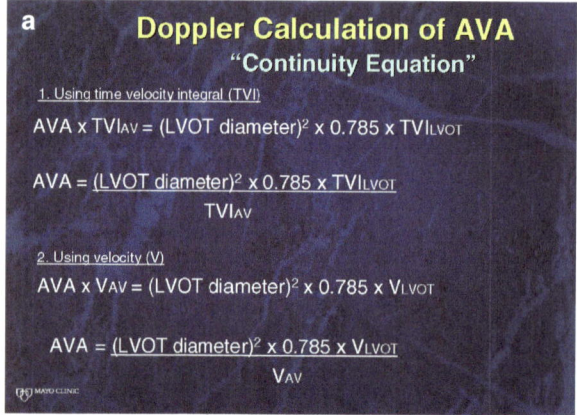

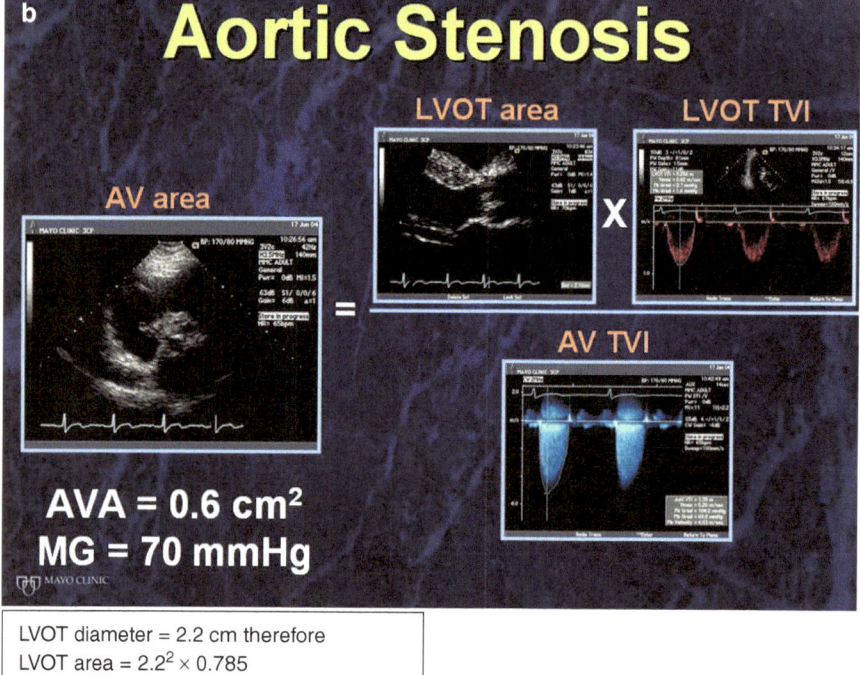

LVOT diameter = 2.2 cm therefore
LVOT area = $2.2^2 \times 0.785$
LVOT TVI = 21 cm
AV TVI = 139 cm

AV area × AV TVI = LVOT area × LVOT TVI
AV area = $\dfrac{\text{LVOT area} \times \text{LVOT TVI}}{\text{AV TVI}}$
AV area = $\dfrac{0.785 \times (2.2 \text{ cm})^2 \times 21 \text{ cm}}{139 \text{ cm}}$
AV area = 0.6 cm^2

Fig. 16.1 Measurement and calculation of AVA using the continuity equation. (**a**) Formulas, (*AV* aortic valve, *AVA* aortic valve area, *LVOT* left ventricular outflow tract, *A* left ventricular outflow tract area, *TVI* time velocity integral), (**b**) Example using time velocity integral (TVI)

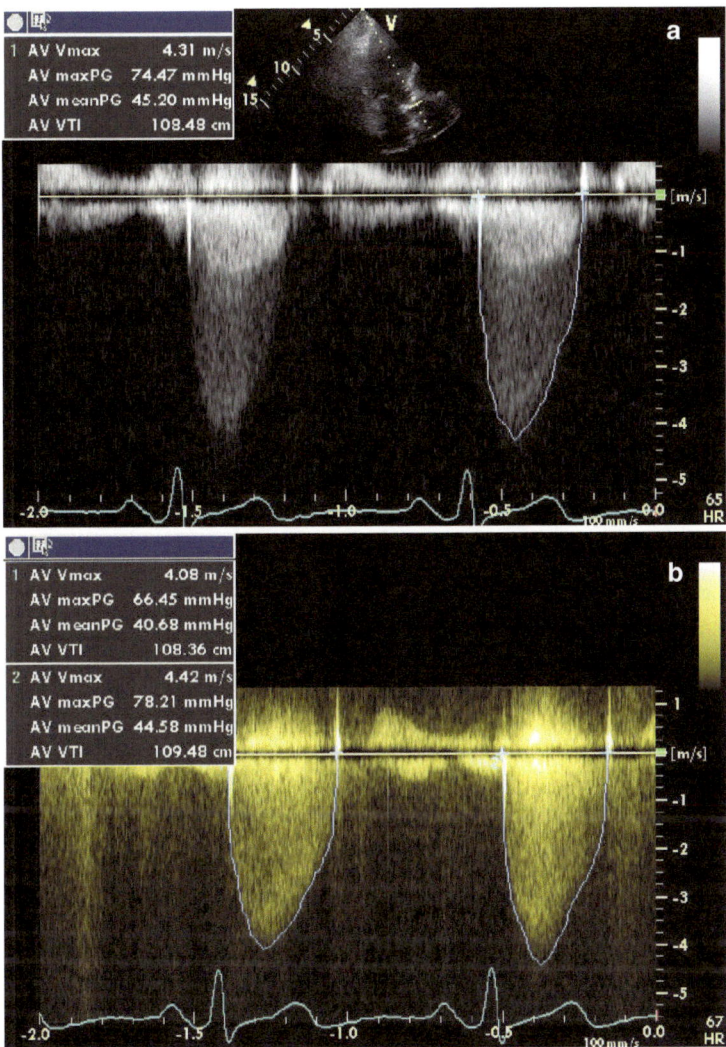

Fig. 16.2 Comparison of jet profiles from aortic stenosis, mitral regurgitation, and dynamic left ventricular outflow tract obstruction as in hypertrophic obstructive cardiomyopathy. The signal of aortic stenosis (**a** and **b**) has a shorter ejection time than that of mitral regurgitation and the mitral regurgitation signal extends beyond ejection and culminates in the mitral inflow signal during onset of diastole (**c** and **d**). The duration and peak velocity of aortic stenosis is shorter than that of MR. Dynamic left ventricular outflow tract obstruction may absent at rest (**e**) and brought on by Valsalva maneuver or amyl nitrite (**f** and **g**). Mitral regurgitation is frequently associated with dynamic LVOT obstruction and mitral regurgitation signal may contaminate the signal from LVOT (**h**). The velocity from mitral regurgitation will always be higher than the velocity from dynamic LVOT obstruction. (**a**) Aortic stenosis continuous wave signal with guided probe. (**b**) Aortic stenosis continuous wave signal with non-guided probe. (**c**) Mitral regurgitation continuous wave signal (*arrow*) with guided probe. (**d**) Mitral regurgitation continuous wave signal (*arrow*) with non-guided probe with mitral inflow signal above baseline (*arrowhead*) consistent with presence of concomitant mitral stenosis. (**e**) LVOT continuous signal without dynamic LVOT obstruction at rest. (**f**) Dynamic LVOT obstruction with Valsalva maneuver. (**g**) Dynamic LVOT obstruction with amyl nitrite. (**h**) Dynamic LVOT obstruction signal contaminated with MR signal

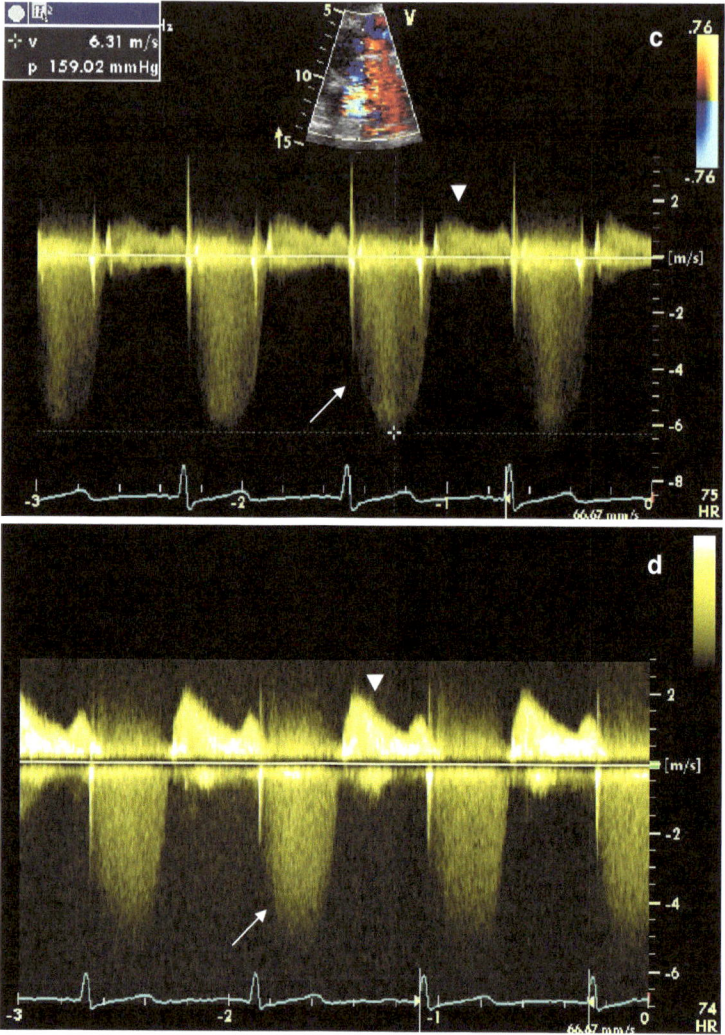

Fig. 16.2 (continued)

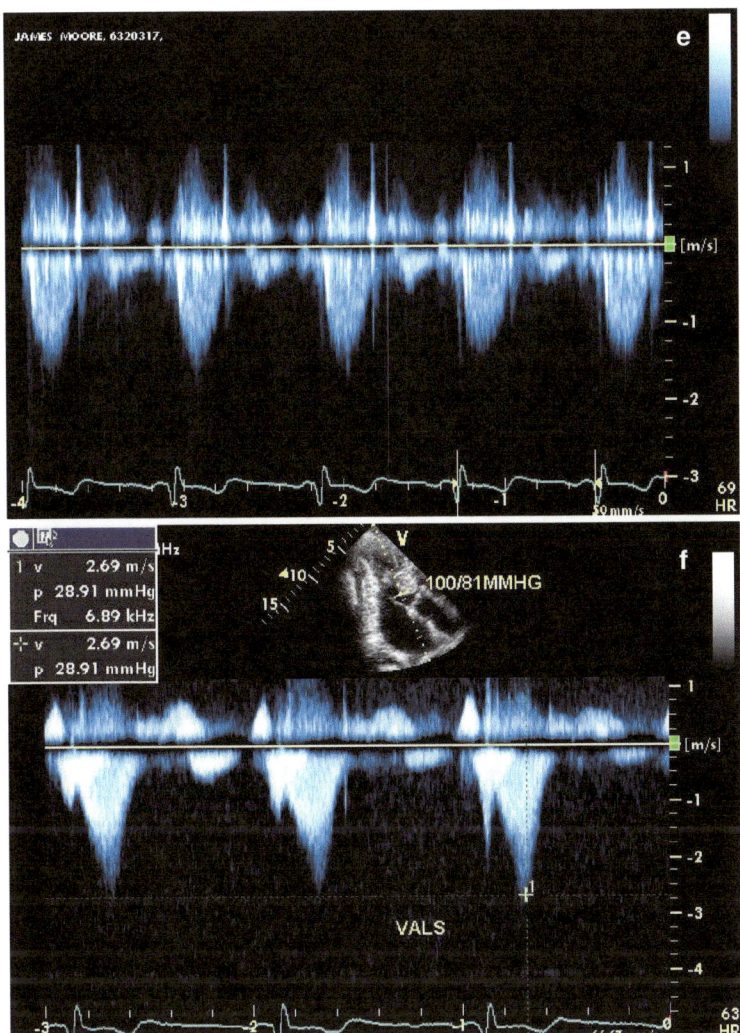

Fig. 16.2 (continued)

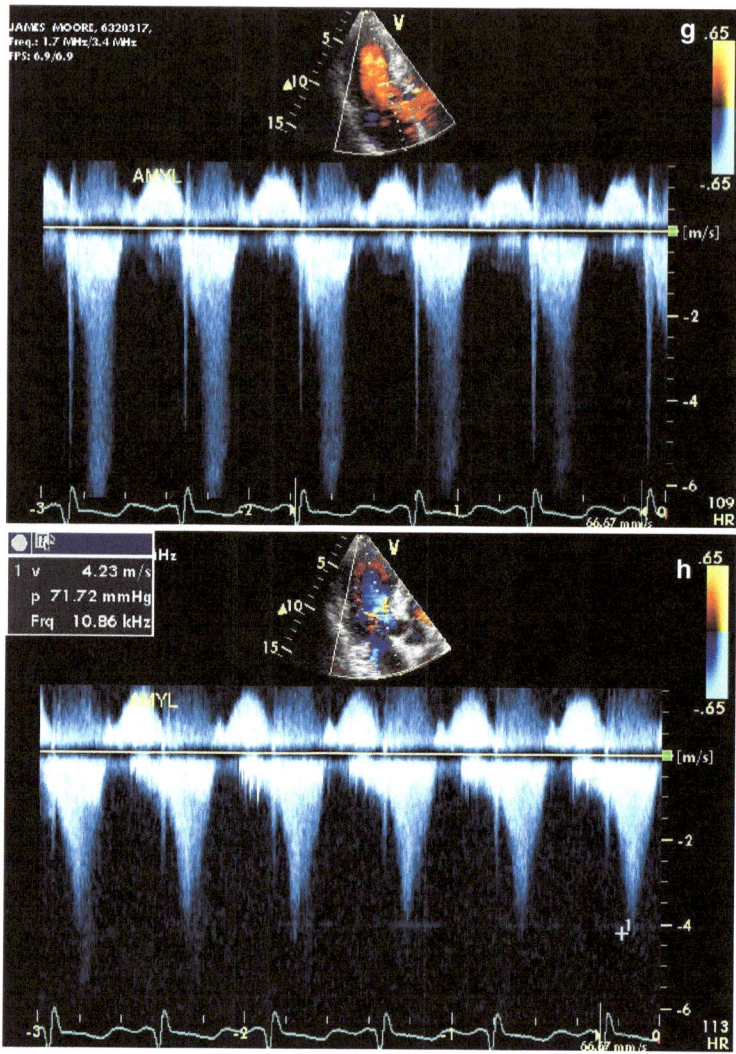

Fig. 16.2 (continued)

Fig. 16.3 (**a–c**) Low gradient, low output aortic stenosis and evaluation

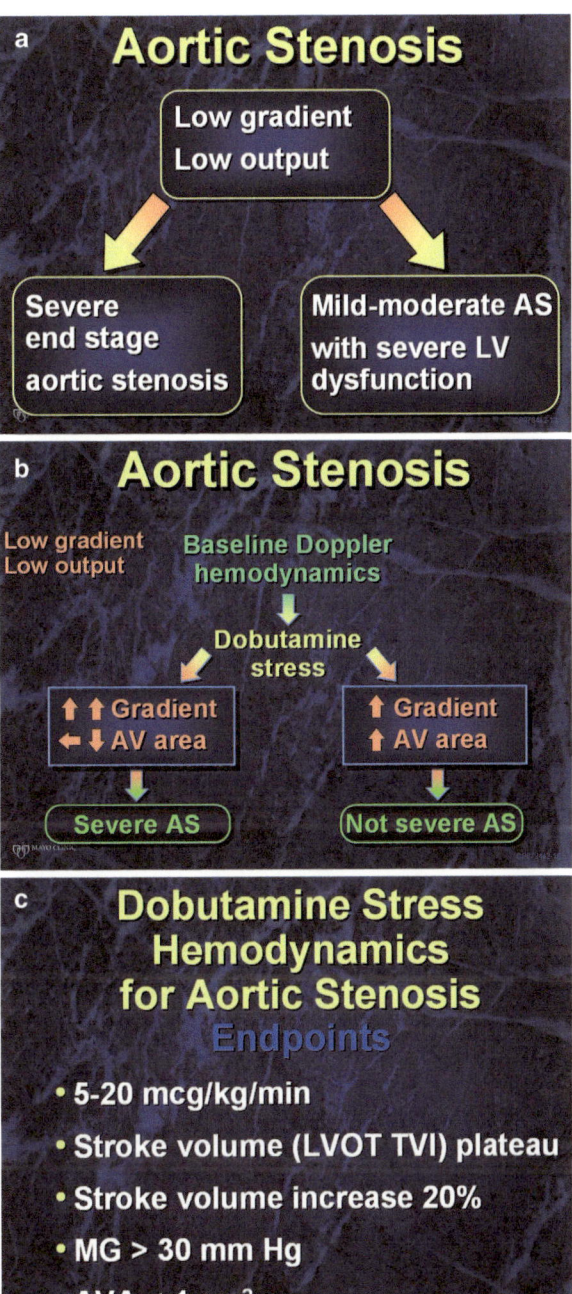

Table 16.1 Etiologies of stenosis and associated lesions

Aortic stenosis	• Valvular
	• Subvalvular
	• Supravalvular
Causes of aortic valve stenosis	• Valve calcification
	• Congenital malformation
	• Rheumatic disease
	• Radiation-induced VHD
	• Mucopolysaccharidoses
Unicuspid aortic valve	• Fatal aortic stenosis in children under 1 year
	• Rare in adults ~0.02%
	• Uni- or acommissural
	• Causes aortic stenosis
	• Associated with aorta dilatation
Bicuspid aortic valve	• 1–2% of general population
	• From fusion of two cusps
	• Aortic stenosis/regurgitation
	• Infective endocarditis
	• Sinus of Valsalva aneurysm
	• Ascending aorta dilatation/aneurysm
	• Aortic coarctation
Subvalvular aortic stenosis	• Discrete fibrous membrane (90%)
	• Muscular narrowing
	• Prevalence ~6.5% in adults CHD
	• Iatrogenic after VSD patch repair
	• Associated aortic regurgitation
Supravalvular aortic stenosis	• Focal or diffuse narrowing starting at the sinotubular junction
	• Rare involvement of aortic arch and peripheral vessels
	• Frequently associated with Williams-Beuren syndrome (71%)
	• Aortic valve abnormalities 50% of patients (commonly BAV)

Table 16.2 Grading severity of aortic stenosis (ACC/AHA guidelines 2006)

	AVA (cm^2)	Indexed AVA (cm^2/m^2)	MG (mmHg)	Velocity (m/s)	Velocity ratio (no units)
Mild	>1.5	>0.85	<25	<3	>0.50
Moderate	1–1.5	0.60–0.85	25–40	3–4	0.25–0.50
Severe	<1	<0.60	>40	>4	<0.25

Table 16.3 Etiologies of aortic regurgitation (*Circulation.* 2006;114:422–429)

Valve 46%	Nonvalve 54%
• Congenital malformation	• Aortic dissection
Bicuspid	• Marfan or forme fruste
Quadricuspid	• Aortitis
Tricuspid	• Cause unclear (maybe associated with hypertension)
• Endocarditis	
• Rheumatic	
• Miscellaneous	

Table 16.4 Assessment and grading of aortic regurgitation (American Society of Echocardiography Guidelines 2003)

	Mild	Moderate	Severe
Qualitative and semi-quantitative			
Jet width in LVOT	<25%	25–64%	≥65%
Jet area in LVOT	<5%	5–59%	≥60%
Vena contracta width	<3 mm	3–6 mm	>6 mm
Color flow reversal in aorta (thoracic descending aorta)	Brief	Intermediate	Holodiastolic
Pressure half-time	≥650 ms	280–650 ms	<280 ms
Qualitative			
Regurgitant volume	<30 cc	30–59 cc	≥60 cc
Effective regurgitant orifice area (EROA)	<0.1 cm^2	0.1–0.29 cm^2	≥0.30 cm^2
Regurgitant fraction	<30%	30–49%	≥50%

Mitral Prolapse Regurgitation and Mitral Stenosis

17

Nuasheen Akhter and Issam A. Mikati

The assessment of mitral regurgitation requires an understanding of the complex anatomy of the mitral valve. The mitral valve complex includes the leaflets, annulus, chordae tendineae, papillary muscles, underlying myocardium, left atrium, and left ventricle.[1] Understanding the interaction of these elements is crucial for determining the mechanism of mitral regurgitation. To facilitate communication, the following classification of MR mechanism is widely used. Type I refers to structurally normal valve leaflet mobility, for example, dilated annulus, perforation, or cleft. Type II refers to valves with excessive leaflet mobility as in patients with mitral valve prolapse. Type III refers to restricted leaflet motion. Type IIIa refers to systolic and diastolic restriction of leaflet motion as in cases of rheumatic MR or MR secondary to radiation, connective tissue disorders, or degenerative calcific disease. Type IIIb refers to systolic restriction of leaflet motion as in ischemic MR.[2]

Mitral valve prolapse is said to occur when there is valve leaflet prolapse of 2 mm or more above the mitral annulus in the long-axis parasternal view.[3] MVP occurs as a clinical entity with or without thickening (5 mm or greater, measured during diastasis) and with or without MR. Prediction of reparability of the valve is possible with transthoracic echocardiography TTE (97% of cases) and transesophageal echocardiography (TEE).[4]

Identification of involved scallops is possible by TEE[5] (see Fig. 17.5). Incorporation of jet direction information helps in identification of involved leaflet. The jet is directed in the opposite direction of the prolapsing leaflet. In cases of restriction of leaflet motion the jet moves in the direction of the involved leaflet (which is usually the posterior leaflet). Three

N. Akhter (✉)
Division of Cardiology, The Feinberg School of Medicine,
Chicago, IL, USA
e-mail: n.akhter@northwestern.edu

T.P. Abraham (ed.), *Case Based Echocardiography*,
DOI: 10.1007/978-1-84996-151-6_17, © Springer-Verlag London Limited 2011

dimensional TTE and 2D TEE were more accurate (90% and 87%) than 2D TTE (77%) in identifying involved scallop.[6] A thorough exam is essential to identify all the pathologies; in one report 5% of patients had more than one mechanism of MR.[7] TEE was able to identify risk factors for post-repair complications such as systolic anterior motion of the anterior leaflet of the mitral valve (tall posterior leaflet > 1.9 cm, posterior leaflet/anterior leaflet < 1, and coaptation distance to septum distance < 2.5).[8,9]

Assessment of the severity of MR should incorporate indirect measures of MR severity (such as LA size, pulmonary venous flow) as well as direct measures for optimal accuracy; reliance on one parameter can often lead to errors. One should question the presence of chronic severe MR if left atrial size is normal or if the mitral inflow shows A-wave dominance. Semiquantitative measures of MR severity (such as jet area by color Doppler, vena contracta, intensity of continuous wave Doppler signal) offer a quick and time-efficient assessment (Table 17.1). Color Doppler techniques assume holosystolic flow; this assumption does not always hold especially in conditions such as mitral valve prolapse and hypertrophic cardiomyopathy in which MR may be a late systolic event. Reliance on color Doppler in these instances may result in overestimation of MR severity.

Quantitative methods improve accuracy and have been shown to predict prognosis even in asymptomatic patients.[10] These include regurgitant volume and fraction as determined by continuity equation and effective regurgitant orifice area (EROA) by proximal isovelocity area (PISA) method. Regurgitant volume can also be derived from EROA using the PISA method. A combination of these parameters is used to grade MR severity as mild, moderate, or severe (Table 17.2 and 17.3).[11]

The 2D assessment of the stenotic mitral valve helps in diagnosis and management. Most common etiology is still rheumatic heart disease resulting in the typical appearance of hockey stick deformity of the anterior leaflet of the mitral valve (secondary to preferential involvement of leaflet tips) and chordal shortening and fusion (see Fig. 17.12a.)

The most commonly used score to predict the potential success of balloon valvotomy is the Wilkins score[12] (see Table 17.4). Others favor scores based on commissural anatomy.[13] No clear superiority of one technique over another has ever been established. Three Dimensional echo is probably superior for visualization of commissures.[14]

Mitral valve area (MVA) measurement by planimetry is considered the reference measurement for assessment of the severity of mitral stenosis.[15,16] Optimization of the image is critical (see Fig. 17.13). Three-dimensional echocardiography facilitates this optimization especially for less experienced sonographers.[17,18]

Mitral valve area can be obtained using the formula MVA = 220/Pressure Half Time. This method is limited in patients with abnormal relaxation (severity of stenosis is overestimated[19]) and in patients with changing compliance (immediately post-valvotomy[20,21])

MVA can also be obtained using the continuity equation. This method suffers from the multiple measurements required with potentially compounding error.

The PISA method can be used to obtain MVA.[22] This method is limited by technical demands.

Another useful measure of mitral stenosis is the mean gradient across the mitral valve (Table 17.5). This has been validated against the gradient obtained invasively in the cath lab using a transseptal approach.[23] The heart rate at which the gradient is obtained should be reported consistently.

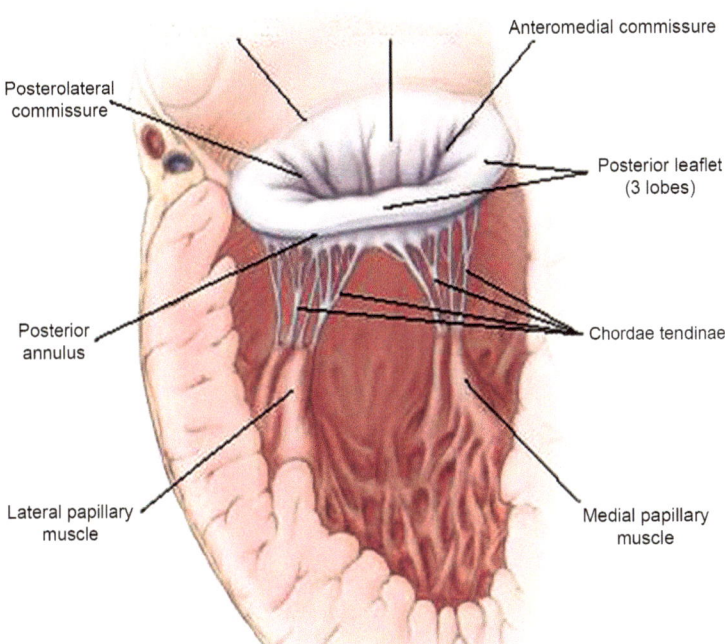

Fig. 17.1 Normal MV anatomy.[1] The mitral valve MV is composed of several elements. The annulus has a saddle shape in three dimensions. It integrates with the fibrous continuity of the mitral valve anterior leaflet and anterior annulus. The intertrigonal distance is fixed. The anterior leaflet has 60% MV area but subtends only a third of the circumference of the MV. An area of coaptation of 3–5 mm is expected normally. Each leaflet is divided into three scallops that are labeled 1–3 going from lateral to medial: lateral (A1, P1), middle (A2, P2), and medial (A3, P3) (See Fig. 17.6). Primary chordae extend from papillary muscles to leaflet edge. Secondary chordae extend from papillary muscle to mid undersurface of leaflets. Tertiary chordae extend from posterior LV wall to base of posterior leaflet. Chords from anterolateral papillary muscle supply lateral part of both anterior and posterior leaflets. Similarly chords from posteromedial papillary muscle supply medial part of both leaflets

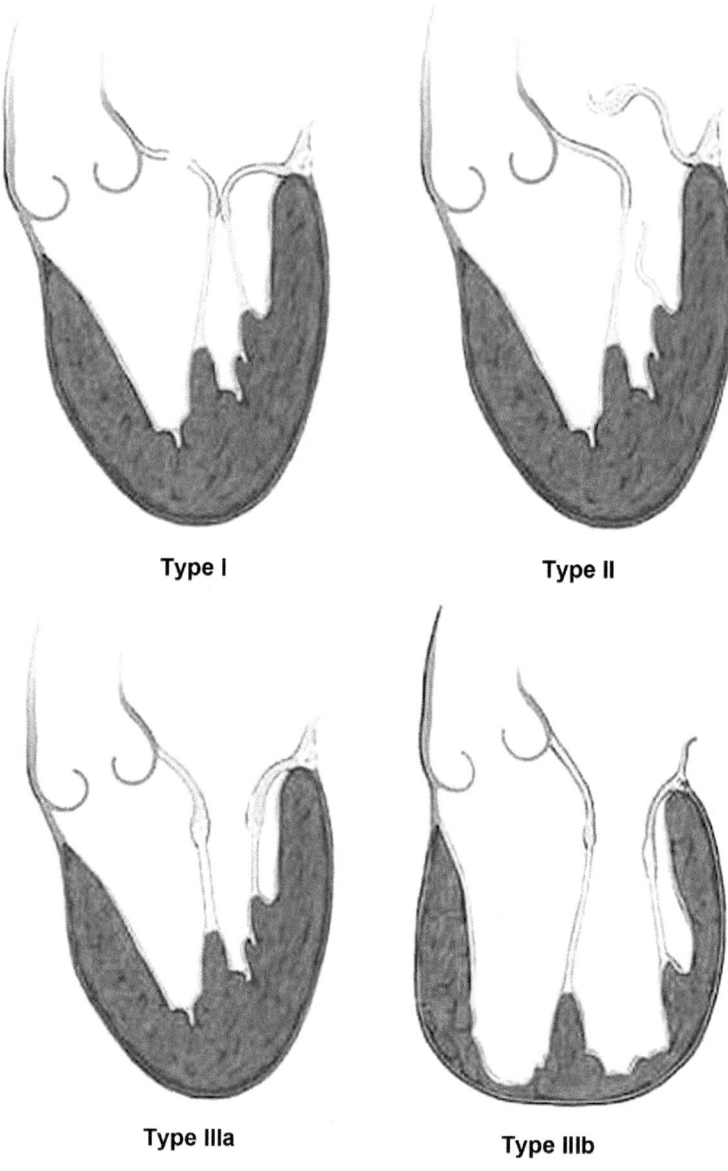

Fig. 17.2 Mechanisms of mitral regurgitation.[2] A commonly used system for classification of MR was developed by Dr Alain Carpentier. It relates function/motion of the leaflets to structure. It facilitates communication between cardiologist and surgeon so that feasibility and type of repair can be determined. Three types have been identified. Type I is characterized by normal leaflet length and motion. Examples, annular dilation or leaflet perforation, such as with endocarditis. Type II MR is caused by excessive leaflet motion (most commonly prolapse or flail) usually from myxomatous disease, or by papillary muscle rupture or elongation (See Fig. 17.5) Type III MR is caused by restricted leaflet motion. Type IIIa is classically caused by rheumatic disease with sub-valvular involvement (See Fig. 17.12b). Type IIIb is usually caused by ischemic or idiopathic cardiomyopathy with ventricular dilation causing tethering and restricted motion of the leaflets

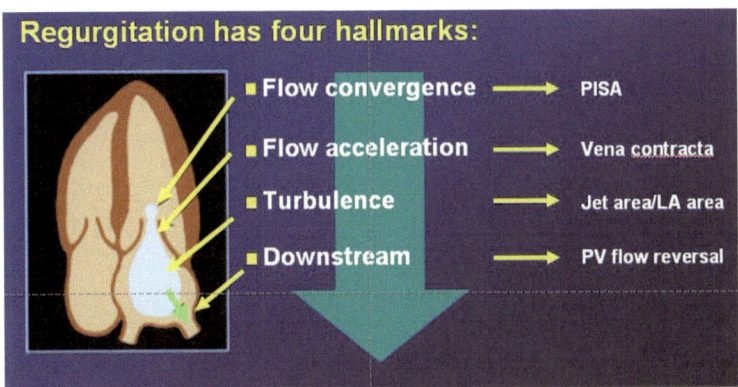

Fig. 17.3 Fluid dynamics and measures of mitral regurgitation severity.[24] (Adapted from www. echoincontext.com/images/anat_pisa003.jpg). Several concepts of fluid dynamics that apply to passage of fluid through a narrow orifice can be used to assess severity of mitral regurgitation. As fluid approaches a narrow orifice it accelerates in concentric hemispheres or shells. Fluid particles at the same distance from the orifice have the same velocity. This is the underlying principle for the PISA method. As the fluid passes through the narrow orifice it accelerates. The wider the neck of that flow (vena contracta) the more severe is the MR (see Fig. 17.10).Chronic volume overload of the left atrium LA results in LA dilatation and increase in LA pressures. This results in systolic flow reversal in the pulmonary veins (See Fig. 17.11b)

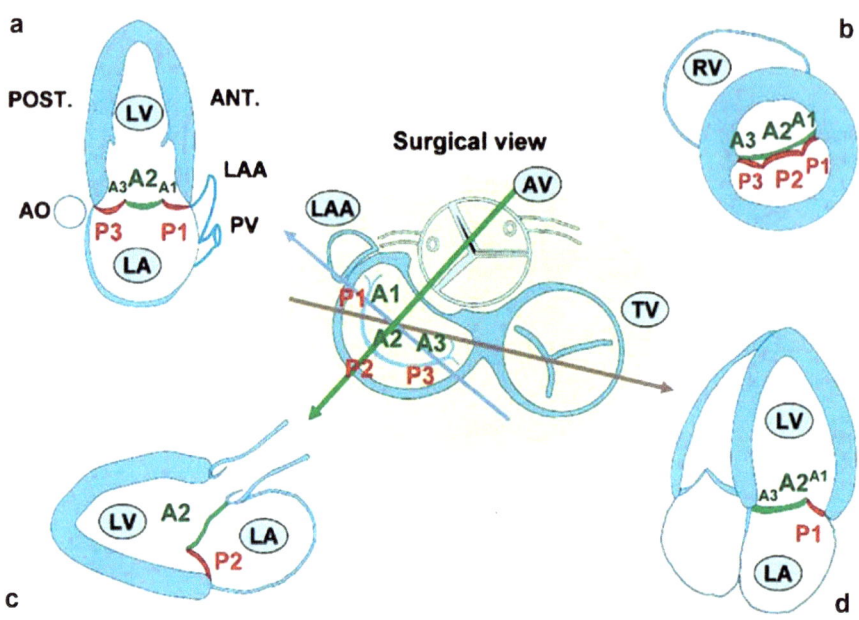

Fig. 17.4 Identification of scallop anatomy of mitral valve by transthoracic echo.[4] Four imaging planes to assess the precise localization of prolapsed or flail segments. (**a**) Inter-commissural plane assessing the continuity of the commissural areas. This is equivalent to vertical midesophageal TEE view with medial angulation (See Fig. 17.5c). (**b**) Parasternal short-axis view showing the anterior leaflet (A1, A2, and A3) and the three scallops of the posterior leaflet (P1, P2, and P3). This is equivalent to horizontal transgastric TEE view (See Fig. 17.5a). (**c**) Parasternal long-axis view showing the middle segments of anterior (A2) and posterior (P2) leaflets. This is equivalent to vertical midesophageal TEE view 120° with medial angulation (See Fig. 17.5d). (**d**) Apical four-chamber view showing the anterior para-commissural zone (between P1 and P2). This is equivalent to horizontal midesophageal TEE (See Fig. 17.5c). *ANT*, anterior; *AO*, descending aorta; *AV*, aortic valve; *LA*, left atrium; *LAA*, left atrial appendage; *LV*, left ventricle; *POST*, posterior; *PV*, pulmonary vein; *RV*, right ventricle; *TV*, tricuspid valve

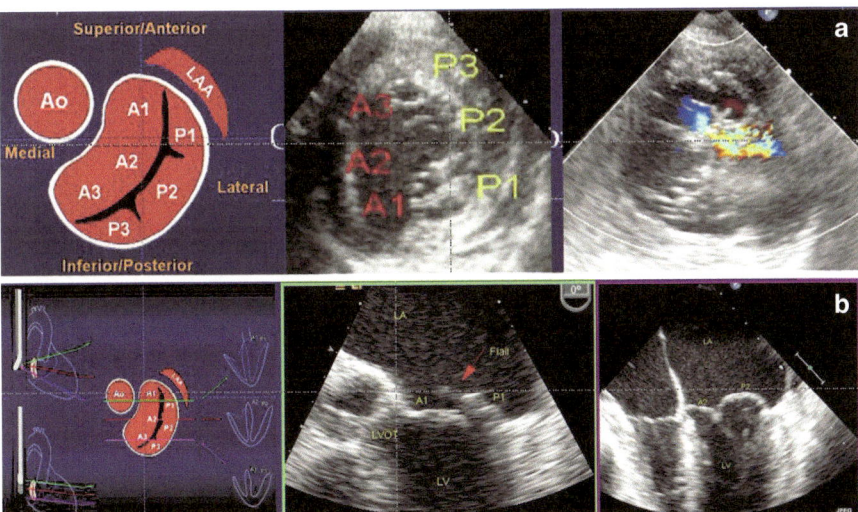

Fig. 17.5 Identification of scallop anatomy of mitral valve by transesophageal echo.[25] (**a**) Foster et al.[25] demonstrated that a systematic approach using TEE is successful in identifying the scallop involved with prolapse/flail. *Left Panel* demonstrates the nomenclature. The lateral, middle, and medial scallops are numbered as follows: A1, A2, A3 and P1, P2, P3 for anterior and posterior leaflets, respectively. The cartoon which is modified from Foster[25] demonstrates the important anatomic relationships. Left atrial appendage is closest to lateral scallops (A1, P1). The aortic valve is closest to medial scallops (A3 and P3). The middle panel demonstrates a basal transverse transgastric TEE view. This is obtained by withdrawing the probe to the proximal part of the stomach. It is difficult to visualize prolapsing/flail segments since the ventricular surface of the mitral valve is seen. It does allow identification of elongated/redundant scallops. Color Doppler in this view allows identification of the origin of the MR jet which also localizes pathology. In right panel color is seen to originate medially in A3, P3 area. (**b**) *Left panel* (Modified from Foster[25]) demonstrates that the lateral scallops of the mitral valve leaflets are cranial to middle and medial scallops. Therefore, when TEE probe is in upper esophagus (*green plane*) one can visualize A1 and P1. The LVOT and aortic valve are important landmarks that help characterize this location. Pushing the probe in (*red plane*) LVOT and aortic valve are no longer visualized and A2 and P2 are now seen. Pushing the probe in further (*purple plane*) A3 and P3 can be examined. An alternative method would be to start at the midesophageal point (*red plane*) and obtain cranial plane (*green*) to visualize A1, P1 by anteflexion. Retroflexion of probe provides caudal view (*purple plane*) and therefore A3, P3. Other planes are needed to confirm findings (see Fig. 17.5c) as individual anatomical variations are common. (**c**) The mid commissural view (60°) can be used to confirm findings from other views (Modified from Foster[25]). Clockwise rotation provides a medial plane (green) cut through anterior leaflet. This allows visualization of A1, A2, and A3 (from *left* to *right* of the screen). Slight counterclockwise rotation (*red plane*) allows visualization of P1, A2, and P3. Further counterclockwise rotation (*purple plane*) provides a view through a lateral plane demonstrating P1, P2, and P3. The *middle panel* (*green frame*) corresponds to a medial vertical cut through mitral valve demonstrating A1 prolapse. The panel on the right (*red frame*) demonstrates a flail (*yellow arrow*) medial scallop of posterior leaflet (P3). (**d**) Other views (30°, 45°, and 120°) can be obtained to confirm findings (See Fig. 17.7)

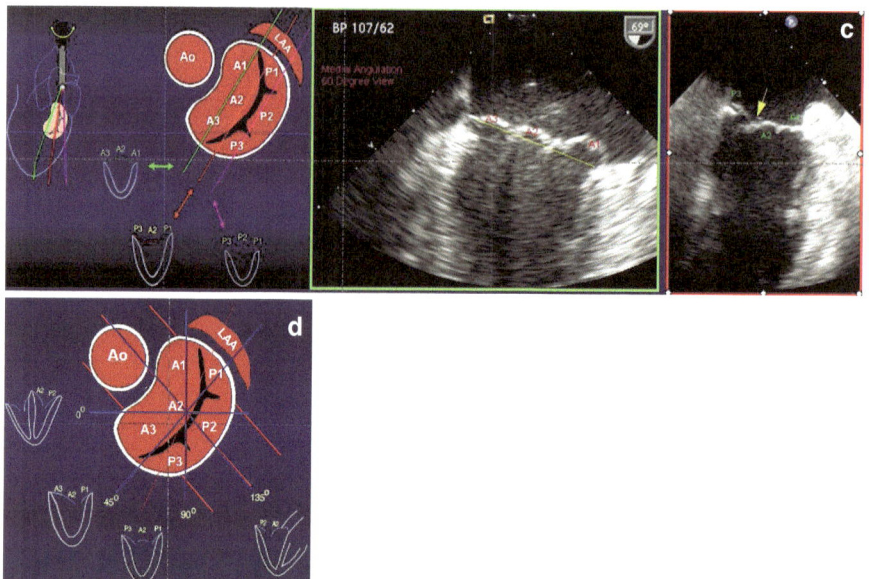

Fig. 17.5 (continued)

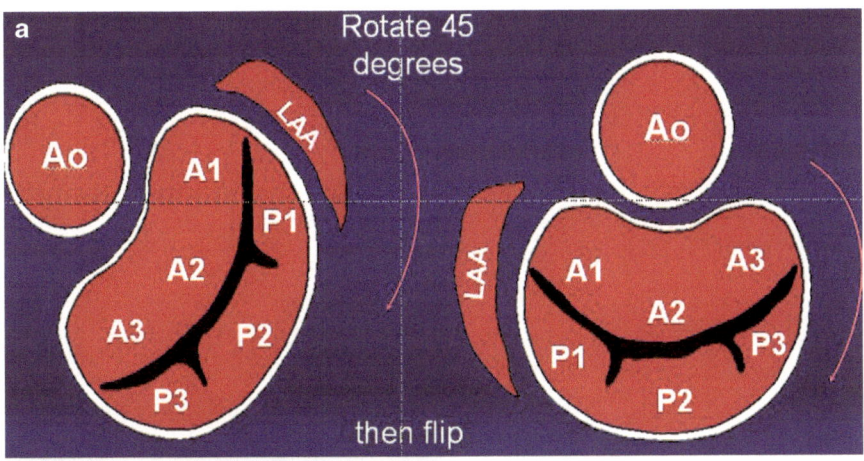

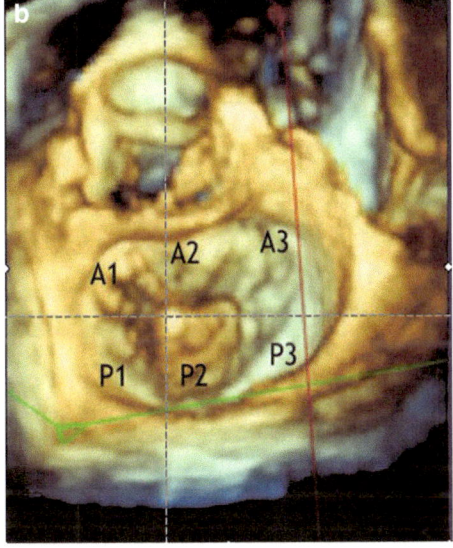

Fig. 17.6 Mitral valve anatomy using real time 3D echocardiography. The 3D image is usually displayed in the surgeon's view. This mimics the orientation of cardiac structures in the surgical field as seen by the surgeon. This can be derived from the reference image by rotating the image by 45° then flipping it (Fig. 17.6a). The full volume is acquired with 4 consecutive heart beats through the MV at a medium density setting in the 2D 0° TEE view, which encompassed the MV annulus and the aortic valve. The next step is image orientation. The MV is displayed from the atrial side with the aortic valve at the 12 o'clock position. In this orientation, the anterior MV leaflet is next to the aortic valve and the posterior MV leaflet is opposite. The scallops are shown from lateral/left (A1/P1) to medial/right (A3/P3). The final step is to optimize the image by cropping the blue short axis plane down toward the MV and decreasing the gain setting. The resulting image is shown in Fig. 17.6b (Image courtesy of Dr Vera Rigolin)

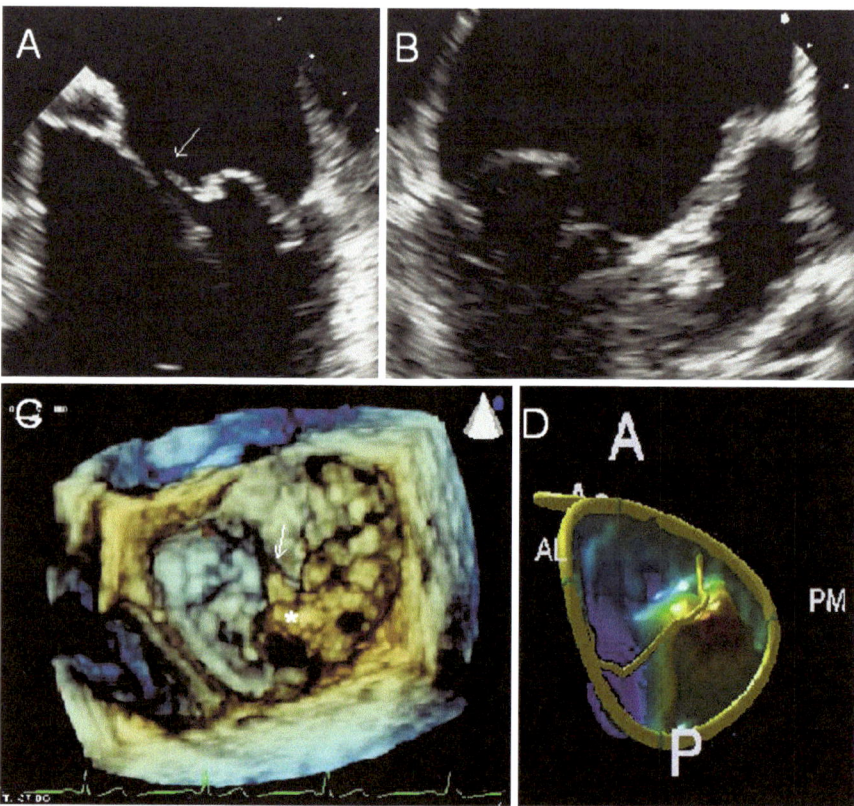

Fig. 17.7 Comprehensive assessment of mitral valve prolapse and flail using 2D TTE, TEE, and 3D echocardiography. (Classic P2 Flail) (**a**) 2D 0° TEE view shows a flail P2 scallop with a ruptured chordae tendinae (*arrow*). (**b**) 2D 120° TEE end-systolic view further demonstrates P2 prolapse. (**c**) 3D TEE live zoom acquisition in from the atrial side with the aortic valve at the 12 o'clock position displays P2 prolapse (*arrow*) with a torn chordae tendinae (*asterisk*). (**d**) A 3D rendering of the P2 prolapse can be created with Philips Mitral Valve Quantification (MVQ) software. The area coded red indicates part of the mitral valve that is breaking the annular plane and encroaching on the atrial side. This clearly demonstrates that prolapse is occurring in middle posterior scallop (P2). The blue color indicates areas of leaflets that are on ventricular side of annular plane and therefore have restricted motion. This facilitates identification of the mechanisms involved in pathophysiology of MR (still a research tool at this point)

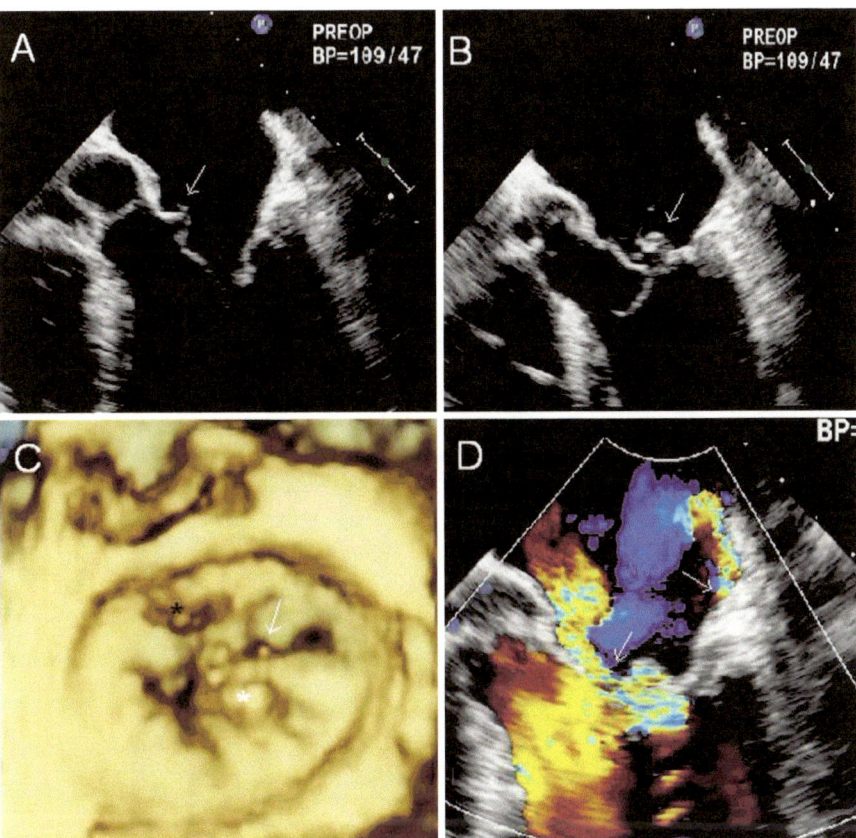

Fig. 17.8 Multiple mechanisms of mitral regurgitation examined by multiple modalities. Although multiple mechanisms of MR are not very frequent[7] they need to be recognized in advance so that complete repair is done to avoid multiple pump runs and residual MR (A2 Perforation, P2 Prolapse). (**a**) This is a 2D 0° esophageal TEE view, which demonstrates an A2 aneurysm and perforation (*arrow*) and (**b**), which shows the P2 prolapse with adjacent flail chordae tendinae. (**c**) The full volume 3D TEE en face view of the MV from the left atrial perspective displays the A2 perforation (*black asterisk*), P2 prolapse (*white asterisk*), and the flail chordae tendinae (*arrow*). 3D echocardiography allows visualization in one view of multiple pathologies that are physically in different planes. (**d**) The presence of multiple MR jets is a clue that multiple pathologies exist and should be looked for. This 2D 0° esophageal TEE view with color Doppler confirms the two jets (*arrows*) of mitral regurgitation, anteriorly from the P2 flail and posteriorly from the A2 perforation

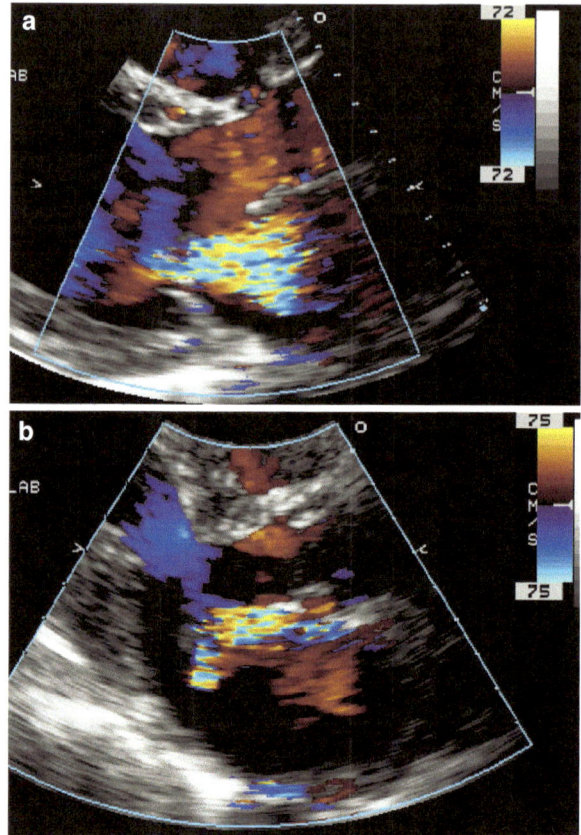

Fig. 17.9 Assessment of mitral regurgitation by color Doppler jet area. (**a**) Color Doppler interrogation of severity of MR can be done semiquantitatively by tracing the area of regurgitant signal or, more commonly, qualitatively by visually assessing the size of the jet and comparing it to left atrial area. Relying on this as a sole criterion for assessment of severity of MR is not recommended. Color display is a velocity map so a high velocity jet may generate same area of turbulence as a larger slower moving jet. This method is very sensitive to velocity map, gain, and filter settings. Setting the Nyquist limit too low will exaggerate severity of MR. Proper Nyquist limit is 50–60 cm/s. High gains as is evidenced in Fig. 17.9a by presence of color pixels overlying LA wall will exaggerate severity of MR. Color Doppler will overestimate severity of central jet similar to one seen in Fig. 17.9a. (**b**) On the other hand eccentric jet (similar to anteromedial jet seen in Fig. 17.9b will be underestimated by color Doppler secondary to entrainment (Coanda effect)

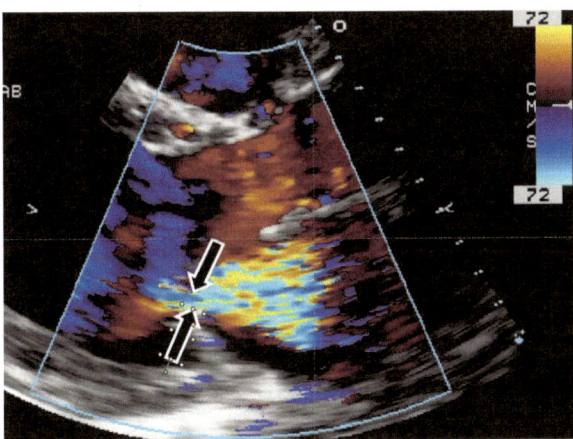

Fig. 17.10 Vena contracta in grading severity of mitral regurgitation. The MR jet as it passes through the regurgitant orifice narrows down before the jet expands in the LA. The width of that neck correlates with severity of MR. Vena contracta width of 8 mm is consistent with severe MR as in Fig. 17.10. The advantage of this method is that it is simple. Its greatest utility is in identifying patients with MR on either end of the spectrum (mild or severe; it is not very useful in patients with moderate degrees of MR). It works in patient with central as well as eccentric jet but not in patients with multiple jets. Technical recommendations: (1) Parasternal views are preferable. Apical two chamber views are to be avoided. (2) Zoomed views should be used. The zoom box should be as small as possible to maximize magnification of the image and minimize measurement error. This will also image line density and frame rate. (3) The position of the focal zone should be placed at the level of the vena contracta. (4) The color sector should be narrowed again if possible and the pulse repetition frequency (color scale) increased to provide the maximum frame rate. (5) Then the image needs to be frozen. Scrolling back through the cineloop will locate the best representative frame for measurement[26]

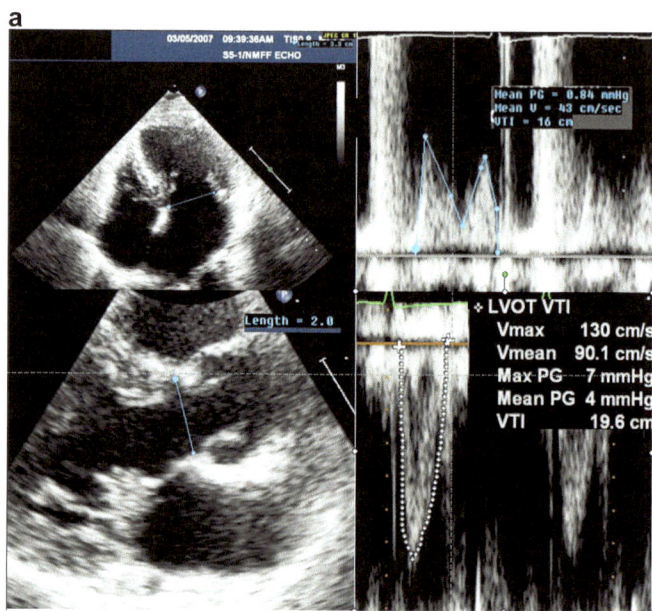

Fig. 17.11 Quantitative measures of mitral regurgitation. (**a**) Mitral regurgitant volume by continuity equation. Advantages of the continuity equation method are that it applies for MR with eccentric jet, late systolic MR jets or even MR with multiple jets. The disadvantages are that numerous measurements are needed. Measurement of annulus is squared resulting in doubling of the relative error. In most cases of severe MR the mitral annulus approaches circular shape. Some practitioners average the four chamber and two chamber diameters. Regurgitant Fraction = $(Flow_{Mitral} - Flow_{LVOT})/$ $Flow_{Mitral}$; $Flow_{Mitral} = (\Pi/4) * D^2 * TVI_{Mitral}$; $Flow_{Aortic} = (\Pi/4) * D^2 * TVI_{Aortic}$; $D_{Mitral} = 33$ mm (4 Chamber) 31 mm (2 Chamber); $TVI_{Mitral} = 16$ cm; $D_{Aortic} = 20$ mm (4 Chamber); $TVI_{Aortic} = 20$ cm; $Flow_{Mitral} = 0.785 * 10.24 * 16 = 128$ mL; $Flow_{Aortic} = 0.785 * 4 * 20 = 62$ mL; Regurgitant volume = $Flow_{Mitral} - Flow_{LVOT} = 128-62 = 66$ mL; Regurgitant Fraction = $66/128 = 52\%$. (**b**) Effective regurgitant orifice area by proximal isovelocity area (PISA) method for grading severity of mitral regurgitation. PISA is based on the continuity principle. When flow converges toward a restrictive orifice, it forms hemispheric isovelocity shells which can be used to calculate an effective regurgitant orifice (ERO) and a regurgitant volume (RV). (A) The aliasing velocity is decreased to approximately 30 cm/s to create the isovelocity shell. The shell area is $2\Pi(R)^2$. The (R) is the radius of the shell. The shell area x the aliasing velocity is the flow on the proximal side of the MV. In this example, R = 0.8 cm and the aliasing velocity = 30 cm/s. The flow is $2 \times \Pi \times (0.815)^2(30) = 125$ cm^3. According to the continuity principle, the flow on the proximal side of the MV = the flow on the distal side of the MV. The distal flow is the area of the effective regurgitant orifice × the maximum velocity of the mitral regurgitation obtained by CW Doppler. (B) In this example, the ERO = 125 cm^3/435 cm/s = 0.29 cm^2. The RV is then calculated by the ERO × mitral regurgitation VTI. In this example, the RV is 0.29 cm^2 × 146 cm = 43 cm^3. This technique is not optimal for eccentric jets, MR with multiple jets, late systolic MR and for patients with deformed valve in whom a proper convergence zone hemisphere cannot be obtained. (C) The PW Doppler of the pulmonary vein demonstrates systolic flow reversal which suggests severe mitral regurgitation

b

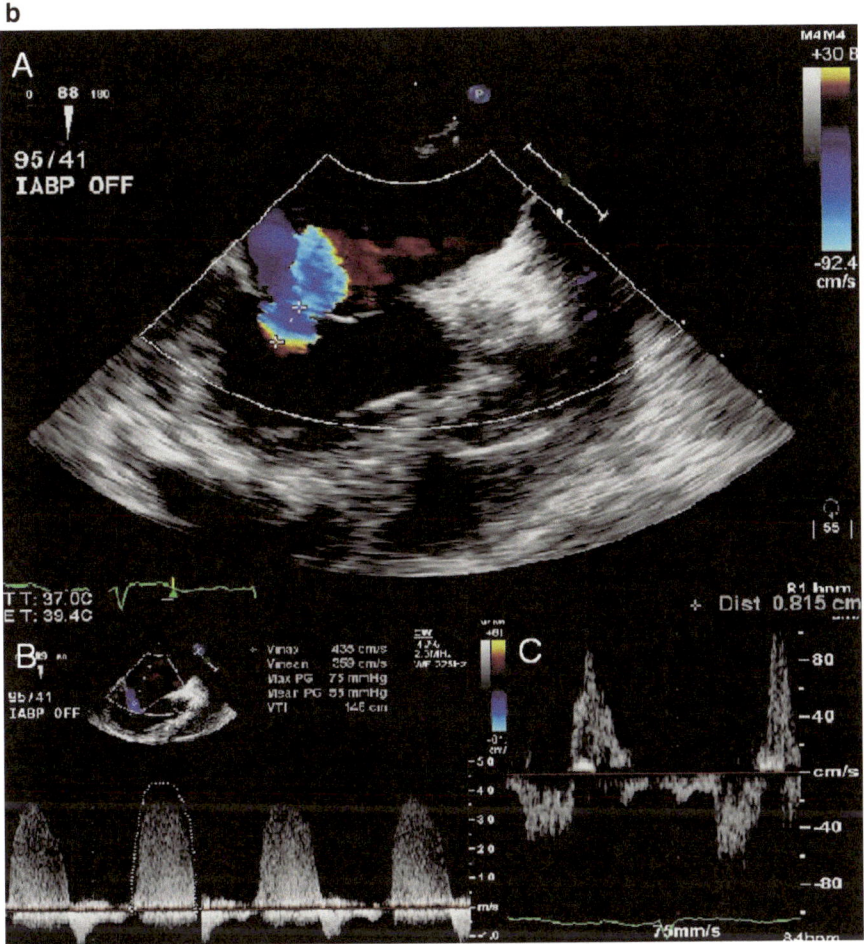

Fig. 17.11 (continued)

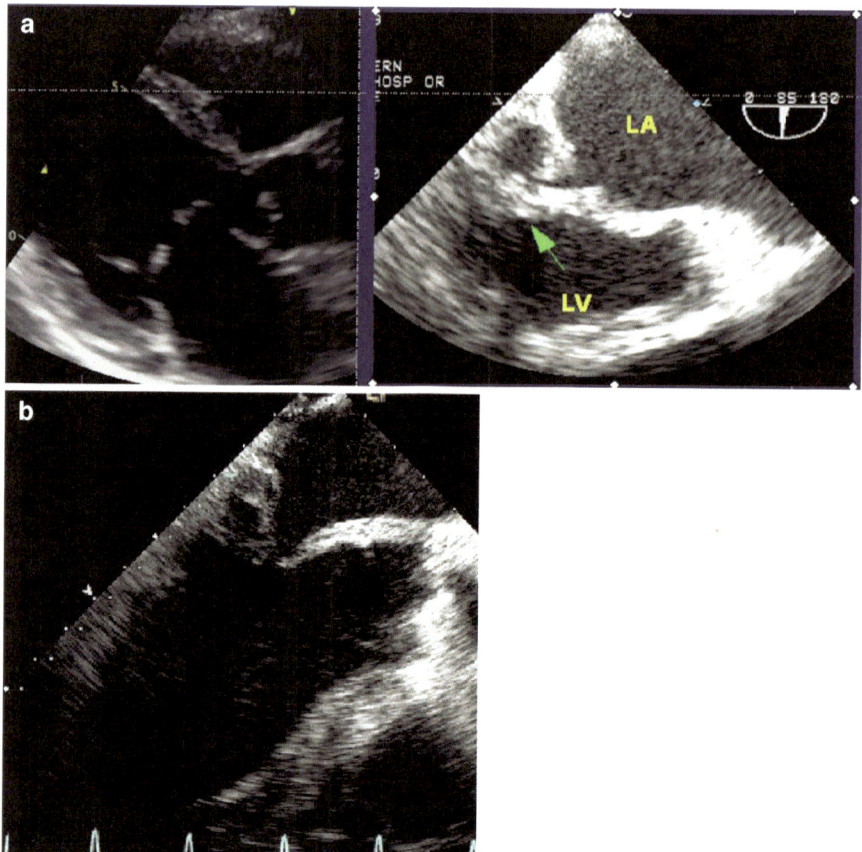

Fig. 17.12 Echocardiographic features of mitral stenosis. (**a**) Rheumatic mitral stenosis. This figure demonstrates typical findings of rheumatic mitral stenosis (MS). The *left panel* shows hockey stick deformity of the anterior leaflet of the mitral valve in diastole. This appearance is a manifestation of the preferential involvement of the tips of the leaflets with the inflammatory/fibrosis process. This leads to relatively preserved mobility of the body with restricted mobility of the tip and the typical appearance. The right panel is a TEE from a different patient. The green arrow shows severe thickening and shortening of the chordae tendinae. Another common feature of rheumatic mitral stenosis is commissural fusion. The presence of commissural fusion may be a good predictor of who will respond to balloon valvuloplasty. (**b**) Other etiologies of mitral stenosis. Other etiologies of mitral stenosis include radiation and connective tissue disorders. Systemic lupus erythematosus causes diffuse thickening of the body of the valve leaflet (see TEE in Fig. 17.12b) as opposed to the tips in rheumatic heart disease

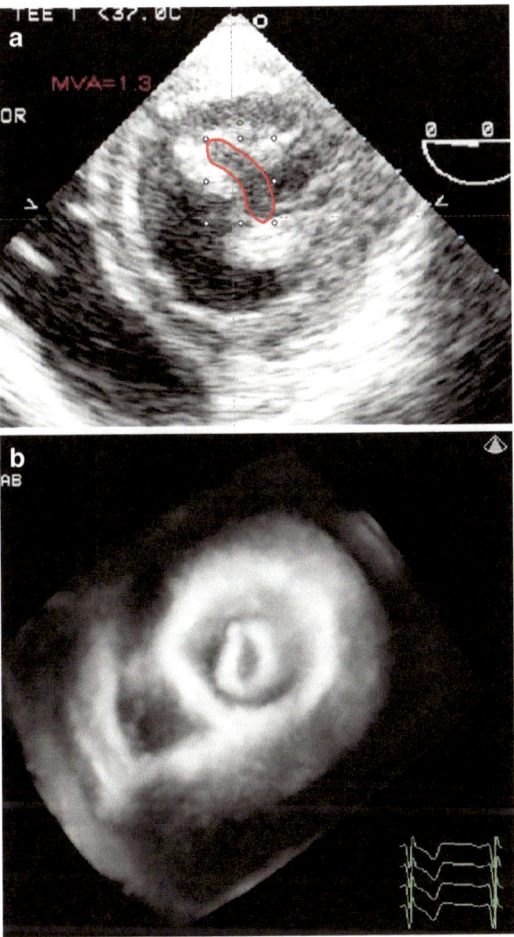

Fig. 17.13 Assessment of mitral stenosis by planimetry. (**a**) Planimetry by 2D echocardiography. Assessment of severity of mitral stenosis by direct planimetry of mitral valve opening is a Level Recommendation[13]. It is direct measurement that does not rely on hemodynamic factors like cardiac output. It can be done on transgastric short axis view (Fig. 17.11a) or parasternal short axis view. To optimize results: (1) a zoomed view of MV is done. (2) It is essential to use proper gains. Over gaining image will result in an area measurement that is smaller than the true mitral valve orifice. (3) A sweep from cranial to caudal helps to ensure the smallest area is obtained. This is usually (but not always) at the leaflet tips. (4) Measurement of area should be done at mid diastole. (5) It is essential to make sure that the plane of the orifice being planimetered is perpendicular to the long axis of LV. An oblique cut will overestimate the area and therefore underestimate severity of MS. (**b**) Planimetry by 3D echocardiography. The main advantage of 3D echocardiography is the ability to achieve a perpendicular en face cut plane of the mitral valve orifice. The measurements are more accurate when performed from the ventricular orientation. Three dimensional derived MVA had better correlation with area calculations derived using the Gorlin formula during cardiac catheterization than 2D and Doppler measurements, such as 2D planimetry, pressure half-time, and flow convergence. 3D measurements have lower intraobserver and interobserver variability. The ease of acquisition and online review of real-time 3D echocardiography facilitates immediate assessment of the mitral valve commissural splitting after percutaneous balloon mitral valvuloplasty in the cardiac catheterization laboratory. This is important since acute changes in compliance make pressure half-time less reliable[27]

Fig. 17.14 Doppler assessment of mitral stenosis by pressure half-time method. (**a**) The pressure half-time PHT method derives from the principle that the decay of the diastolic pressure gradient between the LA and LV is inversely proportional to MVA and therefore is directly related to MS severity.[20] The PHT is the time it takes for the pressure to reach half its original starting value (*red line*). $MVA(cm^2) = 220/PHT$ (ms). Use of this method for assessment of MS receives a Level Recommendation from the American Society of Echocardiography.[13] The advantage of this method is its simplicity. Inadequate recordings may be obtained when there is poor alignment with mitral inflow jet, incorrect gain and filter settings, in presence of aortic regurgitation. Clinical situations in which PHT method does not work well include elderly patients especially in the presence of significant diastolic dysfunction, atrial flutter, and tachycardia and in situations with rapid pressure or compliance changes such as after exercise or balloon valvuloplasty. When the continuous wave signal is not linear or is concave then PHT cannot be measured. (**b**) In some situations the pressure decay is bimodal. There is an early steeper (*red line*) and later shallower pressure decay (*green line*). In these situations the true PHT is reflected by the later slope[28]

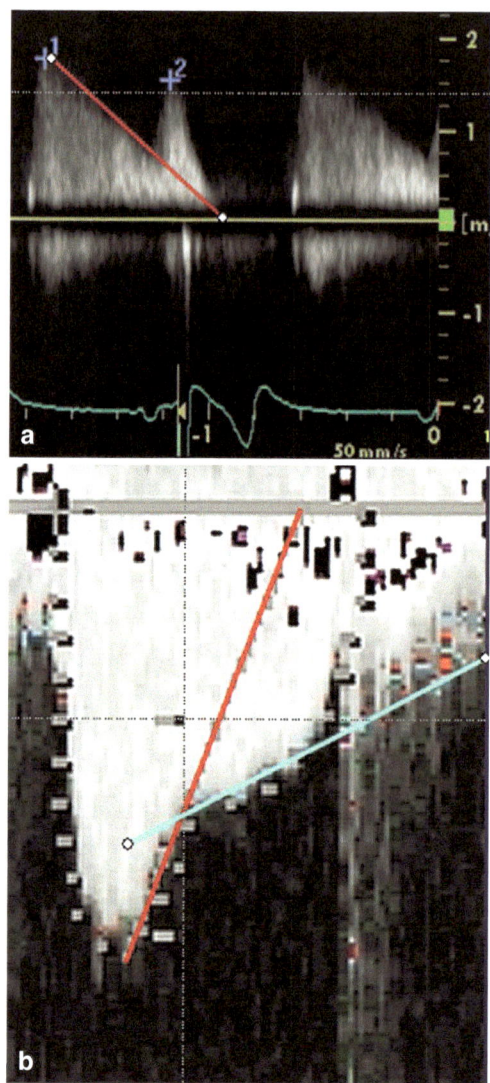

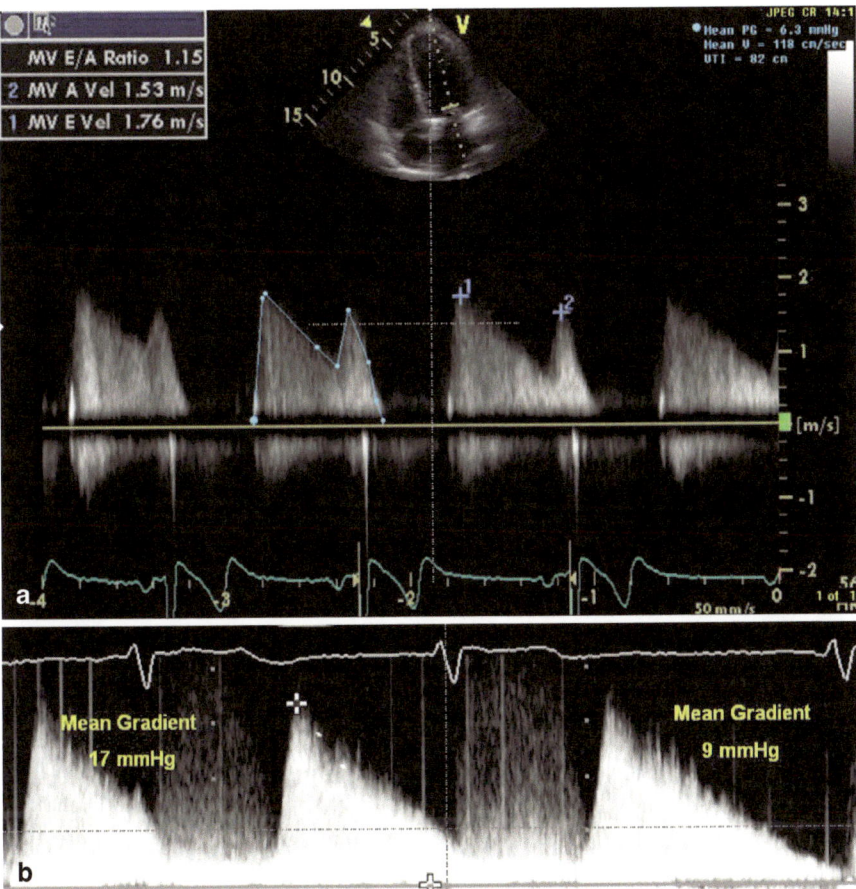

Fig. 17.15 Doppler assessment of mitral stenosis by mean gradient. The mean gradient is a Level Recommendation from the American Society of Echocardiography.[13] The mean gradient depends on the cardiac output. This leads to underestimation of severity of mitral stenosis in patients with low stroke volume and LV dysfunction. Conversely high output states (like mitral regurgitation, anemia, and hyperthyroidism) will lead to overestimation of the severity of MS. Assessment of mean gradient is done through apical windows. Alignment with MR jet is critical. Color Doppler jet may help in patients in whom valve deformity results in eccentric jet. In patients with atrial fibrillation the mean gradient will vary with cycle length. After a short cycle the gradient is higher (Gradient after short cycle in Fig. 17.15b is 17 mmHg) and after long cycles the gradient is lower (Gradient after long cycle in Fig. 17.15b is 9 mmHg). In patients with atrial fibrillation averaging at least five beats is recommended

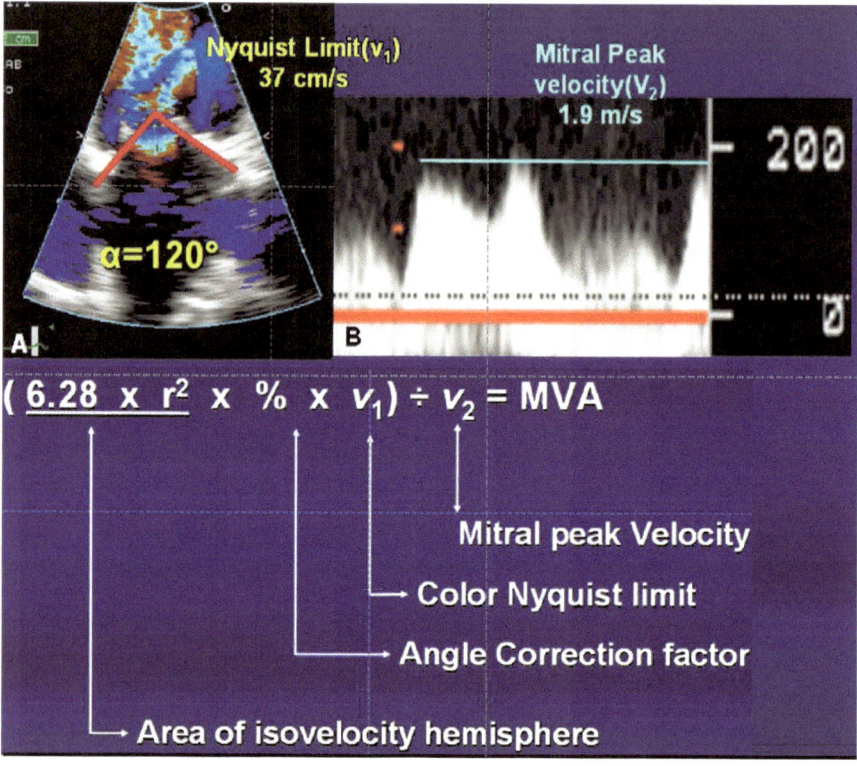

Fig. 17.16 Doppler assessment of mitral stenosis by proximal isovelocity area method. The PISA method can be used to measure MVA. Unlike the case of MR the convergence does not approximate a hemisphere often because of the angle between mitral valve leaflets. This necessitates the correction factor without which flow and therefore MVA would be overestimated. $MVA = (2 \times \Pi \times r^2 \times v_{Nyquist} \times [\alpha / 180]) / v_{Mitral\ CW}$. For the patient in example 16

$r = 1.1$ cm; $v_{Nyquist} = 0.37$ m/s ; $\alpha = 120°$; $v_{Mitral\ CW} = 1.9$ m/s.

$MVA = (2 \times 3.14 \times (1.1)^2 \times 0.37 \times [\alpha 120 / 180]) / 1.9$ $MVA = 1.0$ cm^2. Steps for optimal data

collection for the PISA method include: (1) Zoom on mitral valve. (2) Shift baseline up in direction of flow "toward the LV" or up in case of TTE. The best Nyquist limit is the one that results in a hemispheric convergence zone. This usually is slightly higher than the Nyquist limit used for MR (35–40 cm/s). (3) Radius is measured from the point of color change to leaflet tips. Leaflet tips may be identified using color suppress function. Measurement is usually made in mid diastole. (4) Angle is then measured. (5) Peak diastolic velocity is then measured

Table 17.1 Qualitative and quantitative parameters useful in grading mitral regurgitation severity[11]

	Mild	Moderate	Severe
Structural parameters			
LA size	Normal[a]	Normal or dilated	Usually dilated[b]
LV size	Normal[a]	Normal or dilated	Usually dilated[b]
Mitral leaflets or support apparatus	Normal or abnormal	Normal or abnormal	Abnormal/flail leaflet/ruptured papillary muscle
Doppler parameters			
Color flow jet area[c]	Small, central jet (usually <4 cm² or <20% of LA area)	Variable	Large central jet (usually >10 cm² or >40% of LA area) or variable size wall-impinging jet swirling in LA
Mitral inflow – PW	A wave dominant[d]	Variable	E wave dominant[d]
Jet density – CW	Incomplete or faint	Dense	Dense
Jet contour – CW	Parabolic	Usually parabolic	Early peaking – triangular
Pulmonary vain flow	Systolic dominance[e]	Systolic blunting[e]	Systolic flow reversal[f]

CW, continuous wave; *LA*, left atrium; *LV*, left ventricle; *PW*, pulsed wave; *RF*, regurgitant fraction

[a]Unless there are other reasons for LA or LV dilation. Normal 2D measurements; LV minor axis ≤ 82 mL/m², maximal LA antero-posterior diameter ≤ 2 cm/m², maximal LA volume ≤ 36 mL/m² (2, 33, 35)

[b]Exception: acute mitral regurgitation

[c]At a Nyquist limit of 50–60 cm/s

[d]Usually above 50 years of age or in conditions of impaired relaxation, in the absence of mitral stenosis or other causes of elevated LA pressure

[e]Systolic dominance or blunting or both

[f]Pulmonary venous systolic flow reversal is specific but not sensitive for severe MR

Table 17.2 Quantitative measures of grading MR severity[11]

	Formula	Advantage	Potential Pitfall
EROA (cm²) PISA	$6.28 \times r^2 \times v_{Nyq}/v_{CW}$	Simple, few measurements	Eccentric jets; Non-hemispheric zone of acceleration; Multiple jets
Regurgitant vol. (mL/beat) PISA method	$EROA \times TVI_{CW}$	Simple, few measurements	Eccentric jets; multiple steps
Continuity equation method	$Flow_{Mitral} - Flow_{LVOT}$	Multiple jets, eccentric jets	AF
Regurgitant fraction (%)	$(Flow_{Mitral} - Flow_{LVOT})/Flow_{Mitral}$		Eccentric jets; multiple steps, AF

EROA, effective regurgitant orifice area; *PISA*, proximal isovelocity surface area; V_{Nyq}, velocity of Nyquist limit; v_{CW}, peak velocity of MR continuous wave; D_{Mitral}, diameter of mitral annulus; D_{LVOT}, diameter of LVOT annulus; *AF*, atrial fibrillation;

Table 17.3 Qualitative and quantitative parameters useful in grading mitral regurgitation severity[11]

	Mild	Moderate		Severe
Quantitative parameters[a]				
VC width (cm)	<0.3	0.3–0.69		≥0.7
R Vol (mL/beat)	<30	30–44	45–59	≥60
RF (%)	<30	30–39	40–49	≥50
EROA (cm²)	<0.20	0.20–0.29	0.30–0.39	≥0.40

EROA, effective regurgitant orifice area; *LV*, left ventricle; *PW*, pulsed wave; *RF*, regurgitant fraction; *R Vol*, regurgitant volume; *VC*, vena contracta

[a] Quantitative parameters can help subclassify the moderate regurgitant group into mild-to-moderate and moderate-to-severe

Table 17.4 Assessment of mitral valve anatomy according to the Wilkins score[13]

Grade	Mobility	Thickening	Calcification	Subvalvular thickening
1	Highly mobile valve with only leaflet tips restricted	Leaflets near normal in thickness (4–5 mm)	A single area of increased echo brightness	Minimal thickening just below the mitral leaflets
2	Leaflet mid and base portions have normal mobility	Midleaflets normal, considerable thickening of margins (5–8 mm)	Scattered areas of brightness confined to leaflet margins	Thickening of chordal structures extending to one-third of the chordal length
3	Valve continues to move forward in diastole, mainly from the base	Thickening extending through the entire leaflet (5–8 mm)	Brightness extending into the mid-portions of the leaflets	Thickening extended to distal third of the chords
4	No or minimal forward movement of the leavlets in diastole	Considerable thickening of all leaflet tissue (>8–10 mm)	Extensive brightness throughout much of the leaflet tissue	Extensive thickening and shortening of all chordal structures extending down to the papillary muscles

The total score is the sum of the four items and ranges between 4 and 16

Table 17.5 Recommendations for classification of mitral stenosis severity[13]

	Mild	Moderate	Severe
Specific findings			
Valve area (cm²)	>1.5	1.0–1.5	<1.0
Supportive findings			
Mean gradient (mmHg)[a]	<5	5–10	>10
Pulmonary artery pressure (mmHg)	<30	30–50	>50

[a] At heart rates between 60 and 80 bpm and in sinus rhythm

References

1. Otto CM. Clinical practice. Evaluation and management of chronic mitral regurgitation. *N Engl J Med*. 2001;345(10):740-746.
2. Cohn LH, Edmunds LH. *Cardiac surgery in the adult*. 2nd ed. New York: McGraw-Hill; 2003.
3. Freed LA, Levy D, Levine RA, et al. Prevalence and clinical outcome of mitral-valve prolapse. *N Engl J Med*. 1999;341(1):1-7.
4. Monin JL, Dehant P, Roiron C, et al. Functional assessment of mitral regurgitation by transthoracic echocardiography using standardized imaging planes diagnostic accuracy and outcome implications. *J Am Coll Cardiol*. 2005;46(2):302-309.
5. Enriquez-Sarano M, Freeman WK, Tribouilloy CM, et al. Functional anatomy of mitral regurgitation: accuracy and outcome implications of transesophageal echocardiography. *J Am Coll Cardiol*. 1999;34(4):1129-1136.
6. Pepi M, Tamborini G, Maltagliati A, et al. Head-to-head comparison of two- and three-dimensional transthoracic and transesophageal echocardiography in the localization of mitral valve prolapse. *J Am Coll Cardiol*. 2006;48(12):2524.
7. Stewart WJ, Currie PJ, Salcedo EE, et al. Evaluation of mitral leaflet motion by echocardiography and jet direction by Doppler color flow mapping to determine the mechanisms of mitral regurgitation. *J Am Coll Cardiol*. 1992;20(6):1353-1361.
8. Lee KS, Stewart WJ, Lever HM, Underwood PL, Cosgrove DM. Mechanism of outflow tract obstruction causing failed mitral valve repair. Anterior displacement of leaflet coaptation. *Circulation*. 1993;88(5 Pt 2):II24-II29.
9. Maslow AD, Regan MM, Haering JM, Johnson RG, Levine RA. Echocardiographic predictors of left ventricular outflow tract obstruction and systolic anterior motion of the mitral valve after mitral valve reconstruction for myxomatous valve disease. *J Am Coll Cardiol*. 1999;34(7):2096-2104.
10. Enriquez-Sarano M, Avierinos JF, Messika-Zeitoun D, et al. Quantitative determinants of the outcome of asymptomatic mitral regurgitation. *N Engl J Med*. 2005;352(9):875-883.
11. Zoghbi WA, Enriquez-Sarano M, Foster E, et al. Recommendations for evaluation of the severity of native valvular regurgitation with two-dimensional and Doppler echocardiography. *J Am Soc Echocardiogr*. 2003;16(7):777-802.
12. Wilkins GT, Weyman AE, Abascal VM, Block PC, Palacios IF. Percutaneous balloon dilatation of the mitral valve: an analysis of echocardiographic variables related to outcome and the mechanism of dilatation. *Br Heart J*. 1988;60(4):299-308.
13. Baumgartner H, Hung J, Bermejo J, et al. Echocardiographic assessment of valve stenosis: EAE/ASE recommendations for clinical practice. *J Am Soc Echocardiogr*. 2009;22(1):1-23. quiz 101-102.
14. Messika-Zeitoun D, Brochet E, Holmin C, et al. Three-dimensional evaluation of the mitral valve area and commissural opening before and after percutaneous mitral commissurotomy in patients with mitral stenosis. *Eur Heart J*. 2007;28(1):72-79.
15. Bonow RO, Carabello BA, Chatterjee K, et al. ACC/AHA 2006 guidelines for the management of patients with valvular heart disease: a report of the American College of Cardiology/American Heart Association Task Force on Practice Guidelines (writing Committee to Revise the 1998 guidelines for the management of patients with valvular heart disease) developed in collaboration with the Society of Cardiovascular Anesthesiologists endorsed by the Society for Cardiovascular Angiography and Interventions and the Society of Thoracic Surgeons. *J Am Coll Cardiol*. 2006;48(3):e1-e148.

16. Vahanian A, Baumgartner H, Bax J, et al. Guidelines on the management of valvular heart disease: The Task Force on the Management of Valvular Heart Disease of the European Society of Cardiology. *Eur Heart J.* 2007;28(2):230-268.
17. Zamorano J, Cordeiro P, Sugeng L, et al. Real-time three-dimensional echocardiography for rheumatic mitral valve stenosis evaluation: an accurate and novel approach. *J Am Coll Cardiol.* 2004;43(11):2091-2096.
18. Sebag IA, Morgan JG, Handschumacher MD, et al. Usefulness of three-dimensionally guided assessment of mitral stenosis using matrix-array ultrasound. *Am J Cardiol.* 2005;96(8): 1151-1156.
19. Messika-Zeitoun D, Meizels A, Cachier A, et al. Echocardiographic evaluation of the mitral valve area before and after percutaneous mitral commissurotomy: the pressure half-time method revisited. *J Am Soc Echocardiogr.* 2005;18(12):1409-1414.
20. Thomas JD, Weyman AE. Doppler mitral pressure half-time: a clinical tool in search of theoretical justification. *J Am Coll Cardiol.* 1987;10(4):923-929.
21. Thomas JD, Weyman AE. Fluid dynamics model of mitral valve flow: description with in vitro validation. *J Am Coll Cardiol.* 1989;13(1):221-233.
22. Messika-Zeitoun D, Fung Yiu S, Cormier B, et al. Sequential assessment of mitral valve area during diastole using colour M-mode flow convergence analysis: new insights into mitral stenosis physiology. *Eur Heart J.* 2003;24(13):1244-1253.
23. Nishimura RA, Rihal CS, Tajik AJ, Holmes DR Jr. Accurate measurement of the transmitral gradient in patients with mitral stenosis: a simultaneous catheterization and Doppler echocardiographic study. *J Am Coll Cardiol.* 1994;24(1):152-158.
24. www.echoincontext.com/images/anat_pisa003
25. Foster GP, Isselbacher EM, Rose GA, Torchiana DF, Akins CW, Picard MH. Accurate localization of mitral regurgitant defects using multiplane transesophageal echocardiography. *Ann Thorac Surg.* 1998;65(4):1025-1031.
26. Roberts BJ, Grayburn PA. Color flow imaging of the vena contracta in mitral regurgitation: technical considerations. *J Am Soc Echocardiogr.* 2003;16:1002-1006.
27. Zamorano J, Perez de Isla L, Sugeng L, et al. Non-invasive assessment of mitral valve area during percutaneous balloon mitral valvuloplasty: role of real-time 3D echocardiography. *Eur Heart J.* 2004;25:2086-2091.
28. Gonzalez MA, Child JS, Krivokapich J. Comparison of two-dimensional and Doppler echocardiography and intracardiac hemodynamics for quantification of mitral stenosis. *Am J Cardiol.* 1987;60:327-332.

Right-Sided Heart Valves Assessment in Disease

18

Farouk Mookadam, Julie A. Humphries, Sherif E. Moustafa, and Tahlil A. Warsame

Table 18.1 Etiologies of pulmonic stenosis (PS) and associated cardiac abnormalities

Classification	Causes	Associated cardiac anomalies
Valvular	*Congenital* (most common)	Usually isolated May also occur as part of more complex congenital lesions such as tetralogy of Fallot (TOF), complete atrioventricular canal, double outlet right ventricle, and univentricular heart Peripheral pulmonary artery stenosis may coexist with valvular pulmonary stenosis such as in Noonan's syndrome and Williams syndrome
	Acquired Obstructive tumors Carcinoid heart disease Rheumatic heart disease	–
Subvalvular (infundibular)	*Congenital*	Isolated is rare Usually associated with a large ventricular septal defect (VSD), as seen in TOF
	Acquired Double chamber right ventricle Jet lesion produced by the VSD Severe right ventricular hypertrophy Iatrogenic: prior surgery or intervention Hypertrophic or infiltrative processes such as hypertrophic obstructive cardiomyopathy or glycogen storage disorders Compression from a tumor or vascular structure	–

(continued)

F. Mookadam (✉)
Department of Cardiology, Mayo College of Medicine, Scottsdale, AZ, USA
e-mail: mookadam.farouk@mayo.edu

T.P. Abraham (ed.), *Case Based Echocardiography*,
DOI: 10.1007/978-1-84996-151-6_18, © Springer-Verlag London Limited 2011

Table 18.1 (continued)

Classification	Causes	Associated cardiac anomalies
Supravalvular	*Congenital*	Isolated or in association with other cardiac anomalies Single, involving the main pulmonary artery or either of its branches, or multiple Common associated defects are pulmonary valve stenosis, VSD, and TOF Peripheral pulmonary artery stenosis is often seen in association with congenital syndromes, such as congenital rubella syndrome, Williams' syndrome, Noonan's syndrome, Alagille's syndrome, Ehlers–Danlos syndrome, and Silver–Russell syndrome
	Acquired Iatrogenic: prior surgery or intervention Compression from a tumor or vascular structure Isolated pulmonary artery stenosis	–

Table 18.2 Doppler parameters used in grading pulmonary regurgitation [1]

Parameter	Mild	Moderate	Severe
Pulmonic valve	Normal	Normal or abnormal	Abnormal
RV size	Normal[a]	Normal or dilated	Dilated
Jet size by color Doppler[c]	Thin (usually <10 mm in length) with a narrow origin	Intermediate	Usually large, with a wide origin May be brief in duration
Jet density and deceleration rate – CW[d]	Soft Slow deceleration	Dense Variable deceleration	Dense Steep deceleration, early termination of diastolic flow
Pulmonic systolic flow compared to systemic flow – PW[e]	Slightly increased	Intermediate	Greatly increased

CW continuous wave Doppler, *PR* pulmonic regurgitation, *PW* pulsed wave Doppler, *RA* right atrium, *RF* regurgitant fraction, *RV* right ventricle

[a]Unless there are other reasons for RV enlargement. Normal 2D measurements from the apical four-chamber view; RV mediolateral end-diastolic dimension ≤4.3 cm, RV end-diastolic area ≤35.5 cm^2

[b]Exception: acute PR

[c]At a Nyquist limit of 50–60 cm/s

[d]Steep deceleration is not specific for severe PR

[e]Cut-off values for regurgitant volume and fraction are not well validated

Table 18.3 Etiologies of tricuspid regurgitation (TR)

Classification	Primary TR	Secondary or functional TR (most common)
Congenital	Cleft valve (usually associated with atrioventricular canal defect) Ebstein's anomaly	–
Acquired	Normal variant Rheumatic valve disease Infective endocarditis Carcinoid heart disease Toxic (e.g., Phen-Fen or methysergide) Iatrogenic: pacemaker lead Tricuspid valve irradiation Blunt or penetrating injuries Tricuspid valve prolapse	Right ventricular dilatation Right ventricular hypertension (e.g., pulmonary hypertension) Global right ventricular dysfunction secondary to myocarditis, cardio-myopathy, longstanding pulmonary hypertension with fibrosis Segmental dysfunction secondary to right ventricular ischemia or infarction, arrhythmogenic right ventricular Dysplasia, endomyocardial fibrosis

Table 18.4 Echo parameters of tricuspid regurgitation (TR) severity [1]

Parameter	Mild	Moderate	Severe
Tricuspid valve	Usually normal	Normal or abnormal	Abnormal/flail leaflet/poor coaptation
RV/RA/IVC size	Normal[a]	Normal or dilated	Usually dilated[b]
Jet area-central jets $(cm^2)^c$	<5	5–10	>10
VC width $(cm)^d$	Not defined	Not defined, but <0.7	>0.7
PISA radius $(cm)^e$	≤0.5	0.6–0.9	>0.9
Jet density and contour – CW	Soft and parabolic	Dense, variable contour	Dense, triangular with early peaking
Hepatic vein flow[f]	Systolic dominance	Systolic blunting	Systolic reversal

CW continuous wave Doppler, *IVC* inferior vena cava, *RA* right atrium, *RV* right ventricle, *VC* vena contracta width

[a]Unless there are other reasons for RA or RV dilation. Normal 2D measurements from the apical four-chamber view: RV mediolateral end-diastolic dimension ≤4.3 cm, RV end-diastolic area ≤35.5 cm^2, maximal RA mediolateral and supero-inferior dimensions ≤4.6 and 4.9 cm respectively, maximal RA volume ≤33 mL/m^2

[b]Exception: acute TR

[c]At a Nyquist limit of 50–60 cm/s. Not valid in eccentric jets. Jet area is not recommended as the sole parameter of TR severity due to its dependence on hemodynamic and technical factors

[d]At a Nyquist limit of 50–60 cm/s

[e]Baseline shift with Nyquist limit of 28 cm/s

[f]Other conditions may cause systolic blunting (e.g., atrial fibrillation, elevated RA pressure)

Table 18.5 Etiologies of tricuspid stenosis (rheumatic, carcinoid, congenital, infective endocarditis, Fabry's, Whipple's disease, giant blood cysts)

Classification	Causes
Congenital	Congenital tricuspid stenosis
	Tricuspid atresia
	Ebstein's anomaly
Acquired	Rheumatic valve disease (most common)
	Infective endocarditis
	Carcinoid heart disease
	Toxic (e.g., Phen-Fen or methysergide)
	Pacemaker endocarditis and pacemaker-induced adhesions, lupus valvulitis, mechanical obstruction by benign or malignant tumors
	Fabry's disease
	Whipple's disease

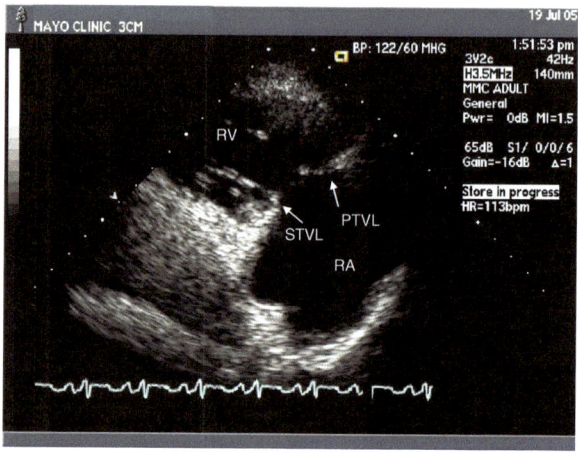

Fig. 18.1 Two-dimensional echocardiogram. Right ventricular inflow view showing thickened and retracted tricuspid valve leaflets due to carcinoid. *RV* right ventricle, *RA* right atrium, *STVL* septal tricuspid valve leaflet, *PTVL* posterior tricuspid valve leaflet

Fig. 18.2 (**a**) Two-dimensional echocardiogram. Right ventricular inflow view showing severe tricuspid regurgitation by color flow Doppler in a patient with carcinoid heart disease. (**b**) Short-axis view showing thickened pulmonic valve leaflets in carcinoid heart disease. *RV* right ventricle, *RA* right atrium, *TR* tricuspid valve, *PV* pulmonic valve, *MPA* main pulmonary artery

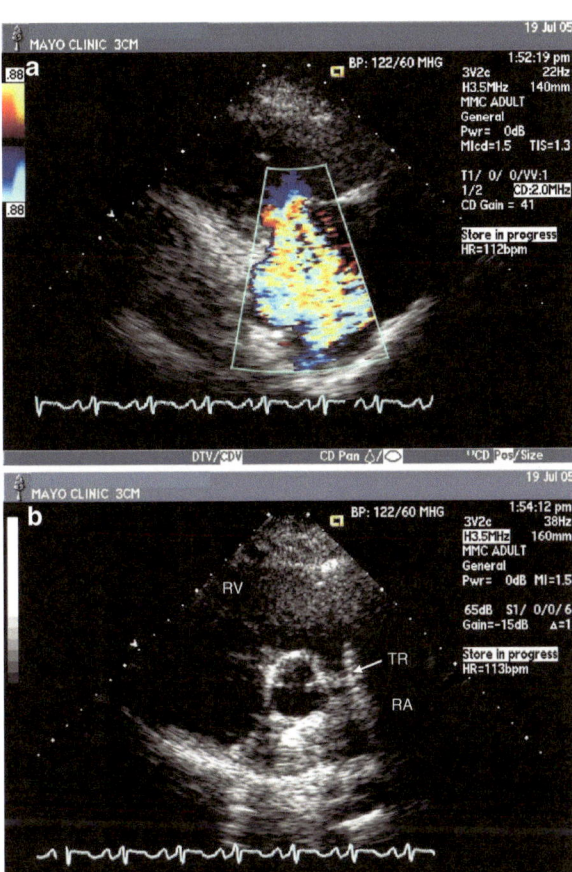

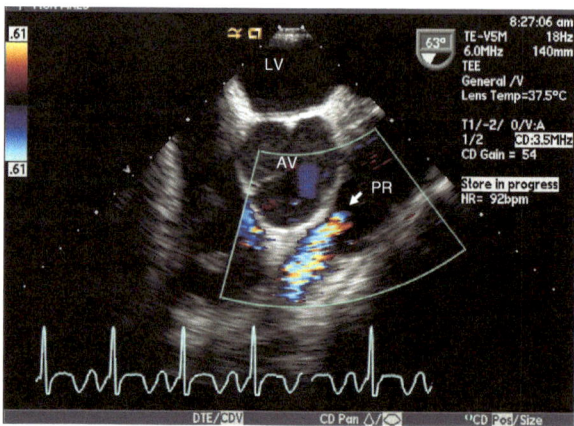

Fig. 18.3 Transesophageal echocardiography showing pulmonary valve thickened and retracted due to carcinoid involvement of the right-sided heart valves. Open pulmonary valve shows doming, *LV* left ventricle, *RV* right ventricle, *RA* right atrium, *PV* pulmonic valve, *MPA* main pulmonary artery, *AV* aortic valve, *AC* anterior cusp, *PC* posterior cusp

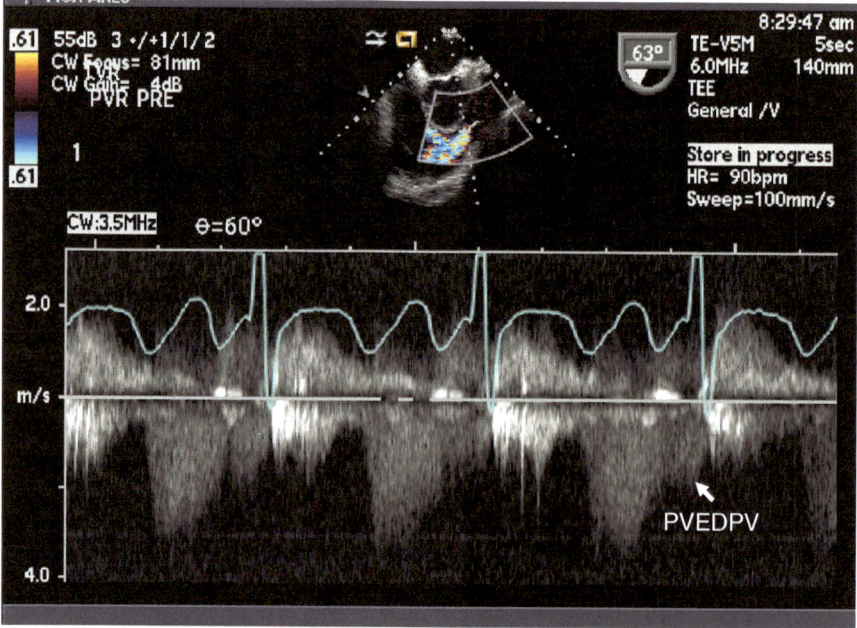

Fig. 18.4 Pulmonary regurgitation Doppler signal showing severe pulmonary regurgitation with a short deceleration time and high pulmonary end diastolic pressures. This is in a case of pacemaker induced tricuspid regurgitation. *PVEDPV* pulmonic valve end diastolic peak velocity, PPM induced TR retraction of septal leaflet

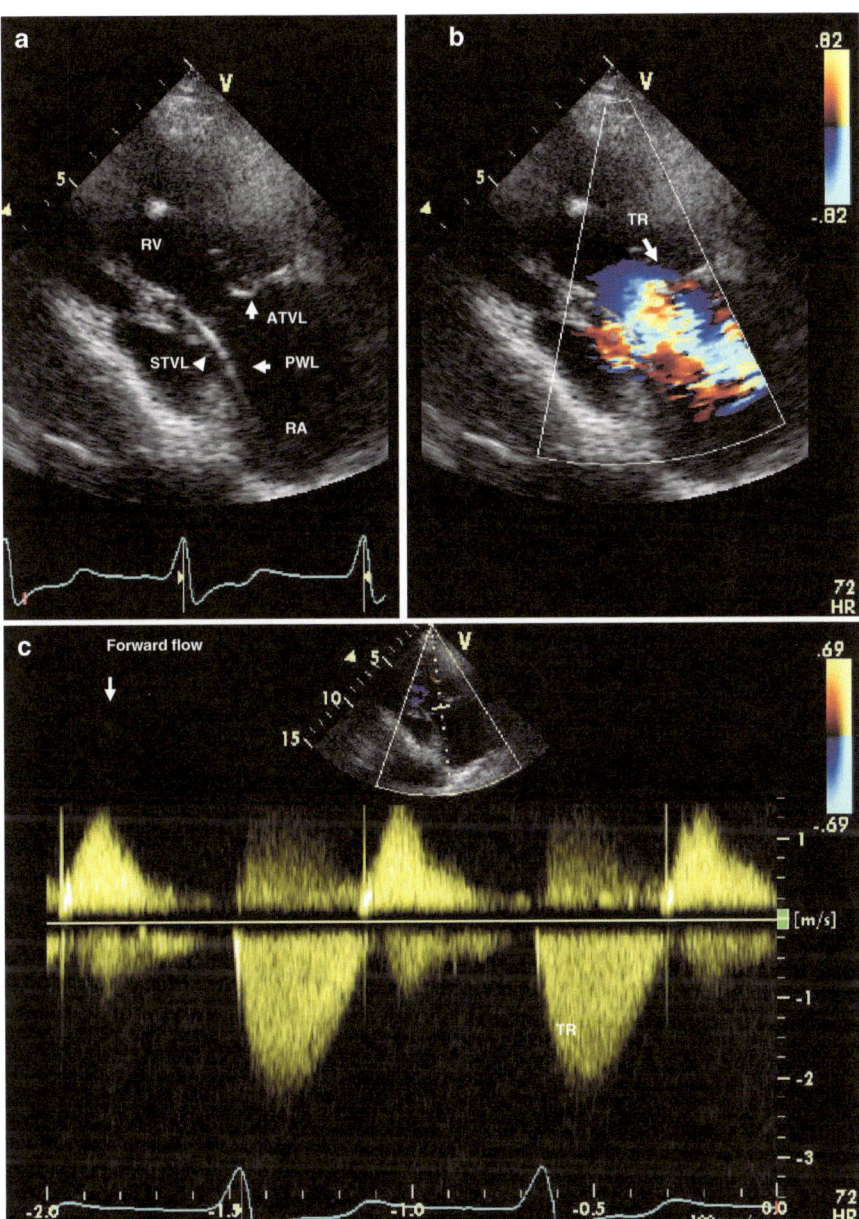

Fig. 18.5 (**a**) Two-dimensional echocardiogram parasternal long axis right ventricular inflow view showing retraction of the septal leaflet by a pacemaker lead, and on the right panel (**b**) severe tricuspid regurgitation from malcoaptation. (**c**) Two-dimensional echocardiogram of the RV inflow view showing tricuspid regurgitation jet velocity Doppler signal showing severe tricuspid regurgitation and low pressure gradient. *RV* right ventricle, *RA* right atrium, *STVL* septal tricuspid valve leaflet, *ATVL* anterior tricuspid valve leaflet, *PML* pacemaker lead, *TR* tricuspid valve

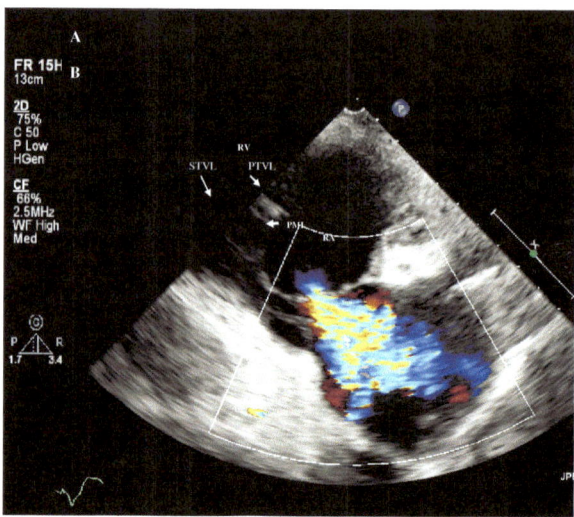

Fig. 18.6 Two-dimensional echocardiogram. (**a**) Right ventricular inflow view showing pacemaker lead obstructing the posterior leaflet of tricuspid valve, *RV* right ventricle, *RA* right atrium, *STVL* septal tricuspid valve leaflet, *ATVL* anterior tricuspid valve leaflet, *PML* pacemaker lead, *TV* tricuspid valve

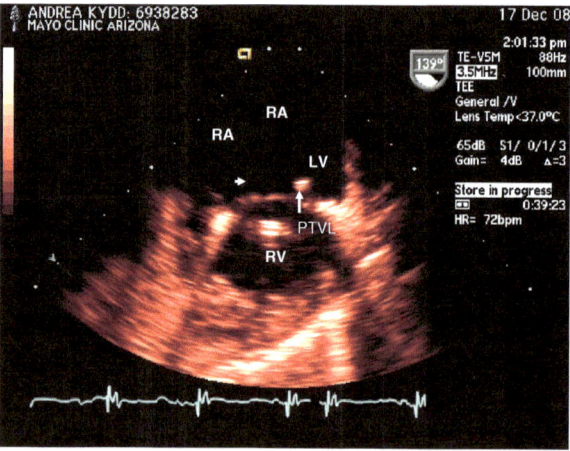

Fig. 18.7 Bioprosthetic tricuspid valve replacement. (**a**) Four-chamber transesophageal view with permanent pacemaker lead externalized to tricuspid ring. *RV* right ventricle, *RA* right atrium, *LV* left ventricle, *LA* left atrium, *PTVL* posterior tricuspid valve leaflet, *TV* tricuspid valve ring

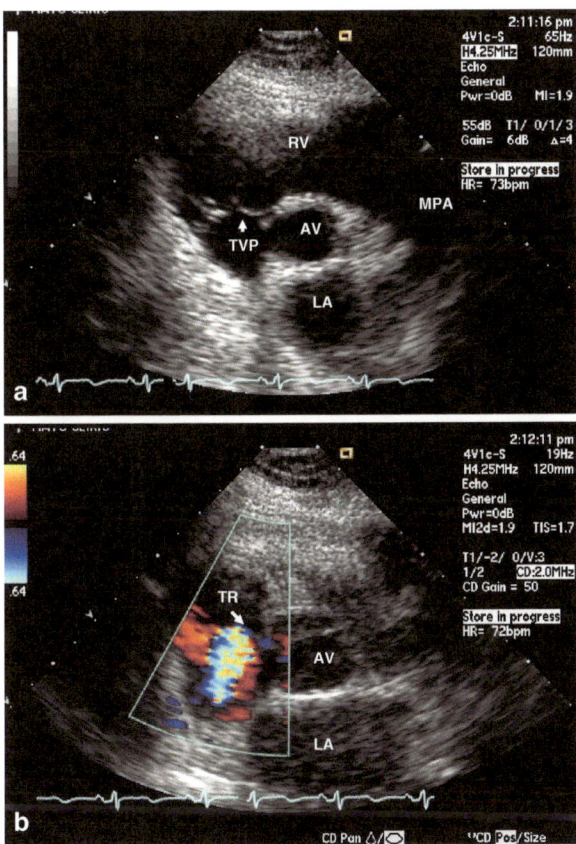

Fig. 18.8 (**a**) Two-dimensional echocardiogram parasternal short axis view at the base of the heart showing tricuspid valve leaflet prolapse. (**b**) Parasternal short axis at the base showing tricuspid valve regurgitation by color. (**c**) Tricuspid regurgitation Doppler signal demonstrates normal RVSP. *RV* right ventricle, *LA* right atrium, *TVP* tricuspid valve prolepses, *AV* aortic valve, *MPA* main pulmonary artery aneurysm, *TR* tricuspid regurgitation, *RPA* right pulmonary artery, *LPA* left pulmonary artery

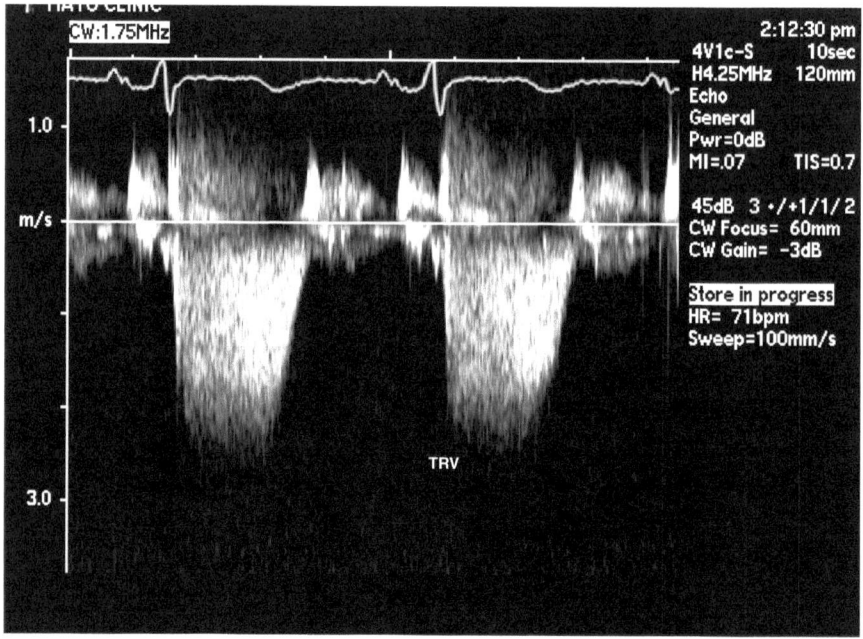

Fig. 18.8 (continued)

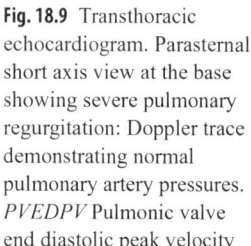

Fig. 18.9 Transthoracic echocardiogram. Parasternal short axis view at the base showing severe pulmonary regurgitation: Doppler trace demonstrating normal pulmonary artery pressures. *PVEDPV* Pulmonic valve end diastolic peak velocity

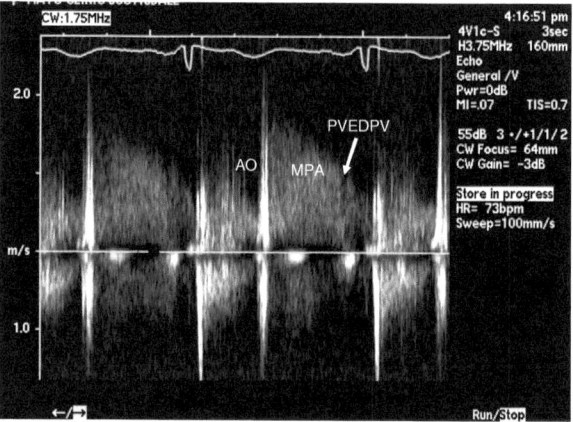

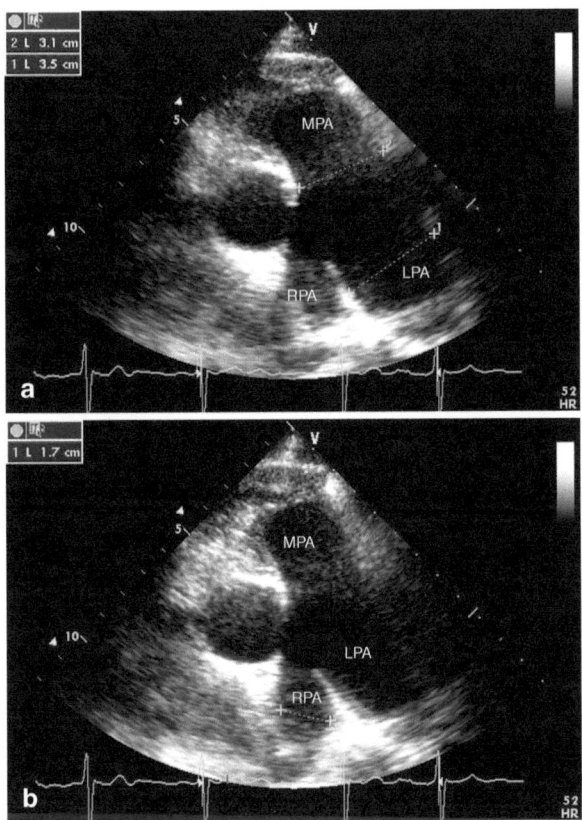

Fig. 18.10 Congenital pulmonary stenosis showing main pulmonary artery and left pulmonary artery dilation. (**a**) Main pulmonary artery measures 3.5 cm and left pulmonary artery measures 3.1 cm, and in comparison, (**b**) right pulmonary artery measures 1.7 cm. *LPA* left pulmonary artery, *RPA* right pulmonary artery

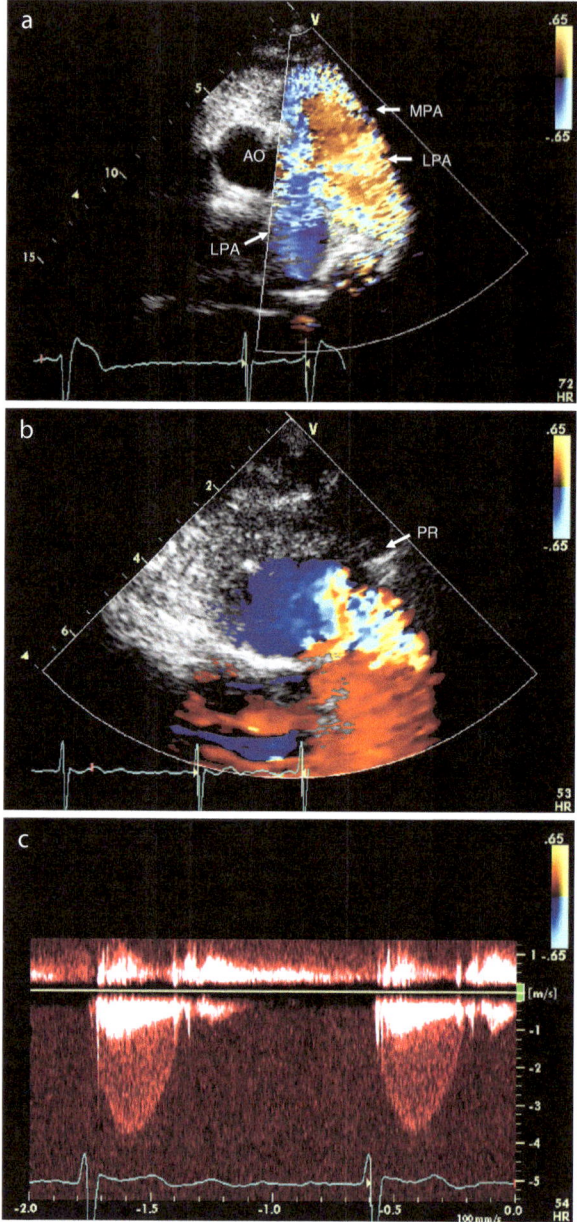

Fig. 18.11 (**a**) Parasternal short axis at the base of the heart showing dilated pulmonary artery and flow acceleration across the stenosed pulmonary valve by color flow Doppler, (**b**) pulmonary stenosis color flow Doppler, (**c**) Doppler trace showing high peak and mean gradient across the pulmonary valve, and (**d**) pulmonary regurgitation showing low pulmonary end diastolic regurgitation velocity indicating mildly raised EDP (8 mmHg + right atrial pressure)

Fig. 18.11 (continued)

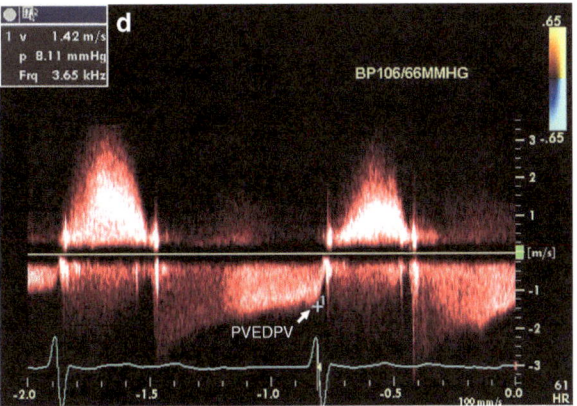

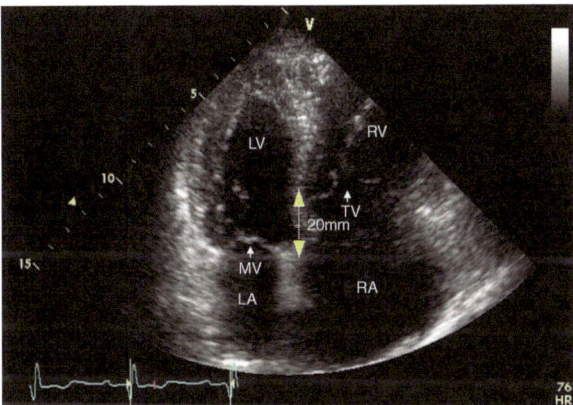

Fig. 18.12 Two-dimensional echocardiogram. Apical four-chamber view showing apical displacement of the septal and anterior tricuspid valve leaflets, leading to atrialization of the right ventricle, moderate size atrialized right ventricle, and severe right atrial enlargement. Crux to TV insertion 20 mm or 1.2 cm/m > 2. Patient has a BSA of 1.7 m. *LA* left atrium, *LV* left ventricle, *RA* right atrium, *RV* right ventricle, *MV* mitral valve, *TV* tricuspid valve

Fig. 18.13 Two-dimensional
echocardiogram. Apical
four-chamber view showing
apical displacement of the
septal and anterior tricuspid
valve leaflets. *LA* left atrium,
LV left ventricle, *RA* right
atrium, *RV* right ventricle,
MV mitral valve, *STVL*
septal tricuspid valve leaflet,
ATVL anterior tricuspid
valve leaflet

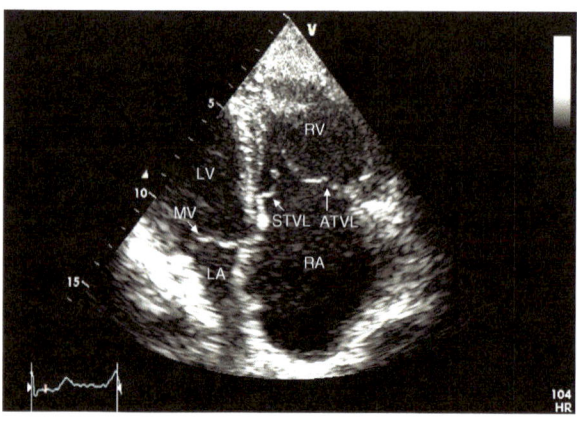

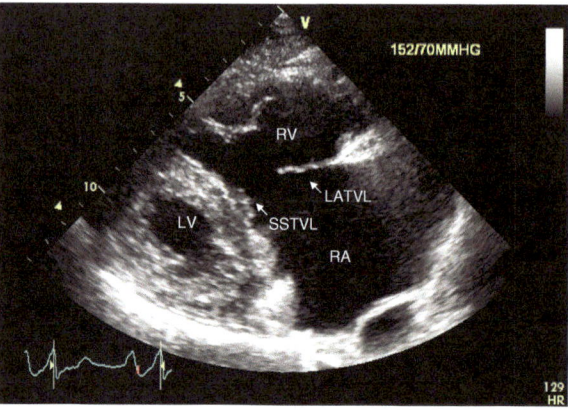

Fig. 18.14 Two-dimensional echocardiogram. Right ventricular inflow view showing thickened, large anterior tricuspid leaflet and short, retracted septal leaflet of the tricuspid valve. *RV* right ventricle, *RA* right atrium, *LV* left ventricle, *SSTVL* short septal tricuspid valve leaflet, *LATVL* large anterior tricuspid valve leaflet

Fig. 18.15 Two-dimensional echocardiogram. Right ventricular inflow view showing large and mobile anterior tricuspid leaflet and short, retracted septal leaflet of the tricuspid valve. *SSTVL* short septal tricuspid valve leaflet, *LATVL* large anterior tricuspid valve leaflet

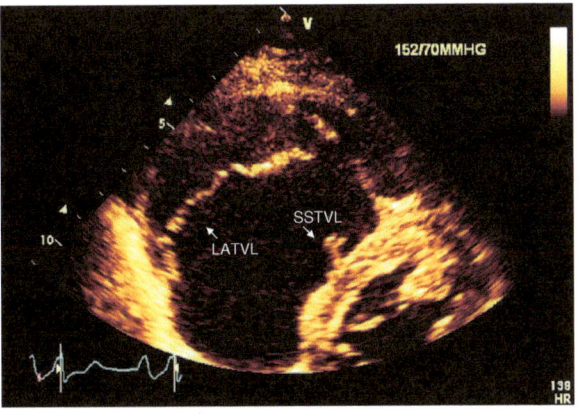

Fig. 18.16 Two-dimensional echocardiogram. Apical four-chamber view showing severe eccentric tricuspid valve regurgitation. *TR* tricuspid regurgitation

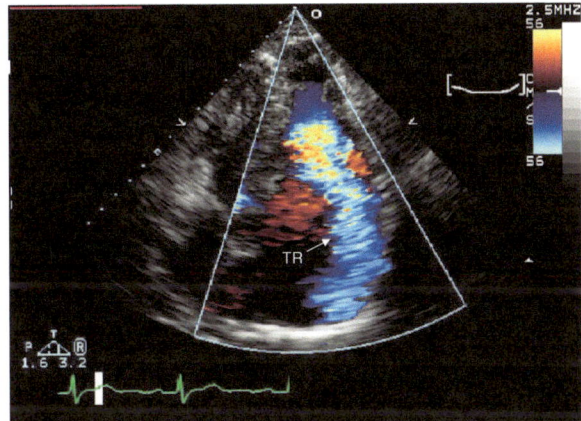

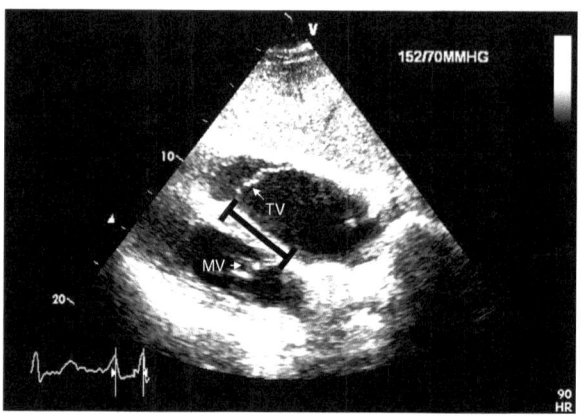

Fig. 18.17 Two-dimensional echocardiogram. Subcostal four-chamber view showing apical displacement of the tricuspid leaflets, leading to atrialization of the right ventricle or Ebstein's anomaly. *MV* mitral valve, *TV* tricuspid valve

Reference

1. Zoghbi WA, Enriquez-Sarano M, Foster E, et al. Recommendations for evaluation of the severity of native valvular regurgitation with two-dimensional and Doppler echocardiography. *J Am Soc Echocardiogr*. 2003;16:777-802.

The Assessment of Prosthetic Valve Function

19

Mengistu Simegn, Anupama Kottam, and Luis Afonso

19.1
Characteristics of Prosthetic Valves: Two General Types (Tables 19.1 and 19.2)

a. Mechanical prosthetic valves:
   i. Composition: Titanium or silicon derived with a sewing ring
   ii. Durability: 25–30 years
   iii. Risk of thromboembolism: 0.1– 5.7 patient-years in mitral valve position
   iv. Obligatory normal regurgitation more common than tissue valves
   v. Types:
      1. Caged-ball (most thrombogenic)
      2. Single tilting disc (intermediate thrombogenicity)
      3. Bileaflet (least thrombogenic)
b. Bioprosthetic valves:
   i. Composition: Intact valve or made of harvested pericardium. Source: Animal (hetero/xenograft), human (allo/homograft), or from patient (autograft)
   ii. Durability: 10–20% of homografts and 30% of heterografts undergo structural degeneration in 15 years (tears, fibrosis, or calcification)
      1. Deterioration more aggressive in those <40 years
      2. Worse with mitral valves than aortic valves due to high closing pressure
   iii. Risk of thromboembolism: equivalent to well anticoagulated mechanical valve (3 months after implantation and endothelialization of sewing ring)
   iv. More resistant than mechanical valves for infection (especially homograft, one reason for their use following endocarditis).
   v. Types:
      1. Stented
      2. Stentless

L. Afonso (✉)
Department of Cardiology, Detroit Medical Centre, Wayne State University, Detroit, MI, USA
e-mail: lafonso@med.wayne.edu

T.P. Abraham (ed.), *Case Based Echocardiography*,
DOI: 10.1007/978-1-84996-151-6_19, © Springer-Verlag London Limited 2011

Table 19.1 Characteristics of mechanical prosthetic valves

Type	Examples	Description	Hemodynamic profile	Image
Caged-ball	Star-Edward's	Bulky and more thrombogenic Oldest; rarely used currently Effective orifice area (EOA) MV = 1.4–3.1 sq cm AV = 1.2–1.6 sq cm	Significant gradient especially in 19–21 mm sizes Higher gradients in AV (as high as 20) than MV Color flow: pair of horns Not suitable for children	
Single-tilting disc	Medtronic Hall, Omniscience, Bjork-Shiley	Single disc that swings 0–80° Effective orifice area (EOA) MV = 1.9–3.2 sq cm AV = 1.5–2.1 sq cm	Hemodynamics better than cage-ball PG < 15 in AV, < 5 in MV Single central orifice 5–10 mL/beat regurgitation	
Bileaflet	St. Jude, CarboMedics	Less bulky and thrombogenic Pivoted two semicircular discs Angle changes from 0° (closed) to 90°(open) The most commonly implanted EOA MV = 2.8–3.4 sq cm AV = 2.4–3.2 sq cm	The best hemodynamic profile among mechanical valves Two larger lateral and one smaller central flow pattern 5–10 mL/beat regurgitation PG < 15 in AV and <4.5 in MV	

Table 19.2 Characteristics of bioprosthetic valves

Type	Examples	Description	Hemodynamic profile	Image
Stented	Heterograft porcine: Carpentier Edwards Hancock Porcine Medtronic Intact Porcine Heterograft bovine pericardial Autograft: Autologous Pericardial	Stent maintains 3D relation between the valve leaflets and facilitates implantation	Hemodynamic profile similar to comparable size mechanical valve Single central flow pattern Regurgitation less than mechanical valve of similar size	
Stentless	Heterografts: St. Jude SPV Medtronic Freestyle Homografts: Harvested from cadavers, could have an aortic conduit Autografts: Pulmonary autograft (Ross procedure)	Less bulky than stented valves Developed only for AV	Lower transvalvular gradients and more laminar flow than stented valves For patients with small aortic root	

19.2
Normal Prosthetic Valve Echocardiograms (Figs. 19.1–19.3)

19.2.1
2D Echo

1. Approach to imaging:
   a. Assess stability of the sewing ring, motion of the leaflets, disk, or occluder mechanism
   b. Identify the type of prosthesis
   c. Evaluate for gross structural abnormalities like thrombus, vegetation, etc.
2. Common features of prosthetic valves:
   a. Clicks: opening and closing dense single-line Doppler signals
   b. Reverberation artifacts: hall mark of mechanical valves. Single with single tilting disc and double in bileaflet
   c. Acoustic shadowing: Echo lucent as well as color flow (CF) bare area behind the valve that limits visualization of leaflets, thrombus, vegetations; the reason why CF alone should not be used for evaluation of regurgitation (part of or all of regurgitation and perivalvular leak may not be seen)
   d. Struts: in stented valves, struts may be seen protruding into the RV/LV cavity or aorta.

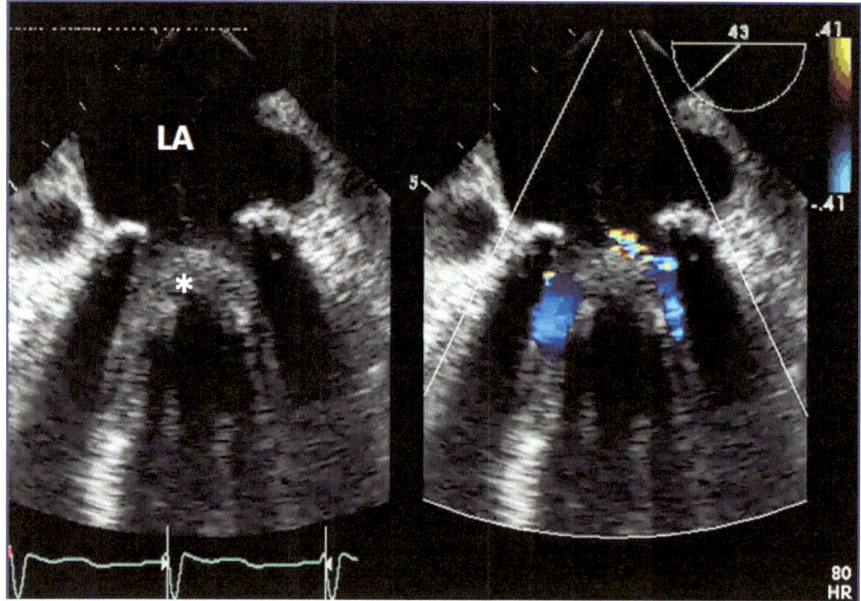

Fig. 19.1 Ball-cage prosthesis (Star Edwards) illustrating poppet (*) and characteristic color flow around it

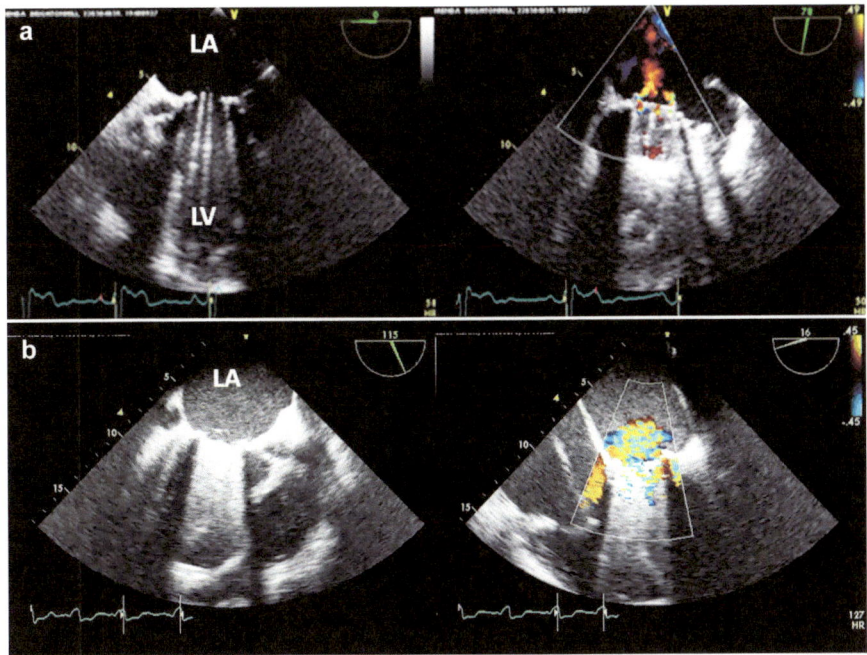

Fig. 19.2 TEE images of a bileaflet mitral prosthesis (St. Jude) showing open leaflets and normal regurgitation wash jets upon valve closure (*Panel A*). Below, an example of a tilting disk prosthesis in mitral position (*Panel B*) and a single central wash jet (normal finding). Note prominent reverberation artifact below disk

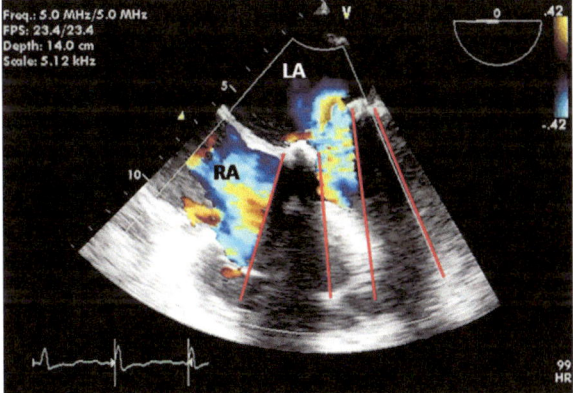

Fig. 19.3 Mechanical mitral prosthesis showing prominent acoustic shadowing originating from valve ring (enclosed between *red bold* lines)

e. In case of prosthetic valve malfunction or endocarditis, TEE is the preferred imaging modality of choice (superior resolution and unobstructed view of atria)

f. All prosthetic valves are inherently stenotic. The degree of obstruction is dependent on the type, size, and site of the prosthetic valve.

19.2.2
Color Flow Doppler

1. Pattern: in general eccentric
2. Single tilting disc: single, eccentric flow
3. Bileaflet: three jets with smaller rectangular central and two larger peripheral
4. Caged-ball: flow bifurcation around the poppet with "pair of horns" appearance
5. Bioprosthetic: single, triangular
6. Prosthetic regurgitation:
   a. Closure backflow: early flow reversal to close the occluding mechanism
   b. Leakage backflow: small, continuous retrograde flow as a washing mechanism to prevent thrombus formation on the upstream side
7. Limitation of color flow Doppler: Flow masking due to acoustic shadowing

19.2.3
Spectral Doppler

1. Normal flow velocity across a valve depends on:
   a. Type of prosthetic valve: caged-ball mechanical valve and heterograft bioprosthesis have the smallest effective orifice areas and therefore higher gradients, whereas homografts have the largest diameter and hence gradients similar to those of native valves
   b. Size of the prosthetic valve: pressure gradients inversely proportional to valve size
   c. Location: For mitral and tricuspid valves, gradient increases with increasing heart rate and flow rate, whereas for aortic and pulmonic valves, gradient increases with flow and contractility
   d. Cardiac output
   e. Heart rate
2. Increased flow velocity may be due to stenosis or regurgitation
3. All prosthetic valves are inherently stenotic except for homografts, i.e., flow velocity across prosthetic valve is higher than native valve
4. Prosthetic valves also have inherent regurgitation
5. All echos should be compared with *prosthetic valve echo fingerprint*; an echo done within 3 months of valve replacement

19.3
Prosthesis Malfunction

Cinefluoroscopy should be recognized as a simple, rapid, inexpensive technique for evaluating prosthetic-valve function, particularly mechanical valves.

19.3.1
Prosthetic Valve Stenosis

Causes
- Outgrowing of prosthetic valve size implanted during childhood with age
- Prosthesis–patient mismatch: Minimal acceptable effective orifice area for AV (below which prosthesis–patient mismatch is common) = Body surface area (BSA) × 0.85 cm².
- Stenosis in mechanical valves: thrombus, pannus, vegetation (seen typically attached at the base or sewing ring)
- Stenosis in bioprosthetic valves: cusp degeneration and calcification

19.3.2
Prosthetic Valve Regurgitation

a. Types:
   - Perivalvular: usually associated with dehiscence
   - Valvular
b. Causes:
   i. Mechanical valves: thrombus, pannus, poppet variance, and endocarditis
   ii. Bioprosthetic valves: cusp degeneration, endocarditis, and torn leaflet (angry bee murmur on Doppler)
c. General principles:
   i. TTE not adequate for evaluation of mitral, tricuspid, and anterior aortic regurgitation
   ii. Normal regurgitation(wash jets):
      - Regurgitant jet area of <2 cm² for MV and <1cm² for AV
      - Regurgitant jet length of <2.5 cm for MV and <1.5 cm for AV
   iii. Various flow patterns

19.3.3
Evaluation of Prosthetic Aortic Valve (Table 19.3)

1. Aortic valve stenosis (Table 19.4):
   a. Determine maximum velocity and peak gradient
   b. Determine mean gradient
   c. Estimate velocity or TVI ratio: LVOT/AV TVI ratio (sewing ring outer diameter may be substituted for LVOT diameter)
   d. Calculate EOA by continuity equation: 0.785 × (sewing ring outer diameter)² × LVOT TVI/AV TVI
2. Prosthetic aortic regurgitation: considered severe if
   a. PHT ≤ 250 ms
   b. Mitral inflow pattern (restrictive pattern in acute regurgitation)
   c. Holodiastolic reversals in descending aorta
   d. Regurgitant fraction of ≥55%

Table 19.3 Doppler hemodynamic profiles of 609 normal aortic valve prosthesis

Type of prosthesis	Peak velocity (m/s)	Mean gradient (mmHg)	LVOT-TVI/ AV-TVI
Heterograft	2.4±0.5	13.3±6.1	0.44±0.21
Ball-cage	3.2±0.6	23.0±8.8	0.32±0.09
Bjork-Shiley	2.5±0.6	13.9±7.0	0.40±0.10
Jude Medical	2.5±0.6	14.4±7.7	0.41±0.12
Homograft	1.9±0.4	7.7±2.7	0.56±0.10
Medtronic-Hall	2.4±0.2	13.6±3.3	0.39±0.09
Total	2.6±0.7	15.8±8.3	0.40±0.16

AV, aortic valve; *LVOT*, left ventricular outflow tract; *TVI*, time velocity integral
From Miller et al.[1]

Table 19.4 Approach to prosthetic aortic valve assessment

Condition	Peak velocity (m/s)	Mean PG (mmHg)	LVOT/Ao TVI ratio	Comment
Normal	≤3	<25	>0.35	Normal output state
Stenosis	>3	>25	<0.3	Pannus or thrombosis, TEE/ fluoroscopy
Patient–Prosthesis mismatch	>3	>25	<0.3	Moderate: EOA: 0.6–0.85 cm²/m² Severe: EOA ≤0.6 cm²/m²
Regurgitation	>3	>25	>0.3	TEE to evaluate
High-output state	>3	>25	>0.3	Confirm the absence of regurgitation

19.3.4
Pulmonic Prosthetic Valve

The hemodynamic profiles are similar to that of aortic valve (Table 19.5).

19.3.5
Evaluation of Prosthetic Mitral Valve (Table 19.6)

1. Prosthetic mitral valve stenosis: (Table 19.7, Fig. 19.4)
   a. E velocity: measure 5 cycles in atrial fibrillation
   b. Mean gradient by Bernoulli equation using the entire continuous wave inflow spectrum during diastole
   c. End-diastolic gradient
   d. PHT: overestimates MVA (not recommended)

Table 19.5 Doppler echocardiographic data for pulmonary valve prosthesis

Type of prosthesis	Size (mm)	Peak velocity (m/s)	Mean gradient (mmHg)	Trivial/mild prosthetic regurgitation (No.)
Carpentier-Edwards	26.5±1.8	2.4±0.5	12.1±5.3	7
Pulmonary homograft	24.2±1.8	1.8±0.6a	8.4±4.8	15
Aortic homograft	22.3±1.8	2.5±0.4	14.4±3.4	3
Hancock	26.0±1.8	2.4±0.5	14.0±5.7	1
Ionescu-Shiley	25.0±1.8	2.4±0.4	12.5±3.5	2
St. Jude Medical	25	2.6	12.0	1
Bjork-Shiley	25	2.0	7.0	1

Compared with all heterografts combined, $P = 0.002$
From Novaro et al.[4]

Table 19.6 Doppler hemodynamic profiles of 456 normal mitral valve prosthesis

Type of prosthesis	Peak velocity (m/s)	Mean gradient (mmHg)	Effective area (cm²)
Hetergraft	1.6±0.3	4.1±1.5	2.3±0.7
Ball-cage	1.8±0.3	4.9±1.8	2.4±0.7
Bjork-Shiley	1.7±0.3	4.1±1.6	2.6±0.6
St. Jude Medical	1.6±0.4	4.0±1.8	3.0±0.8

From Lengyel et al.[2]

    e. MVA by continuity equation: $0.785 \times$ LVOT diameter $^2 \times$ LVOT TVI/MV TVI
    f. TR velocity
    g. MV/LVOT TVI ratio
2. Prosthetic mitral regurgitation:
    a. Mitral inflow peak velocity of >2.5 m/s
    b. PHT of $\leq$ 150 ms
    c. Density of MR continuous-wave Doppler jet
    d. PISA from TEE
    e. Effective regurgitant orifice area of ≥ 0.35 cm^2
    f. Systolic flow reversal in pulmonary vein Doppler

19.3.6
Tricuspid Prosthetic Valve Evaluation (Table 19.8)

1. Follow similar assessment to that of mitral valve.
2. Cutoff normal parameters are slightly different because of the larger average area; peak E < 1.3 m/s, mean PG < 4 mmHg, P1/2t < 140 ms, and TV-TVI to PV-TVI ratio <2.5.

Table 19.7 Approach to prosthetic mital valve assessment

Condition	Peak E velocity	Mean gradient	$P_{1/2}t$	$\dfrac{MV\text{-}TVI}{LVOT\text{-}TVI}$	Comment
Normal	≤1.9 m/s	≤5 mmHg	<130 ms	<2.5	HR 55–90, normal output state
Obstruction or stenosis	≥2 m/s	>5 mmHg	>>130 ms	<2.5	TEE for thrombus pannus formation, and malfunction
Patient-Prosthesis mismatch	Similar to obstruction (above) but is seen at the "Echo finger-print," in the absence of alternative explanation				
Prosthetic valve regurgitation	≥2 m/s	>5 mmHg	<130 ms	>2.5	E>1.9 & TVI ratio >2.5 specific for MR
					When both are normal; specific for absence of MR
					TEE for the rest
High output state	≥2 m/s	>5 mmHg	<130	<2.5	Flow across all valves increased

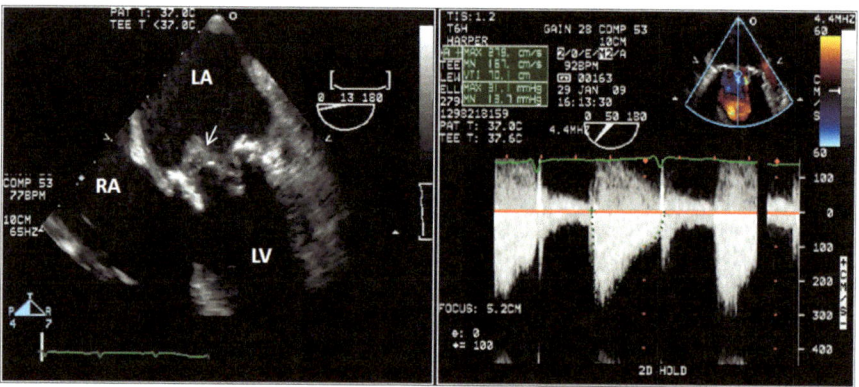

Fig. 19.4 TEE images of mitral bioprosthesis endocarditis. Note thickened leaflets and echogenic mass consistent with a vegetation (*arrow*) obstructing mitral inflow. CW Doppler recorded elevated transmitral velocities and gradient (mean gradient: 12 mmHg). Findings indicative of prosthetic stenosis

19.4
Pannus vs. Thrombus

The echocardiographic differentiation of pannus and thrombus can be challenging.
In general:

Table 19.8 Doppler hemodynamic profiles of 82 normal tricuspid valve prosthesis

Type of prosthesis	Peak velocity (m/s)	Mean gradient (mmHg)	Pressure half-time (ms)
Heterograft	1.3±0.2	1.3±1.1	146±39
Ball-cage	1.3±0.2	3.1±0.8	144±46
St. Jude Medical	1.2±0.3	2.7±1.1	108±32
Bjork-Shiley	1.3	2.2	144
Total	1.3±0.2	3.1±1.0	142±42

Modified from Connolly et al.[3]

- Thrombus
  - Sudden dyspnea, new murmur should raise suspicion
  - Presentation acute or subacute
  - Doppler typically reveals elevated transvalvular gradients
  - Cinefluoroscopy very useful for assessment of leaflet mobility
  - Thrombi tend to be mobile, somewhat less echo-dense, and associated with spontaneous echo contrast (SEC or smoke). INR may be subtherapeutic.
- Pannus
  - Onset generally more insidious; affects mainly mechanical valves
  - Reported as early as 6 months but usually occurs 5–6 years post operation
  - In more than 60% of cases variable amounts of thrombus can be found overlying pannus and contribute to the obstruction
  - May encroach into valve orifice and lead to stenosis/elevated gradients
  - Intermittent valve dysfunction should raise suspicion
  - Ultimately, pannus is a diagnosis of exclusion, and surgical exploration is the gold standard
  - Pannus is highly echogenic, consistent with its fibrous composition, and is usually firmly fixed to the valve apparatus

19.5
Other Complications

A. Infective prosthetic endocarditis

Prosthetic-valve infection occurs at some time in 3–6% of patients (0.2–0.5%/year all valve types)

Early endocarditis (occurring less than 60 days after valve replacement) usually results from perioperative bacteremia arising from skin or wound infections or contaminated intravascular devices.

Late endocarditis (occurring more than 60 days after valve replacement) is usually caused by the organisms responsible for native valve endocarditis

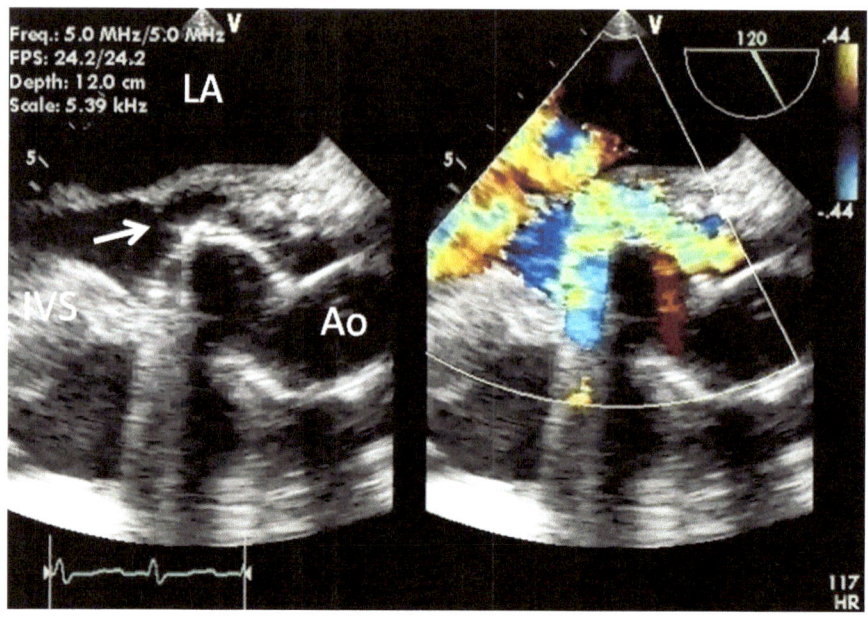

Fig. 19.5 Long-axis TEE view showing dehiscence of mechanical AV prosthesis from posterior aortic root (*arrow*) and resulting torrential paraprosthetic aortic regurgitation

Vegetations
- Mechanical valves: sewing rings are commonly affected (unusual on the disc surface).
- Bioprosthesis: leaflets more than the sewing ring.

B. Perivalvular leak and valve dehiscence (Fig. 19.5)

Disruption of one or more sutures can affect mechanical and bioprosthetic valves resulting in valve regurgitation

Predisposing factors
- Endocarditis (should be considered in all patients with valve dehiscence)
- Marfans syndrome
- Annular calcification
- Atherosclerotic roots

C. Hemolysis:

Typically suggests paravalvular leakage due to partial dehiscence of the valve or infection. Patients with a caged-ball valve or with multiple prosthetic valves have an increased incidence and more severe degree of hemolysis than those with tissue valves. It is more common in men and in patients with heart failure. Beta blockers attenuate degree of hemolysis (by reducing the dp/dt).

Lab findings:
- ↑ LDH
- ↓ Haptoglobin
- Schistocytosis

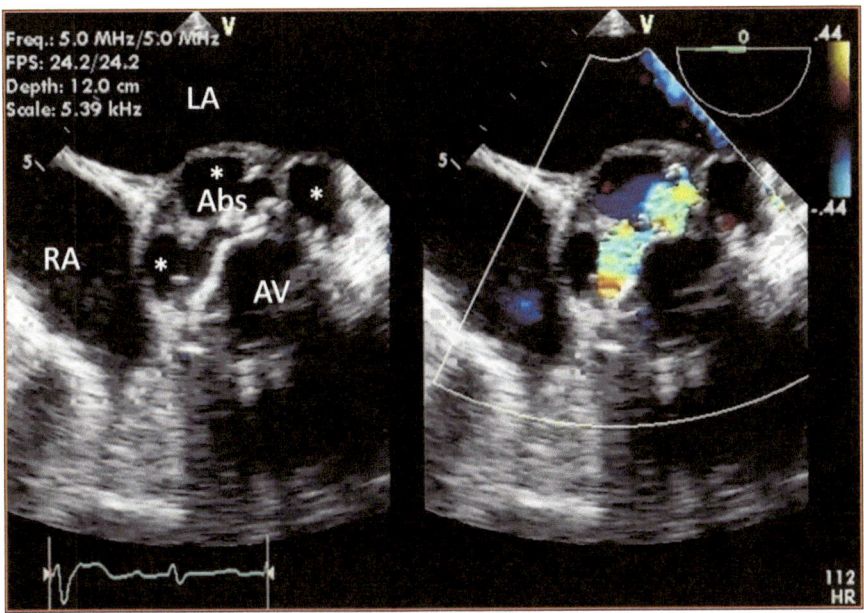

Fig. 19.6 Short-axis TEE views at the level of AV prosthesis showing a large loculated abscess with multiple septate cavities (*asterisks*)

- Reticulocytosis
- Hemosiderinuria/hemoglobinuriasis

D. Valve bed abnormalities (pseudoaneurysm, ring abscess)

TEE is superior to TTE for the detection of endocarditis and invasive complications such as paravalvular abscesses, myocardial abscess, pseudoaneurysms, valve dehiscence, or leaflet perforations (Fig. 19.6).

19.6
Miscellaneous/Caveats

A. Microcavitation: Not an uncommon finding and needs to be recognized (Fig. 19.7).
- As the local pressure drops below the vapor pressure of the liquid, vapor-filled microbubbles are formed.
- This phenomenon has been observed only on the tilting disc type and bileaflet valves.
- No evidence of bubble formation on bioprosthetic valves.
- Has no clinical implications(benign finding).

B. Pressure Recovery (Fig. 19.8)

Pressure recovery is the variable increase in lateral pressure downstream from a stenotic orifice. Downstream from the orifice, flow expands and decelerates with a cor-

Fig. 19.7 Parasternal long-axis view in a patient with tilting-disk aortic valve prosthesis illustrating microcavitation/microbubble (Mcav) formation in the LV outflow tract and aortic root (*arrows*) during valve closure

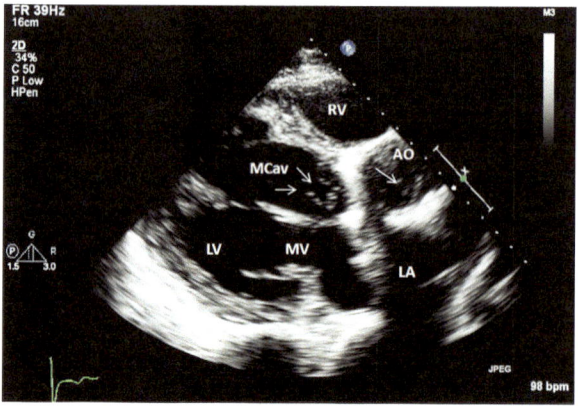

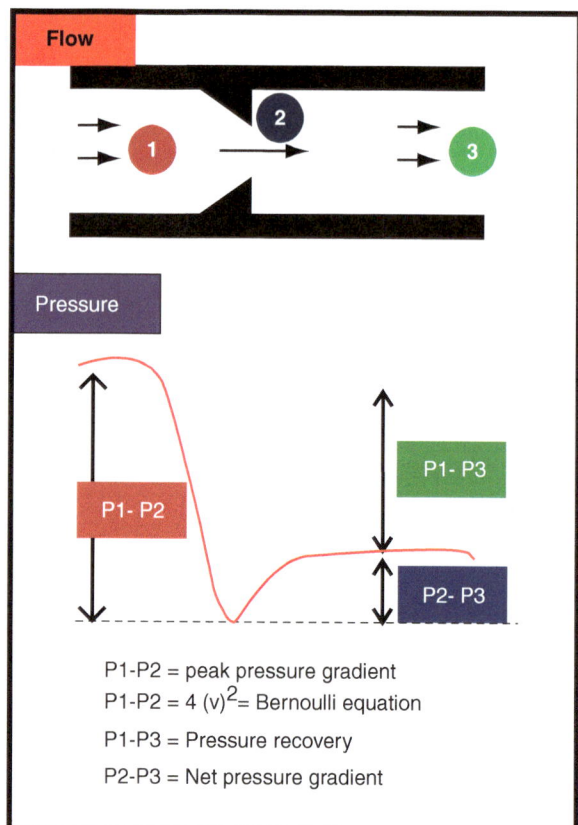

P1-P2 = peak pressure gradient
P1-P2 = 4 (v)^2= Bernoulli equation
P1-P3 = Pressure recovery
P2-P3 = Net pressure gradient

Fig. 19.8 Schematic explaining the pressure recovery phenomenon. Pressure recovery distal to the aortic valve orifice leads to lower cath-derived gradient (P1–P3) relative to gradient obtained with spectral Doppler (P1–P2)

responding decrease in kinetic and increase in potential energy, a phenomenon called "pressure recovery."

Clinical implications:

- Aortic pressure measured by cath distal to the orifice (mid ascending aorta) is higher than at the orifice (pressure recovery)

- Aortic valve gradient measured by catheterization is LOWER than that measured by Doppler (which measures "unrecovered pressure")
- Aortic valve area calculated by catheterization may be "larger"
- Phenomenon more relevant in patients with small or normal (not dilated) roots
- In prosthetic valves, it is a peculiar feature of bileaflet mechanical valve in the aortic position primarily because of measurement of velocity across the *small central orifice* that over estimates the pressure gradient.

C. Patient–Prosthesis Mismatch (PPM)

PPM describes a state in which the effective orifice area (EOA) of a normally functioning heart valve prosthesis is too small in relation to the patient's body size; this situation results in high transvalvular pressure gradients in the setting of a structurally normal valve.

Typically PPM is observed with aortic replacements but may also occur with MV prosthesis.

For example: A patient with a BSA of 1.3 m^2 should get a valve with minimum EOA of 1.1 cm^2

Minimal acceptable effective orifice area for AV (where prosthesis–patient mismatch is common) = BSA × 0.85 cm^2 (corresponding value for mitral valve is BSA × 1.2 cm^2)

- Severe mismatch = EOA of ≤ 0.6 cm^2/m^2
- Moderate mismatch= $> 0.6 \leq 0.85$ cm^2/m^2
- Mild mismatch = >0.85 cm^2/m^2

Clinical implications: Patients with severe PPM have

- ↓ Functional and exercise capacity
- ↓ Regression of LVH
- ↓ Recovery of coronary flow reserve
- Impaired blood coagulation status
- ↑ Late mortality
- ↑ Adverse cardiac events after AVR

Stentless valves provide larger EOA and more favorable hemodynamic profiles compared to their stented counterparts.

References

1. Miller F Jr, Callahan J, Taylor C, et al. Normal aortic prosthesis hemodynamics; 609 prospective Doppler examinations. *Circulation*. 1989;80(Suppl 2):II-169.
2. Lengyel M, Miller F Jr, Taylor C, et al. Doppler hemodynamic profile in 456 clinically and echo normal mitral prosthesis. *Circulation*. 1990;82(Suppl 3):III-43.
3. Connolly HM, Miller FA Jr, Taylor CL, Naessens JM, Seward JB, Tajik AJ. Doppler hemodynamic profiles of 82 clinically and echocardiographically normal tricuspid valve prostheses. *Circulation*. 1993;88:2722-2727.
4. Novaro GM et al. Doppler hemodynamics of 51 clinically and echocardiographically normal pulmonary valve prostheses. *Mayo Clin Proc*. 2001;76:155.

The Aorta: Diseases of the Aorta

20

Mary C. Corretti

20.1
Aorta

- Largest vascular structure in the body
- Vessels are multicellular, and serve numerous dynamic biologic, physiologic, and anatomic functions
- Numerous conditions affect the aorta and branch vessels
- Numerous consequences from various disease processes and environmental exposures.

M.C. Corretti
Division of Cardiology, Johns Hopkins University, Baltimore, MD, USA
e-mail: mcorre+1@yhmi.edu

T.P. Abraham (ed.), *Case Based Echocardiography*,
DOI: 10.1007/978-1-84996-151-6_20, © Springer-Verlag London Limited 2011

20.2
Anatomy of the Thoracic Aorta

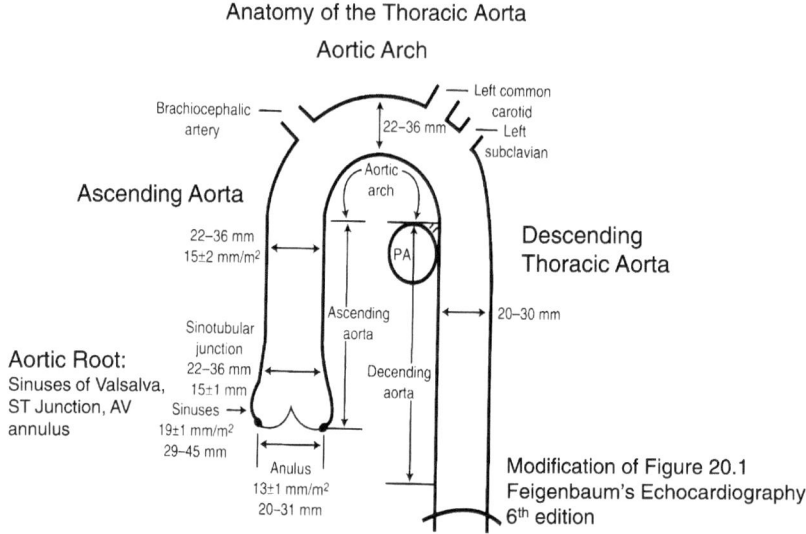

Anatomy of the Thoracic Aorta

Aortic Arch

Brachiocephalic
artery

Left common
carotid

22–36 mm

Left
subclavian

Aortic
arch

Ascending Aorta

22–36 mm
15±2 mm/m²

PA

Descending
Thoracic Aorta

Ascending
aorta

20–30 mm

Sinotubular
junction
22–36 mm
15±1 mm

Decending
aorta

Aortic Root:
Sinuses of Valsalva,
ST Junction, AV
annulus

Sinuses →
19±1 mm/m²
29–45 mm

Anulus
13±1 mm/m²
20–31 mm

Modification of Figure 20.1
Feigenbaum's Echocardiography
6th edition

20.3
Conditions Affecting the Aorta

- Atherosclerosis
- Hypertension
- Inflammatory diseases
- Infection
- Trauma
- Aortic valve disease
- Genetic collagen vascular conditions: Marfan's, Ehler's Danlos, Loeys-Deitz, Sinus of Valsalva aneurysm
- Iatrogenic injury

20.4
Aorta-Atherosclerosis

- Atherosclerotic disease can manifest in the aorta in a variety of ways:
  - Aneurysmal dilitation
  - Atherothrombic plaque
  - Dissection
  - Intramural hematoma
  - Penetrating ulcer in the aortic plaque/or vessel wall
  - Rupture-transection of the aorta
  - Pseudoaneurysm

20.5
Imaging of the Aorta

- Transthoracic echo exam should include full view of the aortic root, mid ascending aorta, and arch view displaying the upper ascending and proximal descending aorta
- TEE also provides similar views with exception of the blind spot due to tracheal interference at the level of the aortic arch
- CT and MRI are gold standards to evaluate the full extent of the aorta and disease processes.

Aorta
Transthoracic Suptrasternal Notch View
Normal

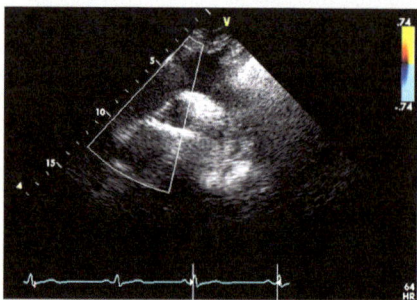 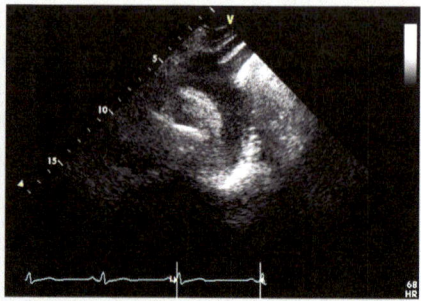

Aortic Arch with upper ascending aorta in box view, and branch vessels

Aortic arch with upper descending aorta and branch vessels off the arch

Bicuspid Valve and Mid Ascending Aortic Dilitation due to Associated Aortopathy

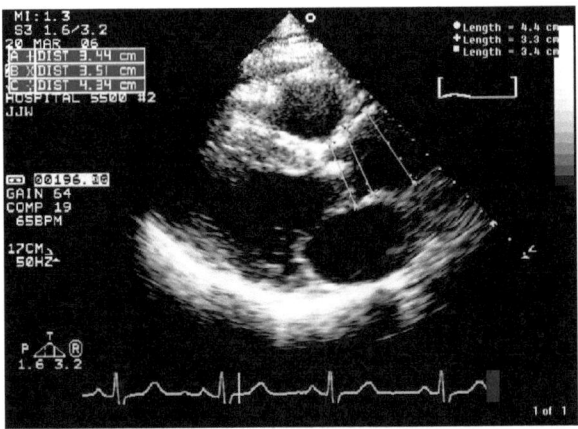

Transthoracic Parasternal Long Axis View

Marfan's Syndrome
Dilated Sinuses of Valsalva-ST Junction
Normal AV

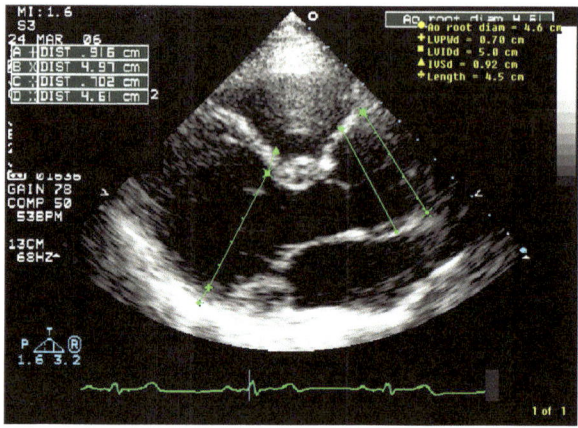

Transthoracic Parasternal Long Axis View

20.6
Aortic Plaque

20.6.1
General Classification as Noted on TEE

- Mild: plaque or intimal thickening: ≤1 mm
- Moderate: 2–3.9 mm
- Severe: >4 mm
- Severe/complex: ≥4mm with ulceration and/or superimposed thrombi

Aortic Arch with Severe Atherosclerotic Plaque

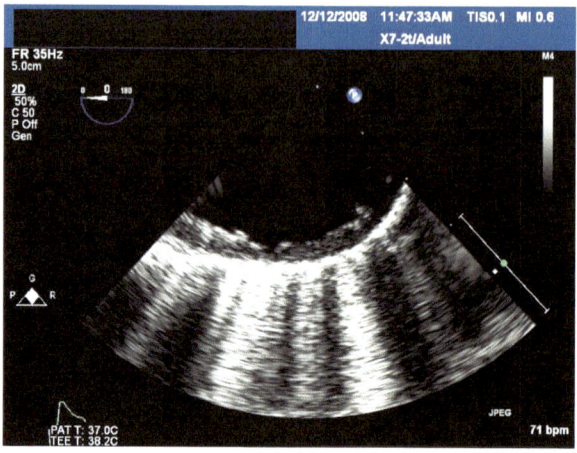

Transesophageal Echo View of the Aortic Arch

20.7
Classification of Aortic Dissection

- DeBakey classification
  - Type I – proximal and descending aorta
  - Type II – proximal only
  - Type IIIa – proximal descending
  - Type IIIb – complete descending and abdominal aorta
- Stanford classification
  - Type A – proximal and descending aorta
  - Type B – descending aorta

Aortic Dissection

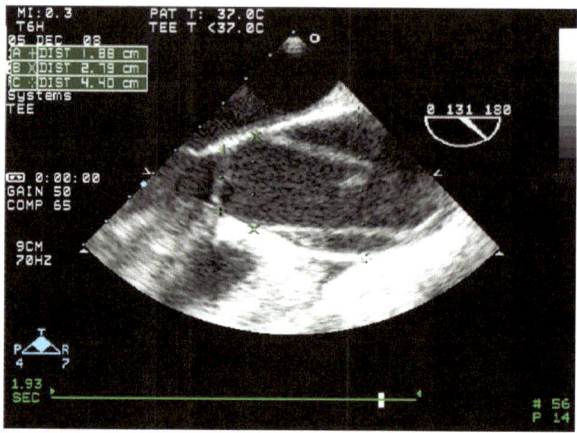

Type A Proximal Aortic Dissection.
Circumferential dissection flap beginning at the ST junction.
Dilitation (aneurysm formation) of the mid ascending aorta.
Transesophageal view

Aortic Dissection

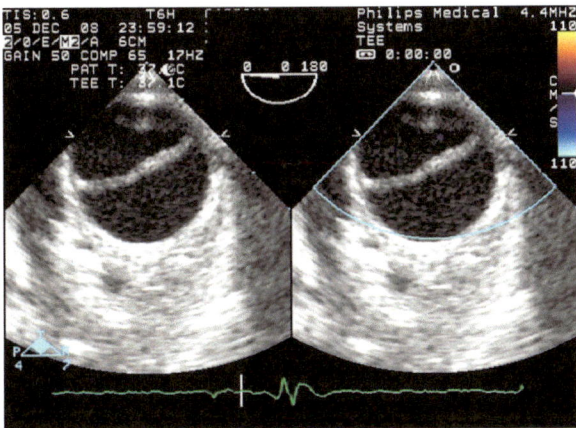

Type B Cross-section of a Descending Aortic Dissection

Aortic Dissection

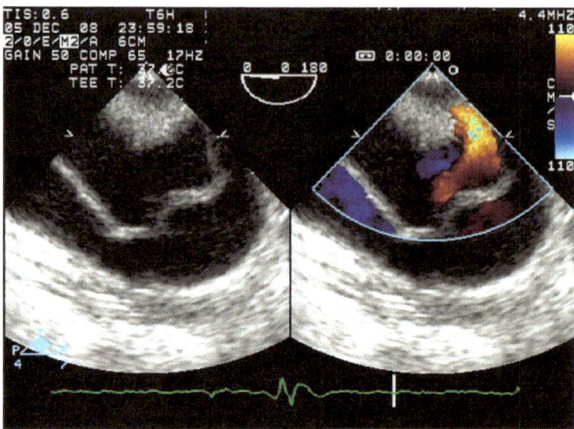

Transesophageal echo view of the arch with color flow Doppler.

Aortic Dissection with Thrombus in the False Lumen

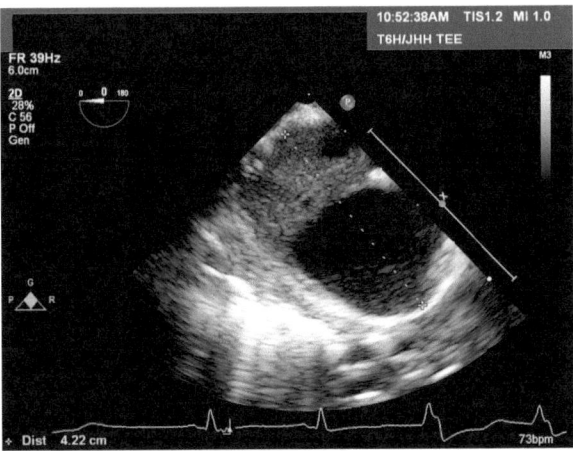

Transesophageal Echo View of a section of the descending aorta.

The aorta is aneurysmal with discrete dissection flap and organized thrombus in the false lumen.

20.8
Functional Assessment of Aorta and Other Vascular Structures

- Numerous imaging modalities to assess vascular structures
- Various invasive and noninvasive testing modalities offer some degree or aspect of function
- Vascular function is complex and requires assessment beyond intraluminal occlusion assessment in the over-all evaluation of structure and function in health and disease states.

20.9
Vascular Function

- Ultrasound-evaluations structure and flow assessment
- Artery tonometry – noninvasive acquisition of arterial waveforms to measure parameters of arterial stiffness

20.10
Pulse Waveform Velocity Analysis

- Each pulsation of the heart generates a velocity of the pressure wave that is transmitted throughout the peripheral vascular system. The waveform biomechanical properties of the arterial system includes arterial wall stiffness.
- Ascending aortic pressure waveform can be measured from the carotid artery, femoral artery or radial artery using noninvasive techniques such as applanation tonometry and Doppler ultrasound.
- The peak systolic pressure is represented by Ps. Pd is the minimum diastolic pressure. An inflection point Pi in the waveform identifies the merging point of the beginning upstroke of the reflected pressure wave. *AIx*, augmentation index; *AP*, augmented pressure; *Pi*, inflection point; *PP*, pulse pressure.

Aortic Pulse Velocity Waveform

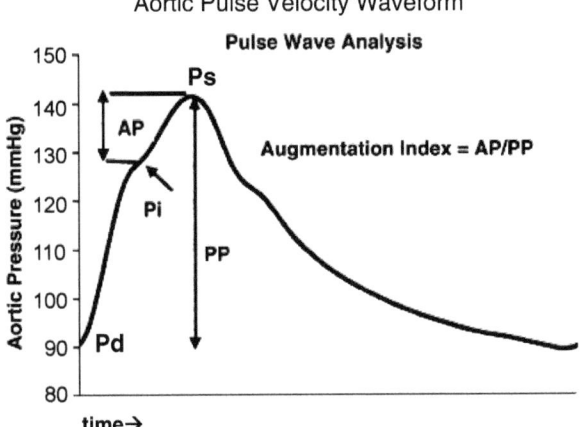

Aortic Pulse Velocity Waveform

Hypertrophic Cardiomyopathy

21

Allison G. Hays and Aurelio C. Pinheiro

21.1
Introduction

- Hypertrophic cardiomyopathy (HCM): relatively common genetically heterogeneous disease characterized by myocardial hypertrophy with myocyte disarray and impaired LV performance (Fig. 21.1).
- HCM is characterized by asymmetric left ventricular hypertrophy typically involving the septum, but may involve other segments.
- Diagnostic criteria for asymmetric septal hypertrophy on echocardiography: septal thickness >15 mm, and septal to posterior wall ratio >1.3.
- Asymmetric septal hypertrophy is not pathognomonic for HCM and may be seen in other conditions such as glycogen storage disease.

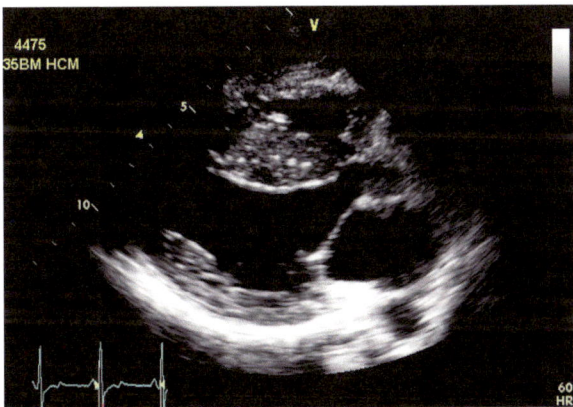

Fig. 21.1 Hypertrophic obstructive cardiomyopathy. The ventricular septum is markedly thickened

A.G. Hays (✉)
Division of Cardiology, Johns Hopkins University, Baltimore, MD, USA
e-mail: ahays2@jhmi.edu

T.P. Abraham (ed.), *Case Based Echocardiography*,
DOI: 10.1007/978-1-84996-151-6_21, © Springer-Verlag London Limited 2011

21.2
Patterns of Hypertrophy

- Anterior portion of LV septum (96%)
- Basal septum (15%)
- Concentric variant (1–5%)
- Apical hypertrophic variant (1–3%)
- Midventricular septal variant (1%)

21.3
Obstructive Gradients/Provocative Maneuvers

- Resting LV Outflow Tract (LVOT) obstruction defined as a peak gradient >30 mmHg.
- Resting LVOT obstruction in HCM patients has important prognostic value and predicts death and advanced heart failure.
- Many HCM patients do not have resting LVOT obstruction, and provocative maneuvers should be performed such as amyl nitrite, Valsalva or upright exercise.
- Mid cavitary or apical cavitary obstruction is not uncommon in rare HCM variants.

21.4
LVOT Obstruction: Echocardiographic Features

- Mid systolic notching
- Early aortic valve closure
- Course systolic fluttering of the aortic valve
- Fibrotic septal changes at the level of leaflet-septal contact
- Doppler signal across the LVOT: characteristic signal with a late-peaking dagger-shaped appearance
- Severe obstruction: mid-systolic drop in LV velocity → characteristic "lobster claw" Doppler tracing abnormality

21.5
Systolic Anterior Motion (SAM)

- SAM (Figs. 21.2–21.4) of the anterior mitral valve leaflet with or without LVOT gradient is indicative of HCM and with a high specificity (Fig. 21.5).
- Characterized by mid-late systolic posterolaterally directed mitral regurgitation.
- Dominant mechanism may be due to hydrodynamic "drag" or the pushing force of flow, rather than due do a "Venturi" effect.
- Leaflet elongation and anterior/inward displacement of papillary muscles also contribute to SAM.

Fig. 21.2 Hypertrophic cardiomyopathy. (**a**) Systolic anterior motion (SAM) of the anterior mitral valve leaflet is shown, contributing to the obstruction of the left ventricular outflow tract. (**b**) Color flow imaging showing posteriorly- directed mitral regurgitation secondary to SAM

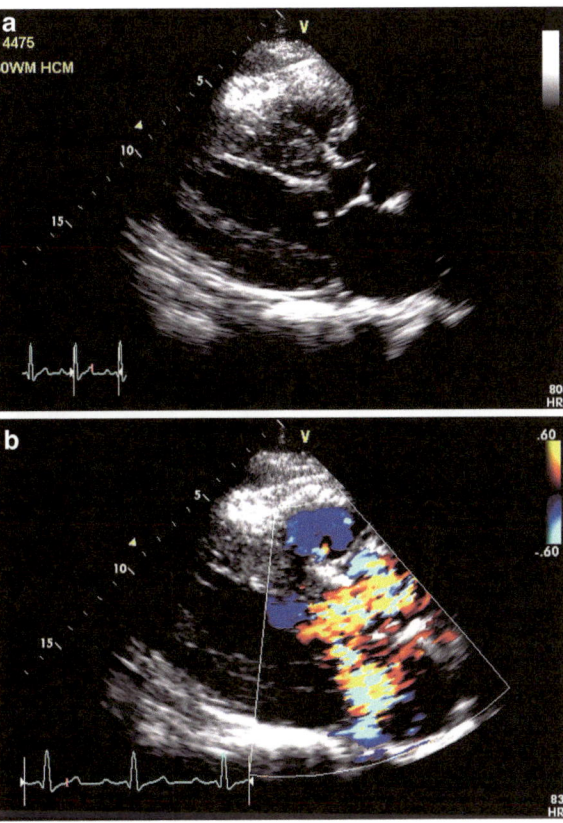

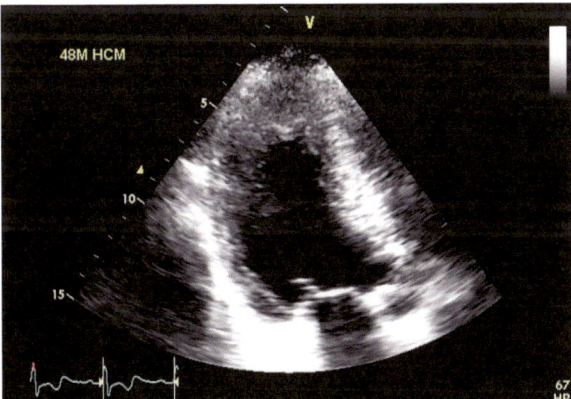

Fig. 21.3 Apical hypertrophic cardiomyopathy. Apical four-chamber view during systole showing markedly increased apical wall thickness

Fig. 21.4 Continuous wave Doppler from the left ventricular outflow tract illustrating a late peaking "dagger-shaped" signal indicating a dynamic outflow obstruction

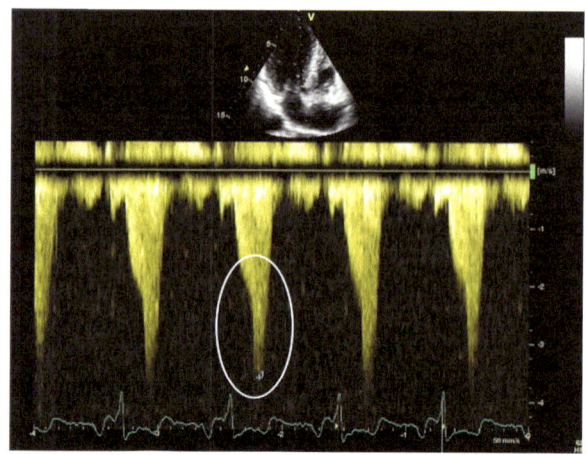

Fig. 21.5 M-mode echocardiography of the mitral valve (MV) in the parasternal short axis view. Example of systolic anterior motion of the MV leaflet

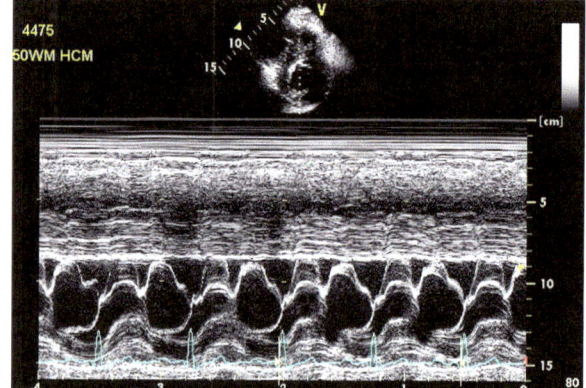

21.6
Ejection Dynamics

- Systolic function typically normal or hyperdynamic.
- Ejection fraction usually preserved despite significant decrease of longitudinal contractile function as assessed by strain and strain rate.
- Diastolic dysfunction often present with impaired relaxation.
- A reduction in chamber compliance, increased stiffness, and heterogeneity of relaxation contribute to diastolic dysfunction.
- In late stages of the disease, progressive myocardial fibrosis results in impaired systolic function, myocardial thinning and cavity dilation.

21.7
Conditions Mimicking HCM

- Hypertensive heart disease and athletic heart may mimic HCM.
- Long term exercise training causes LV remodeling and physiologic LVH, making the diagnosis of HCM difficult.
- The presence of wall thickness >12 mm (males) and >11 mm (females) in a trained athlete suggests HCM.
- In athletic LVH, hypertrophy is symmetric and occurs without diastolic dysfunction.
- Typically, cessation of exercise (for 6–8 weeks) causes 2–5 mm regression in wall thickness in athletic LVH but not in HCM.

Stress Cardiomyopathy

22

Jacob Abraham and Ilan S. Wittstein

22.1
Stress Cardiomyopathy: Definition

- Also called Takotsubo cardiomyopathy, transient apical ballooning syndrome, and broken heart syndrome
- Acute heart failure precipitated by sudden, intense emotional or physical stress characterized by:
  - Three distinctive patterns of LV wall motion abnormalities ("ballooning patterns") that extend beyond a single coronary artery distribution
  - Recovery in days to weeks
  - Mild troponin elevation despite severe wall motion abnormalities
  - Evolving ECG abnormalities including ST elevation, T-wave inversion, and QT-prolongation
- Diagnosis is based on clinical criteria and may be difficult to distinguish from myocardial infarction without coronary angiography

22.2
Echocardiographic Evaluation of SCM

- Left ventricular variants
  - Apical
  - Mid-ventricular
  - Basal
- RV involvement
- Apical thrombus

J. Abraham (✉)
Department of Medicine, Johns Hopkins Hospital, Baltimore, MD, USA
e-mail: ja@jhmi.edu

T.P. Abraham (ed.), *Case Based Echocardiography*,
DOI: 10.1007/978-1-84996-151-6_22, © Springer-Verlag London Limited 2011

22.3
Apical Variant (Fig. 22.1)

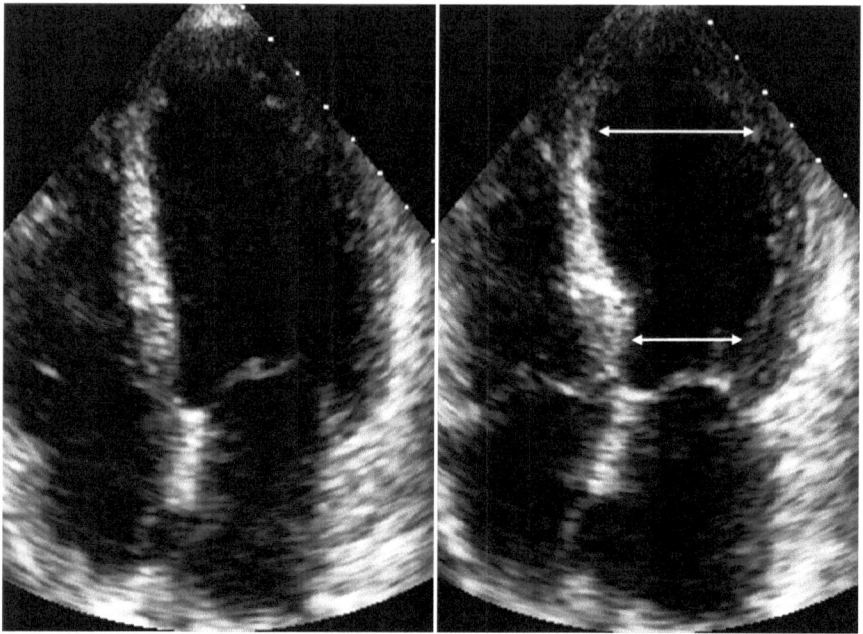

Fig. 22.1 Example of SCM, Apical variant with basal sparing during systole. Diastole (*left panel*) and systole (*right panel*) from apical four-chamber view. Note mid-apical akinesis with normal basal wall motion (*arrows*)

22.4
Mid-Ventricular Variant (Fig. 22.2)

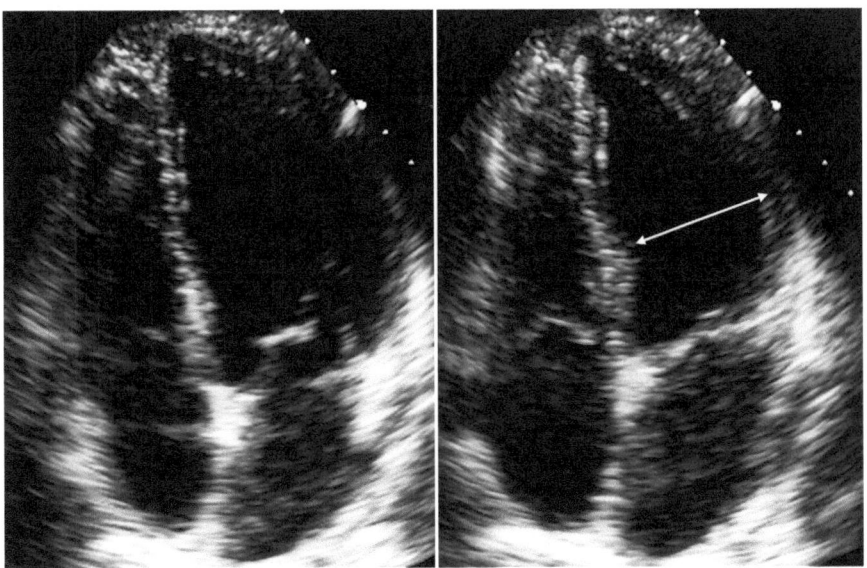

Fig. 22.2 Example of SCM with mid-ventricular sparing during systole. Diastole (*left panel*) and systole (*right panel*) from apical four-chamber view. Note focal hypokinesis of the mid-ventricle (*arrow*)

22.5
Basal Variant (Fig. 22.3)

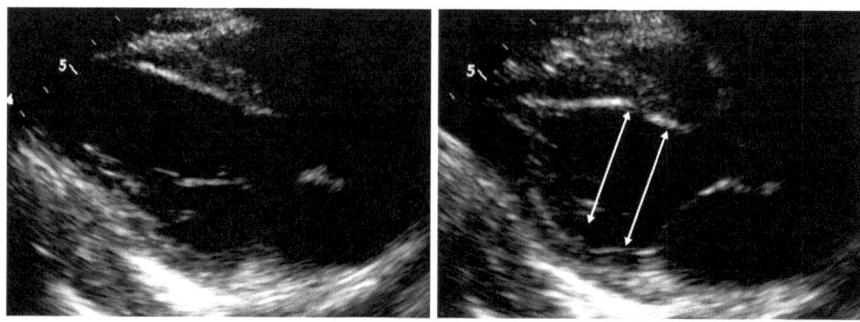

Fig. 22.3 Example of SCM, basal variant with basal ballooning during systole. (Diastole (*left panel*) and systole (*right panel*) from parasternal long-axis view. Note akinesis of mid and basal segments (*arrows*))

22.6
RV Involvement (Fig. 22.4)

- RV involvement in SCM has been associated with greater hemodynamic compromise, longer length of stay, and increased mortality

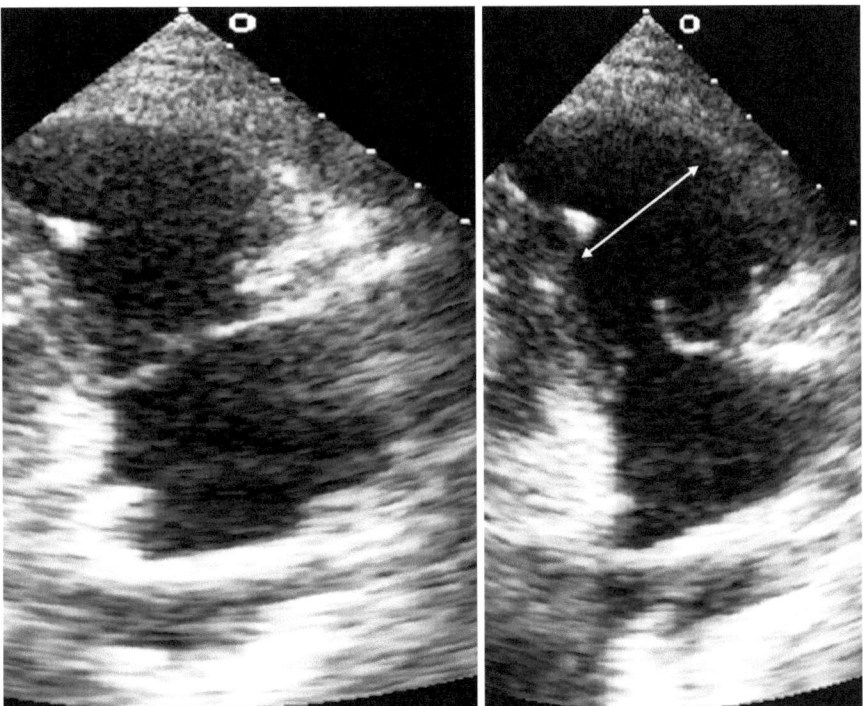

Fig. 22.4 Example of RV involvement during SCM with RV apical dyskinesis. Diastole (*left panel*) and systole (*right panel*) from right ventricular inflow view. Note mid-apical hypokinesis of the right ventricle

22.7
Apical Thrombus (Fig. 22.5)

- May be seen with apical variant
- Recovery of apical wall motion confers high embolic risk
- Anti-coagulation is recommended as prophylaxis until wall motion recovers

Fig. 22.5 Example of Apical
variant SCM with LV mural
thrombus (*arrow*). (Well-
circumscribed thrombus
(*arrow*) present at the apex
in apical ballooning variant.)

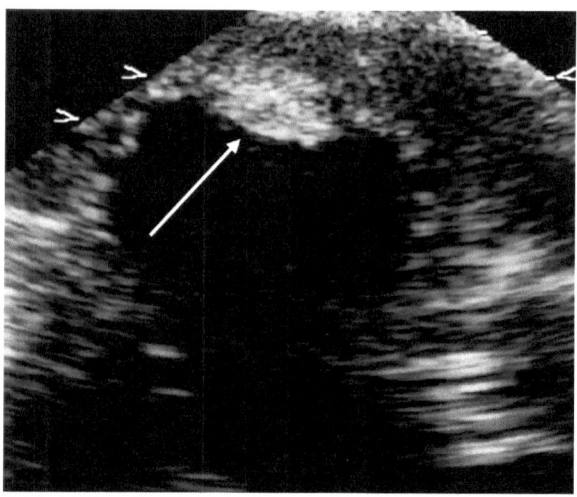

Suggested Reading

Elesber AA, Prasad D, Bybee KA, et al. Transient cardiac apical ballooning syndrome: prevalence and clinical implications of right ventricular involvement. *J Am Coll Cardiol*. 2006;47(5): 1082-1083.

Hahn JY, Gwon HC, Park SW, et al. The clinical features of transient left ventricular nonapical ballooning syndrome: comparison with apical ballooning syndrome. *Am Heart J*. 2007;154(6): 1166-1173.

Wittstein IS, Thiemann DR, Lima JA, et al. Neurohumoral features of myocardial stunning due to sudden emotional stress. *N Engl J Med*. 2005;352(6):539-548.

Wittstein IS. Acute stress cardiomyopathy. *Curr Heart Fail Rep*. 2008;5(2):61-68.

Pericardial Diseases

23

Partho P. Sengupta and Bijoy K. Khandheria

- The diagnosis of pericardial effusion was one of the first clinical applications of echocardiography.
- Transthoracic echocardiography is generally sufficient in the evaluation of patients with pericardial diseases.
- Transesophageal echocardiography is useful in measuring pericardial thickness, in the evaluation of diastolic function, and in detecting loculated pericardial effusion and other structural abnormalities of the pericardium.

P.P. Sengupta (✉)
Cardiovascular Division, University of California, Irvine, USA
e-mail: partho@uci.edu

T.P. Abraham (ed.), *Case Based Echocardiography*,
DOI: 10.1007/978-1-84996-151-6_23, © Springer-Verlag London Limited 2011

23.1
Pericardial Effusion

- Differentiating pleural effusion from pericardial effusion.
- The potential spaces around the heart when filled with fluid or blood is detected as an echo-free space.
- Pleural effusion can be distinguished from pericardial effusion by identifying the descending aorta. The descending aorta is anterior to pleural effusion and posterior to pericardial effusion.
- The reflection of the pericardium around the pulmonary veins tends to prevent collection of pericardial fluid behind the left atrium. Hence an echo-free space behind the left atrium is more likely to be pleural than pericardial effusion.

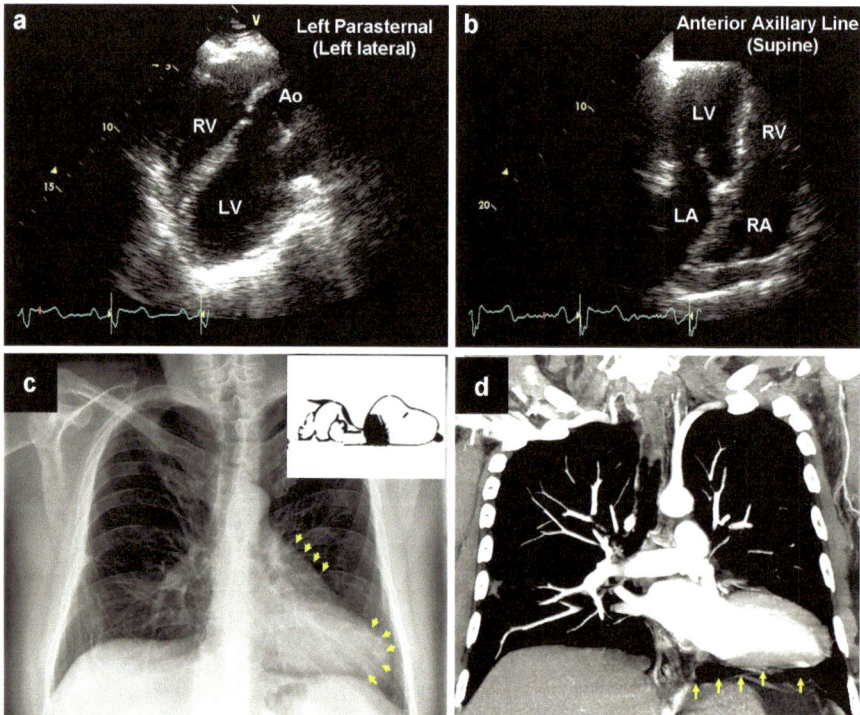

Fig. 23.1 Congenital absence of pericardium. 2D echocardiogram of a 53-year-old male patient with an unusual echo window in the absence of thoracic wall deformity. Note the unusual appearance of the heart on standard parasternal window (**a**) and the need to reach the anterior axillary line for obtaining the apical four-chamber view of the cardiac chambers (**b**). Diagnosis of congenital absence of pericardium is suspected on X-ray which may reveal prominent pulmonary artery contour and flattened elongated contour of LV apex (*snoopy sign*) (**c**) and confirmed by 2D echo and MRI (**d**). Note the absence of parietal and visceral pericardial coverings and interposed lung tissue between inferior wall of the left ventricle and the diaphragm (d)

23.2
Loculated Pericardial Effusions

- Pericardial effusions can be loculated and eccentric, a situation commonly encountered after cardiac surgery.
- The presence of an anterior echo-free space in the absence of a posterior echo-free space should be interpreted with caution since this may result from a large epicardial fat pad.
- The conditions resulting in an anterior echo-free space are listed in Table 23.1.

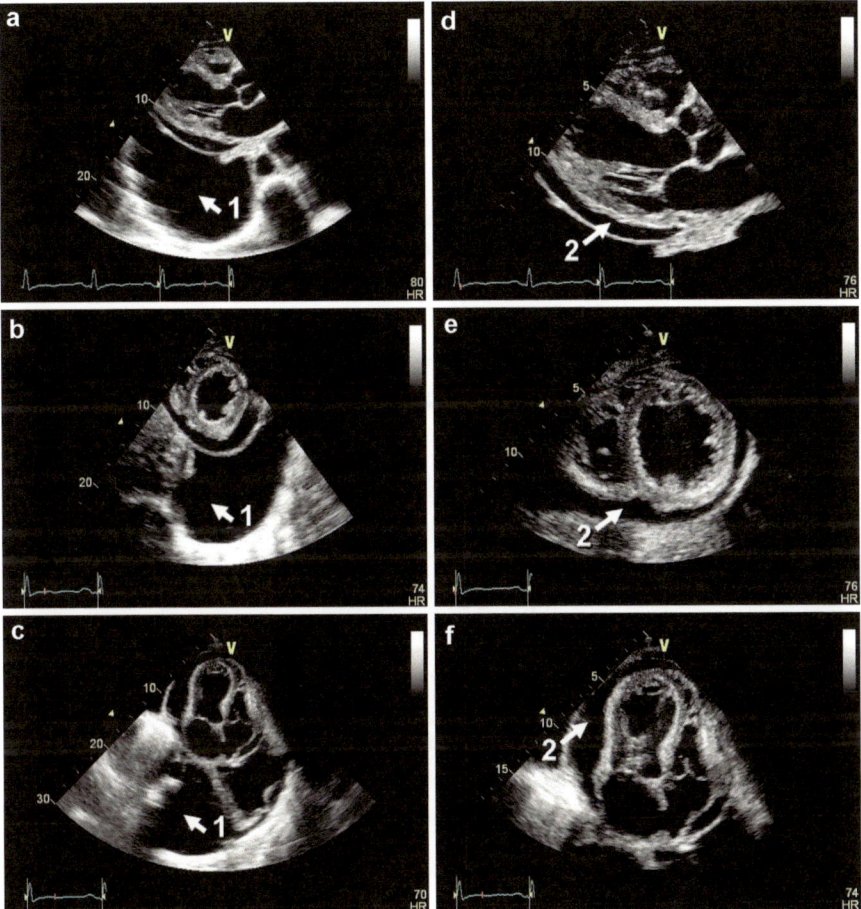

Fig. 23.2 Pericardial effusion. The space around the heart when filled with fluid or blood can be seen as an echo-free space (*arrows*). Note the differences in location of left sided pleural effusion (*arrow 1*, **a–c**) and pericardial effusion (*arrow 2*, **d–f**)

Table 23.1 Conditions producing an anterior echo-free space

Epicardial fat pad

Hernias of foramen of Morgagni

Pericardial cyst

Pericardial tumors

Left atrial enlargement

Thrombus

Massive ascites

23.3
Pericardial Deposits

- Echocardiogram can give clues as to the cause of effusion. Metastatic deposits can be noted on visceral pericardium as echogenic masses in patients with neoplastic pericardial effusion. The presence of fibrinous strands in the pericardial fluid suggest an infective pathology.

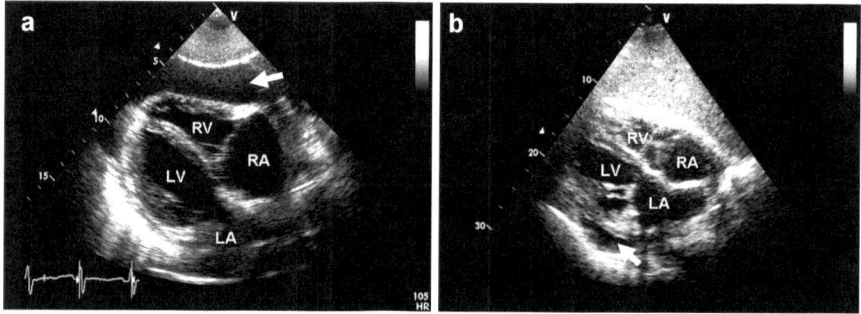

Fig. 23.3 Loculated pericardial effusions image shows the appearance of anterior (**a**) and posterior (**b**) loculated pericardial effusions

23.4
Cardiac Tamponade: Echocardiographic Features of Cardiac Tamponade

- The presence of an effusion even when large does not indicate its hemodynamic significance.
- The presence of an effusion must be correlated with the clinical features and other echocardiographic parameters of cardiac filling and transvalvular flow.
- The earliest echocardiographic sign of hemodynamic compromise is right cardiac chamber diastolic compression, which may precede other signs like pulsus paradoxus.
- The thinner and more compliant right cardiac chambers manifest the first signs of hemodynamically significant effusion as evidenced by compression of these chambers in diastole when their filling volume is lowest and therefore the effects of the external pericardial constraint are greatest. The signs appear first as right ventricular free wall collapse early in diastole.
- The right ventricular collapse may be absent despite cardiac tamponade in patients with preexisting elevated right ventricular pressures because of coexisting pathology. Echocardiographic artifacts and pitfalls seen with large pericardial effusions which may confound the interpretation of features of cardiac tamponade are shown in Tables 23.2 and 23.4.

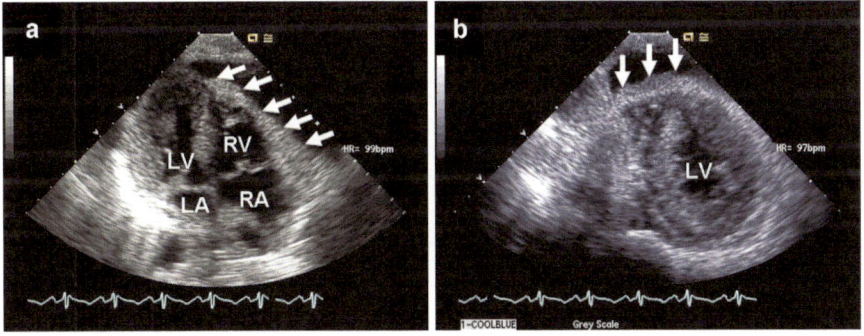

Fig. 23.4 Pericardial deposits. Image showing metastatic deposits on visceral pericardium as echogenic masses (*arrows*, **a** and **b**)

23.5
Transvalvular Flow in Cardiac Tamponade

- The presence of exaggerated respiratory variation in the transvalvular flow is an important indicator of a hemodynamically significant effusion.
- In cardiac tamponade the intrapericardial pressure falls substantially less than intrathoracic pressure.
- The gradient between the pulmonary veins and the left sided cardiac chambers decreases with inspiration, thus reducing early transmitral flow, which on pulsed wave Doppler is seen as decreased early diastolic transmitral velocity. This also results in increased filling during late diastole, with greater dependence on atrial systolic contribution.
- The corresponding increase in tricuspid valve flow and augmented right heart filling during inspiration further compromises left heart filling through diastolic interactions mediated by the septum. These flow variations correlate with pulsus paradoxus and may precede chamber collapse.

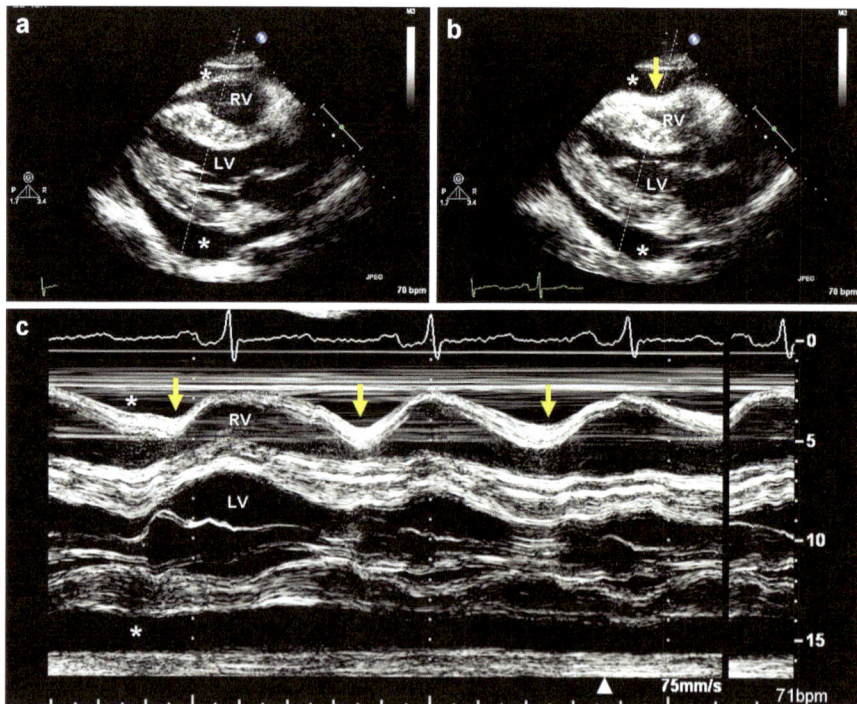

Fig. 23.5 Cardiac tamponade. Image showing the presence of an effusion (**a**). The right cardiac chambers manifest the first signs of hemodynamically significant effusion evidenced by compression in diastole when filling volume is lowest and effect of pericardial constraint is maximum appearing first as right ventricular free wall collapse early in diastole (**b**, *arrows*)

23.6
Pericardiocentesis

- Pericardiocentesis is life saving, but a blind percutaneous pericardiocentesis can result in several complications like pneumothorax, puncture of the cardiac wall, and death.
- Monitoring pericardiocentesis echocardiographically helps in localizing the fluid, optimal site of puncture, depth of the pericardial effusion, and hence the distance from puncture site to the effusion, thus increasing the patient's safety.
- Following initial aspiration of pericardial fluid, injection of saline helps creating a contrast echocardiogram, and if the contrast echoes located in the pericardial space are not intracardiac the needle-tip location is confirmed in the pericardial space.

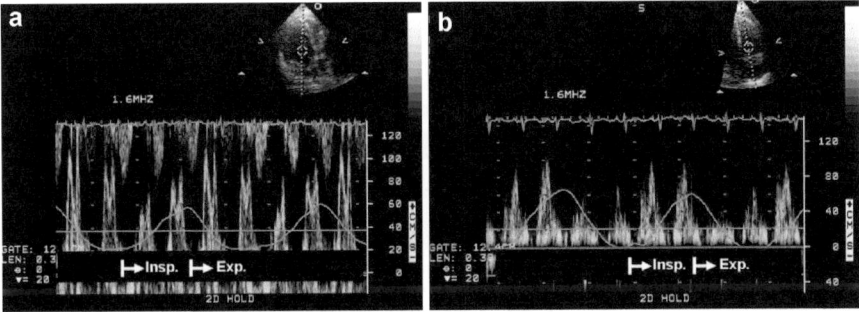

Fig. 23.6 In cardiac tamponade, the gradient between the pulmonary veins and the left sided cardiac chambers decreases with inspiration, thus reducing early transmitral flow seen on pulsed wave Doppler as decreased early diastolic transmitral velocity (**a**). The corresponding increase in tricuspid valve flow and augmented right heart filling during inspiration (**b**) is seen

23.7
Pericarditis

- The echocardiogram may be normal or show thickened parietal and visceral pericardium with either absent or minimal effusion unless pericardial effusion is associated with pericarditis.
- Transesophageal echocardiogram has higher diagnostic yield than transthoracic echocardiogram in assessing the thickness of pericardial layers with the transgastric view reported to give high-quality images of the pericardium useful in diagnosing chronic pericarditis.

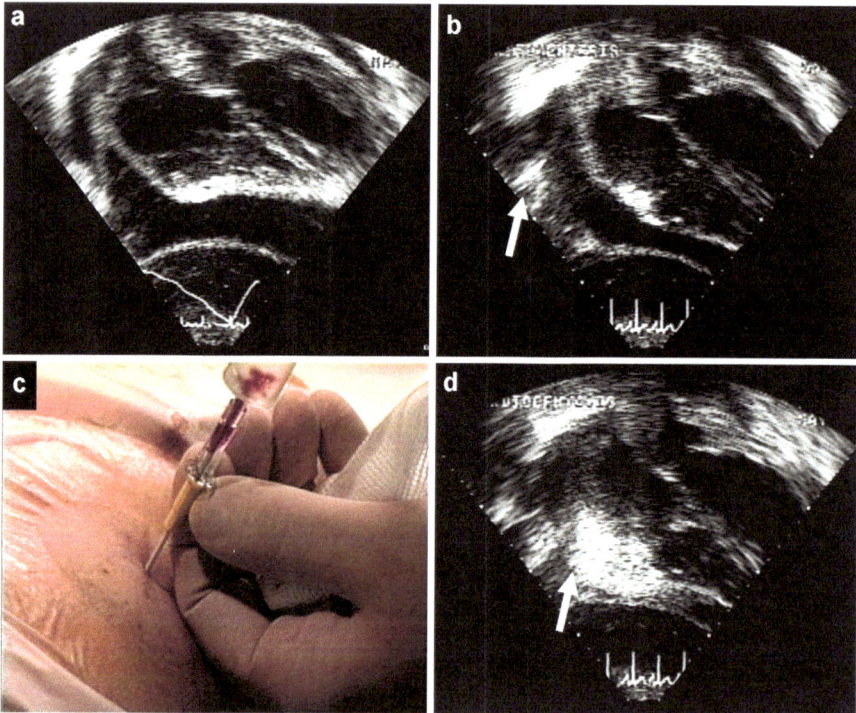

Fig. 23.7 Pericardiocentesis. Echo helps in localizing the fluid, optimal site of puncture, depth of the pericardial effusion (**a**). The shaft of the needle is not difficult to see (**b**), but it is difficult to be certain that the entire needle is being visualized. Following initial aspiration of pericardial fluid (**c**), injection of saline helps creating a contrast echocardiogram (**d**)

23.8
Constrictive Pericarditis

- M-mode signs reflecting rapid early diastolic filling in constrictive pericarditis.
- In presence of thickened pericardium, abrupt anterior or posterior motion of the septum in early diastole is seen in most patients with constrictive pericarditis and reflects a rapid change in transseptal pressure gradient during early diastole caused by unusually vigorous early ventricular filling.
- The left ventricular posterior wall demonstrates a rapid early relaxation with posterior movement during early diastole followed by an abrupt cessation of such movement during mid and late diastole .This flat motion of the left ventricular posterior wall during mid and late diastole corresponds to abrupt transition of rapid ventricular filling in patients with constrictive pericarditis.
- The net diastolic left ventricular posterior wall endocardial movement posteriorly is less than 1 mm in constrictive pericarditis compared to normal where the posterior wall endocardial posterior movement ranges from 1.5 to 4 mm. The abrupt motion of the septum and posterior wall can be discerned on tissue Doppler imaging in the form of high velocities. The hemodynamic and echocardiographic features of constrictive pericarditis compared with restrictive cardiomyopathy are shown in fig. 23.4.

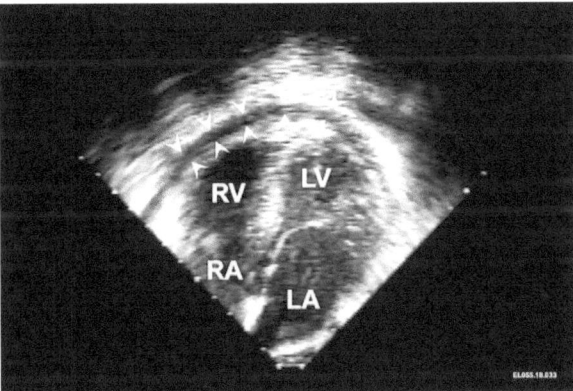

Fig. 23.8 Pericarditis. Transesophageal echocardiogram is very useful in assessing the thickness of pericardial layers (*arrows*)

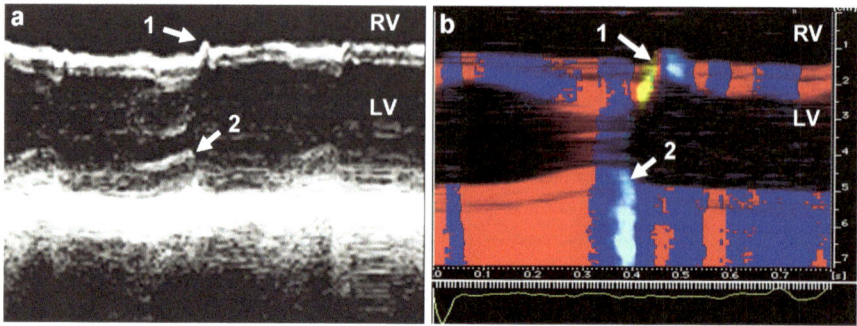

Fig. 23.9 Constrictive Pericarditis. The unusually vigorous early ventricular filling (**a**, *arrow 1*), in presence of thickened pericardium and abrupt anterior or posterior motion of the septum in early diastole is seen in most patients with constrictive pericarditis and reflects a rapid change in transseptal pressure gradient during early diastole. The left ventricular posterior wall demonstrates a rapid early relaxation with posterior movement during early diastole followed by an abrupt cessation of such movement during mid and late diastole (**b**, *arrow 2*)

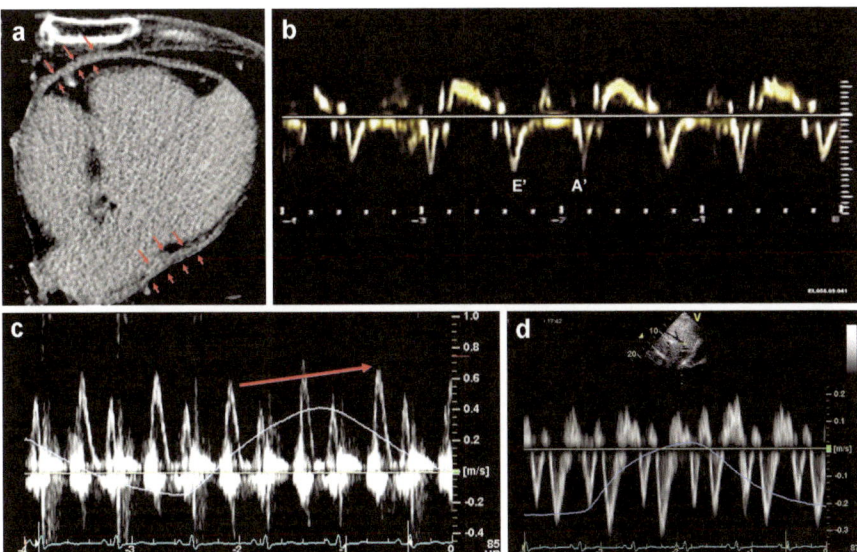

Fig. 23.10 Tissue Doppler and pulsed wave Doppler in constrictive pericarditis. Note the extent of pericardial thickening on cardiac computed tomography (**a**). An early diastolic mitral annular velocities (E' >8 cm/s) at lateral or septal mitral annular corner can distinguish constrictive pericarditis from restrictive cardiomyopathy (**b**). On pulse wave flow Doppler imaging, early diastolic mitral flow is reduced in constriction with the onset of inspiration (**c**), whereas an increase in mitral inflow early diastolic velocity greater than or equal to 25% occurs with expiration. The pulsed Doppler recording of hepatic venous flow mirrors the right atrial pressure tracing. Pulsed wave Doppler recordings from hepatic vein in constriction (**d**) show marked diastolic flow reversal, which increases with expiration compared to inspiration, although it is not unusual to see significant diastolic flow reversals during both inspiration and expiration in patients with advanced constriction

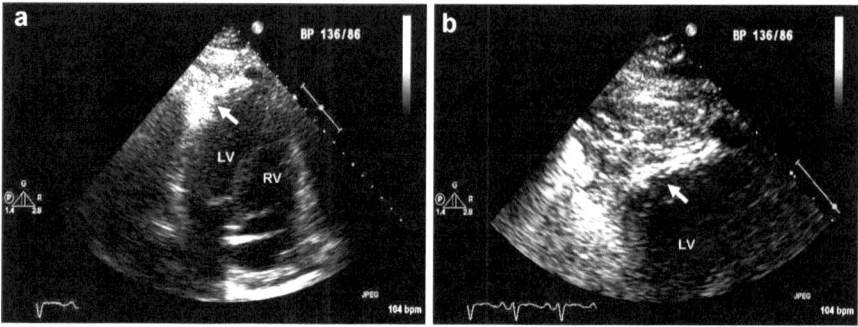

Fig. 23.11 Pericardial masses. Two-dimensional echocardiography can help in identifying pericardial masses. (**a** and **b**) This example shows a solid mass in pericardium (*arrow*) arising from metastatic spread of bronchogenic adenocarcinoma

Table 23.2 Echocardiographic artifacts seen in large pericardial effusions

Mitral valve prolapse
Tricuspid valve prolapse
Systolic anterior motion of the mitral valve
Early systolic closure of the aortic valve
Midsystolic notching of the pulmonary valve
Paradoxical septal motion
Attenuated motion of the posterior wall of the aortic root

Table 23.3 Pitfalls in the diagnosis of pericardial effusion

1. Excess gain settings may mask a pericardial effusion by "filling-in" the echo-free area.

2. The presence of left pleural effusion can make the demonstration of a pericardial effusion difficult. A left pleural effusion may be best demonstrated echocardiographically by placing the transducer in the left axillary line.

3. An anterior echo-free space can be produced by an epicardial fat pad or by a homogenous, localized thrombus or by a pericardial cyst. In general, it is unlikely that an anterior clear space results from pericardial effusion in the absence of a posterior effusion.

4. The presence of a loculated effusion can also cause a false-negative diagnosis, unless the pericardial space is examined carefully in different views.

Table 23.4 Hemodynamic and echocardiographic features of constrictive pericarditis compared with restrictive cardiomyopathy

Feature	Constrictive pericarditis	Restrictive cardiomyopathy
Paradoxical pulse	Present in one-third of cases	Absent
Pericardial knock	Present	Absent
Prominent Y descent in JVP	Present	Variable
Right and left sided filling pressures	Equalized within 5 mmHg	Left sided pressures at least 3–5 mmHg more than right
Filling pressures more than 25 mmHg	Rare	Common
RVSP > 50 mmHg	No	Common
"Square root" sign	Present	Variable
RVEDP/RVSP	≥0.33	<0.3
Discordant respiratory variation of ventricular peak systolic pressures	Right and left ventricular peak systolic pressure variations are out of phase	Right and left ventricular peak systolic pressure variations are in phase
Pericardial thickness	Usually increased	
Atrial size	Mild enlargement, usually of the left atrium	Biatrial enlargement, usually severe
Ventricular wall thickness		Usually increased
Septal bounce	Present	Absent
Mitral or tricuspid regurgitation	Usually absent or mild	Often present
Respiratory variation in left–right pressures or flow	Exaggerated	
Mitral inflow	Inspiratory E less than expiratory E (≥25% change) DT usually ≤160 ms	No respiratory variation of E velocity Increased E/A ratio ≥2.0 DT <160 ms
Tricuspid inflow	Inspiratory E greater than expiratory E (≥40% change)	Mild respiratory variation in E velocity (≤15%)
Pulsed wave Doppler of hepatic vein	Decreased diastolic forward flow with expiration Marked diastolic flow reversal, which increases with expiration compared to inspiration	Systolic forward flow less than diastolic forward flow Diastolic flow reversal in the hepatic vein is more prominent with inspiration

RVSP right ventricular systolic pressure, *RVEDP* right ventricular end-diastolic pressure, *E* early rapid filling wave, *A* filling wave due to atrial systole, *DT* deceleration time

Atrial Septal Defect

24

Naser M. Ammash

The population of adults with congenital heart disease (CHD) is rapidly growing as a result of improvement in diagnostic techniques, medical and surgical expertise. It is estimated that 85% of infants born with CHD survive into adulthood, some of whom have never had any intervention or surgery. This patient population represents a heterogeneous group that includes simple defects such as atrial septal defects, ventricular septal defects, pulmonary stenosis, coarctation of aorta, and complex defects such as Tetralogy of Fallot, Ebstein's anomaly, pulmonary atresia, transposition of the great artery, and univentricular heart. Adults CHD survivors have special needs and require expertise care even after surgical repair since there is usually no cure after repair of CHD and many residua and sequelae are being recognized. The challenges of caring for these adult survivors of CHD can be diagnostic, medical, electrophysiologic, surgical, and psychological. Many of these patients require reoperation that should be performed by surgeons with expertise in that field. The improved outlook for adults with CHD could be best sustained by having adult congenital specialists working in close collaboration with electrophysiologists, cardiac surgeons, cardiac imaging including echocardiography (ECHO), magnetic resonance imaging, computer tomography, as well as obstetricians, psychiatrists, intensivists, transplant service, and medical subspecialists. This multidisciplinary approach toward the care of adults with CHD is the best we can offer for these survivors. This chapter will illustrate the most important echocardiographic features of the common CHD seen before and after repair.

24.1
Atrial Septal Defect

Atrial septal defects (ASD) are common CHD seen in adulthood causing left-to-right shunt across the atrial septum with secondary volume overload of the atria and the right ventricle. Both transthoracic (TTE) and transesophageal (TEE) Echos play a very important role in the assessment of these patients before and after surgical or percutaneous closure. In

N.M. Ammash
Department of Internal Medicine, Mayo Clinic, Rochester, MN, USA
e-mail: ammash.naser@mayo.edu

T.P. Abraham (ed.), *Case Based Echocardiography*,
DOI: 10.1007/978-1-84996-151-6_24, © Springer-Verlag London Limited 2011

addition to the detection of ASD, Echo assesses the degree of shunting, severity of volume overload, and the presence and severity of pulmonary hypertension, tricuspid regurgitation, and associated CHD most commonly partial anomalous pulmonary venous connection (PAPVC) (Figs. 24.1–24.4).

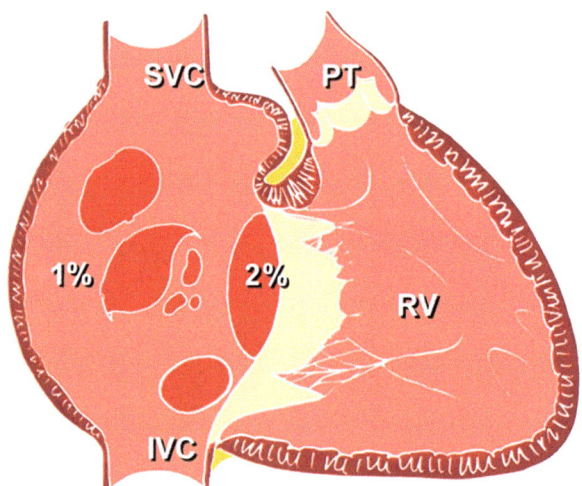

Fig. 24.1 Diagrammatic illustration of the different ASD demonstrating the most common septum secundum ASD (1). Please note the location of the defect in middle of the septum as compared to the septum primum ASD (2) in close proximity to the tricuspid valve, sinus venosus ASD in close proximity to the superior vena cava, and the least common coronary sinus ASD in proximity to the coronary sinus and inferior vena cava

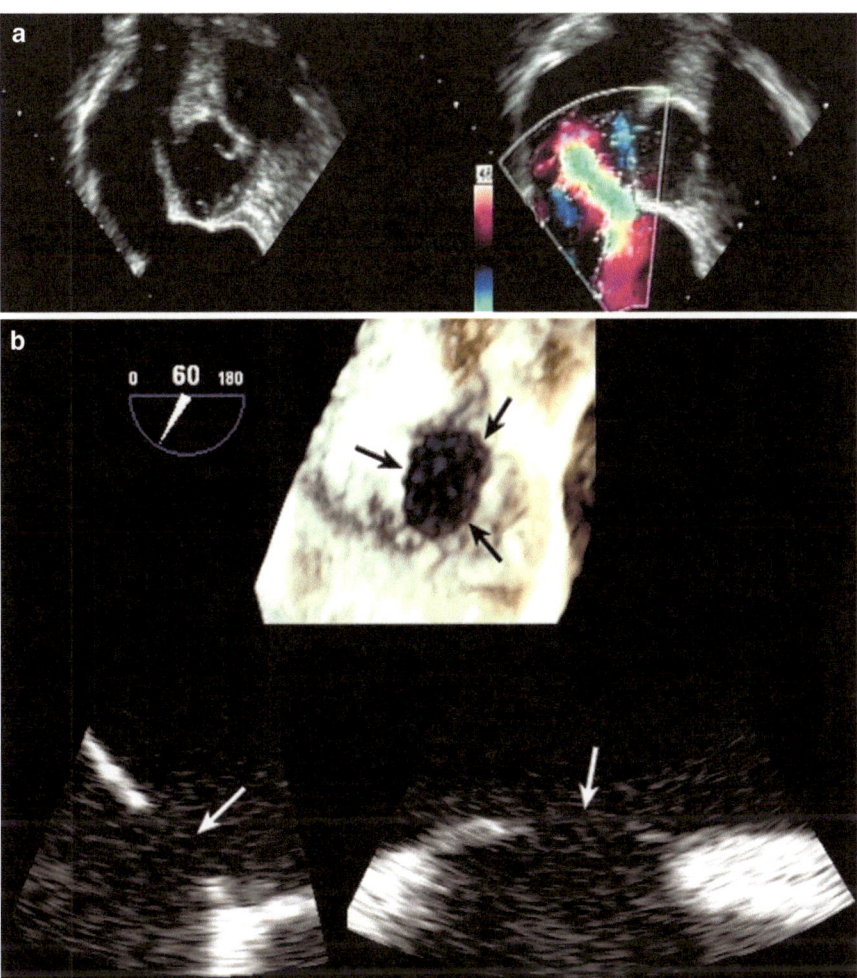

Fig. 24.2 TEE view (**a**) obtained at the base of the heart demonstrating a secundum ASD with left-to-right shunt between the left atrium (LA) and the right atrium (RA). In (**b**), a three-dimensional view of secundum ASD delineating clearly the margins of the defect as compared to the two-dimensional TEE images

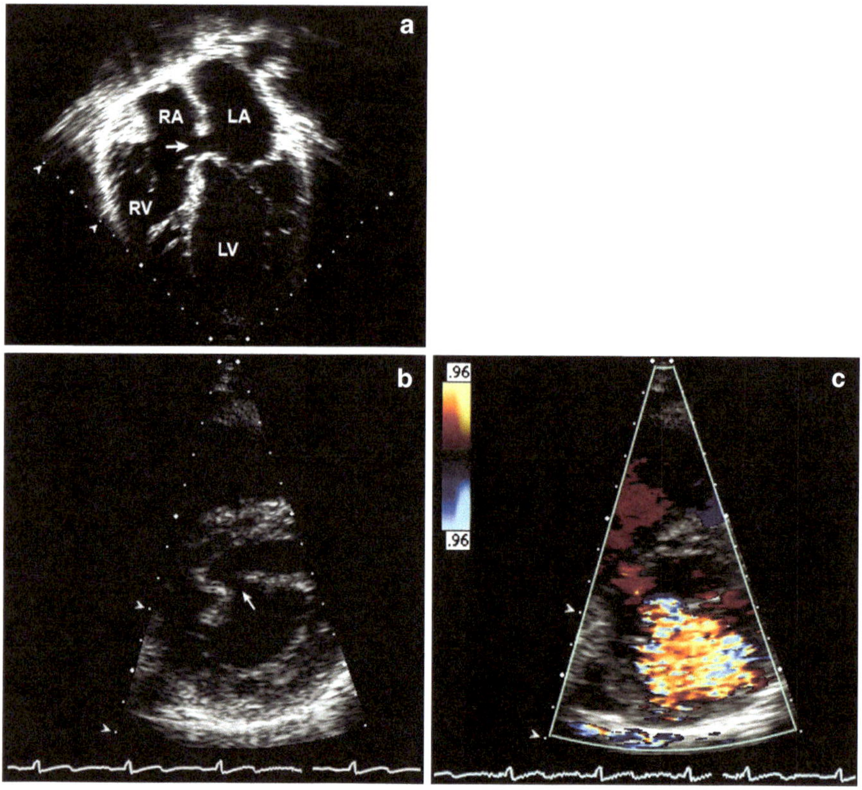

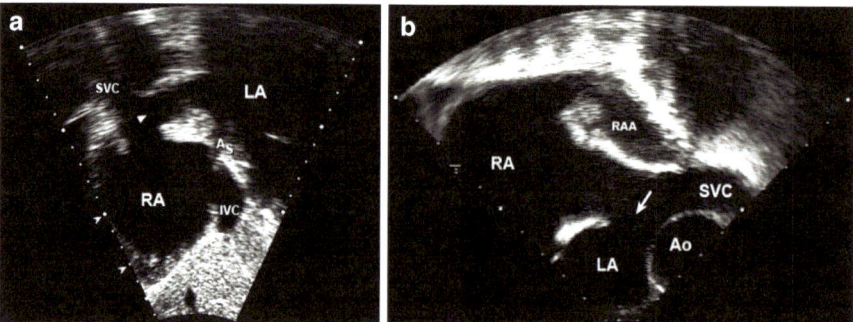

Fig. 24.3 Apical 4 chamber view demonstrating a primum ASD (*arrow*) in close proximity to the mitral and tricuspid valves (**a**). On parasternal short-axis view (**b** and **c**), a cleft in the anterior mitral valve leaflet is seen associated with mitral regurgitation. Typically, these patients have leaflet anterior fascicular block on electrocardiogram. *LA*, left atrium; *RA*, right atrium; *LV*, left ventricle; *RV*, right ventricle

Fig. 24.4 Sinus venosus ASD as noted by TTE (**a**) and TEE (**b**). On both studies, note the defect which is superior to the fatty limbus of the atrial septum (AS) and in close proximity to the superior vena cava (SVC). *RA*, right atrium; *LA*, left atrium; *RAA*, right atrial appendage

Summary

> ASD are common defects of the atrial septum, leading to left-to-right shunt
> ASD cause enlargement of the atria and right ventricle and can lead to pulmonary hypertension
> Imaging of the atrial septum is best done with TEE, as compared to TTE especially in the adult patient

Percutaneous Interventions for Congenital Heart Defects

25

Christian D. Nagy, Richard E. Ringel, and W. Reid Thompson

25.1
Atrial Septal Defect Closure

- Atrial septal defect (ASD) closure leads to improved functional status, reduces the risk of progressive right-sided failure, and prevents the development of severe pulmonary hypertension or paradoxical embolism.
- Percutaneous device closure using a number of different devices has become the treatment of choice for secundum ASDs, whereas other types of ASDs are treated surgically.
- Device closure of ASD is guided by a combination of fluoroscopic and echocardiographic imaging. Intracardiac echocardiography (ICE) is now being used more commonly for adults and transesophageal echocardiography (TEE) employed in special situations and small children.
- Indications for ASD closure are right heart dilation by echocardiography, MRI, or CT (Qp:Qs >1.5:1) in the absence of advanced pulmonary arterial hypertension.
- Patients with an ASD too large for device closure, inadequate atrial septal rims to permit stable device deployment, or those with proximity of the defect to the AV valves, the coronary sinus, or the vena cavae are referred for surgical repair.
- Device closure is a safe and effective procedure in experienced hands, with major complications such as cardiac perforation or device embolization occurring in less than 1% of patients. Successful closure is achieved in up to 95% of patients. Although small residual shunts are often seen on echocardiography at the end of the procedure, these are hemodynamically insignificant, and most will close spontaneously within 1 year.

C.D. Nagy (✉)
Pediatric Cardiology/Adult Cardiology, Johns Hopkins University Medical Center,
Baltimore, MD, USA
e-mail: cnagy3@jhmi.edu

T.P. Abraham (ed.), *Case Based Echocardiography*,
DOI: 10.1007/978-1-84996-151-6_25, © Springer-Verlag London Limited 2011

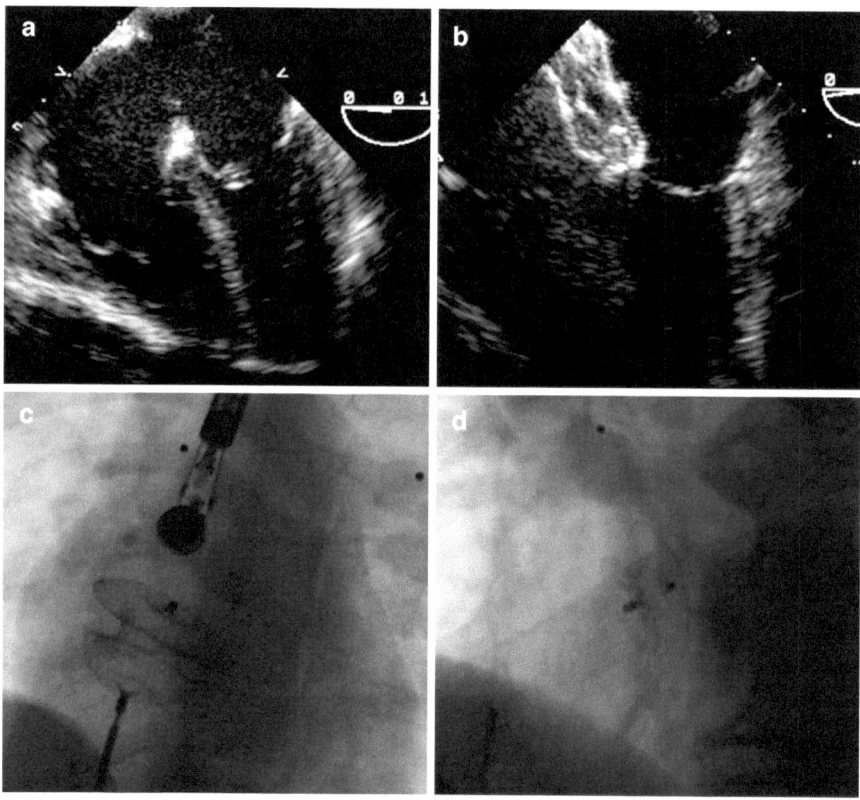

Fig. 25.1 TEE apical 4-chamber view demonstrating a large secundum ASD (**a**). In Fig. 25.1**b** the defect has been closed using an Amplatzer septal occluder. Figure 25.1**c** and **d** show angiographic correlates. Under TEE guidance, the ASD device is positioned across the interatrial septum and then released

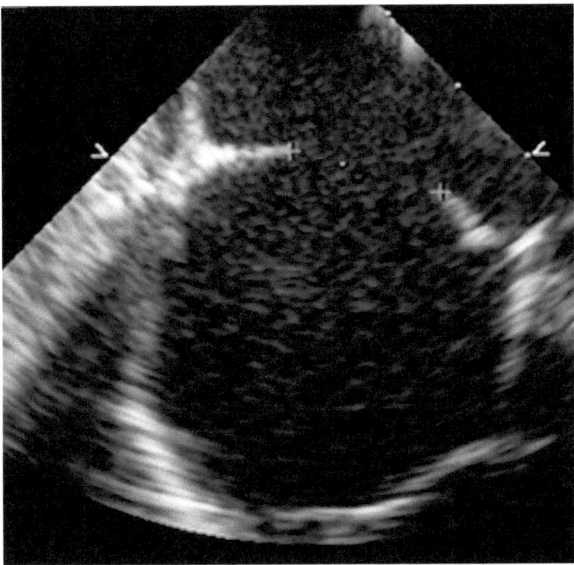

Fig. 25.2 TEE view demonstrating a large secundum ASD. In addition to determining the maximal diameter of the defect and total atrial septal length, measurement of the surrounding rims to the aorta, right upper pulmonary vein, superior vena cava, inferior vena cava, mitral valve, and coronary sinus, is warranted in order to assess candidacy for percutaneous closure

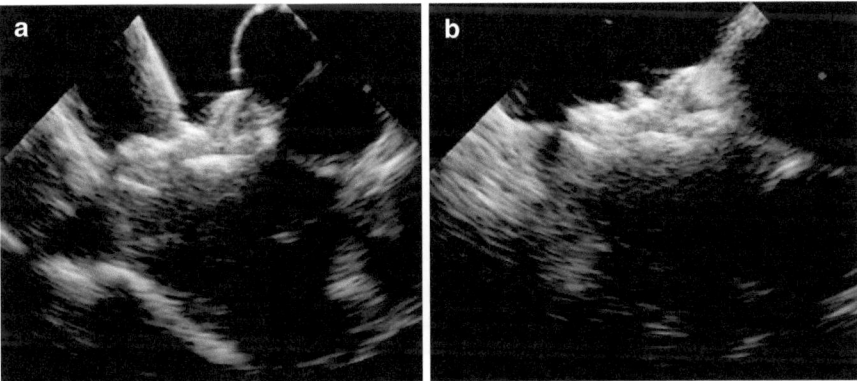

Fig. 25.3 ICE demonstrating ASD closure. In Fig. 25.3**a** both the left and right atrial disks have been deployed; however the device is still attached to the delivery cable. In Fig. 25.3**b** the device has been released. Note the septal occluder in stable position, anchored between the aortic rim and the posterior rim

25.2
Ventricular Septal Defect Closure

- In adults, congenital ventricular septal defect (VSD) device closure in the catheterization lab is relatively uncommon, reserved primarily for defects in the apical muscular septum, which are difficult to close surgically.
- Acquired VSD is a rare, but serious, complication of myocardial infarction occurring in <1% of cases, and mortality is high if untreated.
  - Early surgical cure is difficult, and in selected patients percutaneous closure may be an alternative treatment option.
  - Individuals most likely to benefit from transcatheter VSD occlusion are those with persistent hemodynamic compromise who are medically difficult to manage.

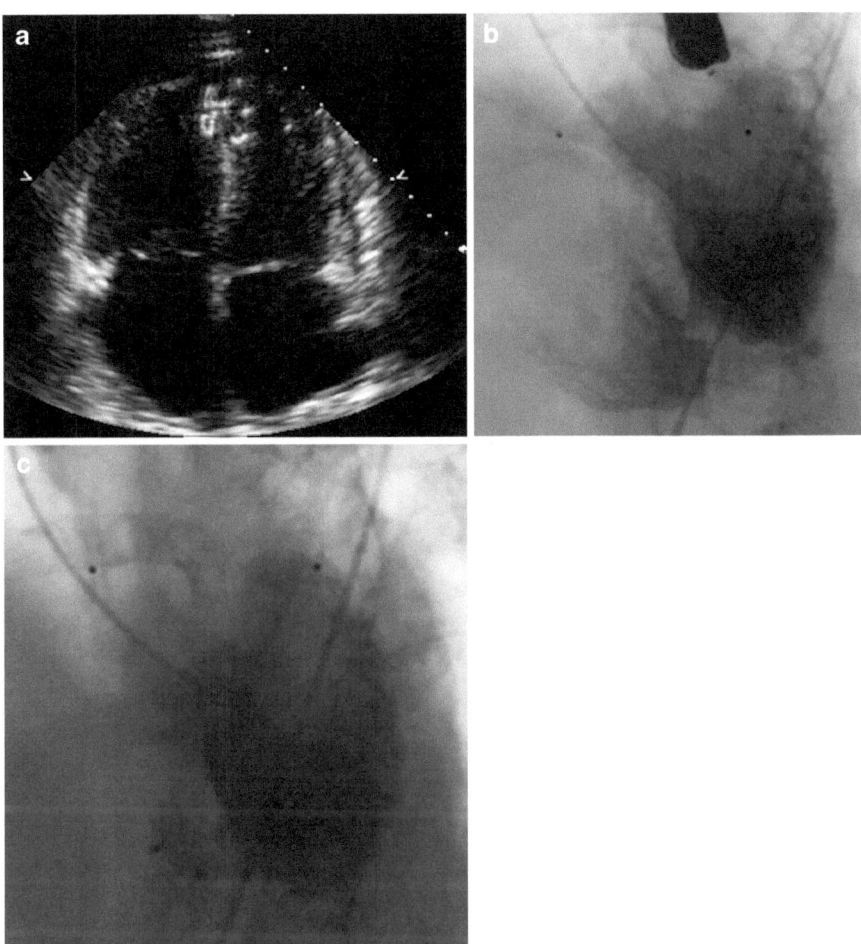

Fig. 25.4 Apical 4-chamber TTE view (**a**) demonstrating device closure of a post-myocardial infarction muscular VSD (in this case using an Amplatzer septal occluder) in the apical interventricular septum. In Fig. 25.4**b** the VSD is visible angiographically and in Fig. 25.4**c** the defect is closed with the VSD device

25.3
Patent Ductus Arteriosus Closure

- Patent ductus arteriosus (PDA) is a congenital cardiac disorder that can be first identified at almost any age.
- The clinical implications vary and can include development of heart failure and pulmonary hypertension.
- Transcatheter techniques have replaced surgical therapy in most patients with PDA and recent advances in echocardiography have resulted in better detection and characterization of PDA and avoiding complications.

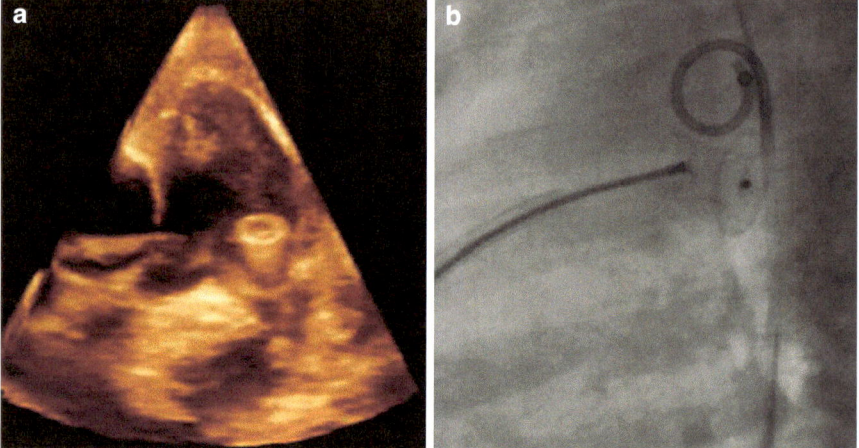

Fig. 25.5 Fig. 25.5**a** shows the 3-D echo image demonstrating an Amplatzer duct occluder closing a PDA. The larger end faces the aorta and the smaller end is positioned toward the pulmonary artery. Figure 25.5**b** shows the angiographic correlate. A catheter is positioned in the aorta. The closure device is deployed in the ductus arteriosus and still attached to its delivery cable and the device is released after confirming the position

Table 25.1 Structural heart conditions amenable to percutaneous cath lab interventions

Secundum atrial septal defect
Patent foramen ovale
Muscular ventricular septal defect
Patent ductus arteriosus
Fenestrated Fontan
Atrial baffle leaks after Mustard/Senning operation for transposition of the great arteries
Aortic to pulmonary artery collaterals
Pulmonary arteriovenous malformations
Venous collaterals
Coarctation of the aorta
Branch pulmonary artery stenosis
Stenosis of the systemic venous baffle after Mustard operation
Balloon atrial septostomy
Percutaneous balloon valvotomy for pulmonary stenosis
Aortic balloon valvotomy for aortic stenosis
Mitral balloon valvotomy for mitral stenosis
Percutaneous pulmonary valve implantation
Percutaneous aortic valve replacement

Table 25.2 Comparison of different echocardiographic techniques

	Transthoracic echocardiogram	Transesophageal echocardiogram	Intracardiac echocardiogram
Indications	Cardiac biopsy	ASD/PFO closure	ASD/PFO closure
	Septostomy	VSD closure	
	Pericardiocentesis	Fenestrated Fontan closure	
Advantages	Noninvasive	High sensitivity	No sedation required
	No sedation required	Posterior structures well imaged	Inferior atrial septum well imaged
	Anterior structures well imaged		
Disadvantages	Inconvenient in cath lab	Deep sedation required	Additional venous access required
	Lower resolution of small structures	May compromise airway	Limited visualization
		Anterior structures difficult to assess	

Summary Box

ASD, VSD, and PDA are congenital defects amenable to percutaneous device therapy. Imaging studies such as echocardiography with its various modalities including TTE, TEE, 3-D echo, and ICE play a crucial role in the diagnosis and management of congenital heart disease.

Recommended Reading

Minette MS, Sahn DJ. Ventricular septal defects. *Circulation*. 2006;114:2190-2197.

Mullen MJ, Dias BF, Walker F, et al. Intracardiac echocardiography guided device closure of atrial septal defects. *J Am Coll Cardiol*. 2003;41:285-292.

Schneider DJ, Moore JW. Patent ductus arteriosus. *Circulation*. 2006;114:1873-1882.

Warnes CA, Williams RG, Bashore TM, et al. ACC/AHA 2008 guidelines for the management of adults with congenital heart disease. *J Am Coll Cardiol*. 2008;52(23):e1-121.

Webb G, Gatzoulis MA. Atrial septal defects in the adult: recent progress and overview. *Circulation*. 2006;114:1645-1653.

Cardiac Tumors and Masses

26

Mary C. Corretti

26.1
Categories of Tumors/Masses

- Primary benign tumors
- Primary malignant tumors
- Intracardiac thrombus
- Intracardiac vegetations/infections
- Degenerative valvular changes creating mass effect
- Pericardial masses or cysts
- Normal variants

26.2
Cardiac Masses: Benign

- Myxoma-most common
- Lipoma
- Fibroma
- Valvular –papillary fibroelastoma
- Hemangioma

M.C. Corretti
Division of Cardiology, Johns Hopkins University, Baltimore, MD, USA
e-mail: mcorret1@jhmi.edu

T.P. Abraham (ed.), *Case Based Echocardiography*,
DOI: 10.1007/978-1-84996-151-6_26, © Springer-Verlag London Limited 2011

26.3
Cardiac Masses: Malignant

- Angiosarcoma – most common in adults
- Rhabdomyosarcoma – more common in children
- Mesothelioma
- Fibrosarcoma
- Lymphoma
- Leiomyosarcoma
- Thymoma

26.4
Myxoma

- Comprise the majority of benign intracardiac tumors
- Usually on a stalk attached to the fossa ovalis (mid portion of the interatrial septum) protruding into the left atrium, or right atrium. They can develop in the ventricules as single masses, or as a multiple presence in the Carney syndrome-genetic defect in the long arm of chromosome 17.
- Tumor is of mesenchymal origin, appears amorphous, gelatinous and usually mobile on a stalk. Sessile myxomas can also occur.
- Potential for embolization is high thus requiring surgical removal upon diagnosis.
- Diagnosis is made often with transthoracic echo and transesophageal echo, if transthoracic echo image quality is limited.

26.5
Atrial Myxoma (Fig. 26.1)

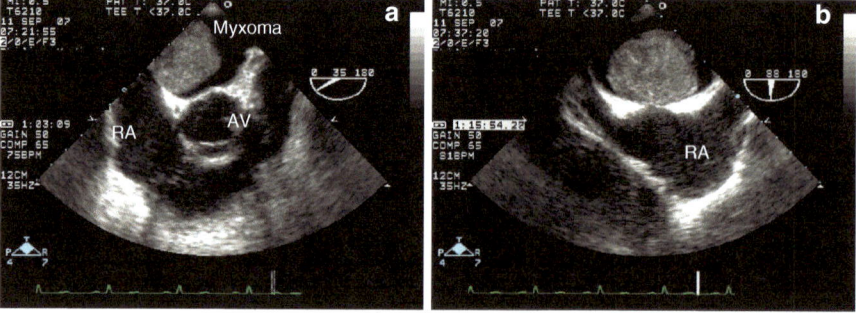

Fig. 26.1 (**a**) TEE-midesophageal short axis aortic valve view. Tumor attached to the left atrial side fossa. Ovalis portion of the interatrial septum. (**b**) TEE-midesophageal bicaval view. Tumor attached to the left atrial side. Interatrial septum

26.6
Papillary Fibroelastoma: Benign Valvular Tumor

- Second most common primary benign tumor in the adult
- Small in size with characteristic stippled or frond-like edge that appears to vibrate in motion at the tumor-blood interface. The tumor emanates from a stalked central core which often arises from a valvular structure (more commonly on the aortic and mitral valves, less so on the tricuspid and pulmonary valves.
- Potential for embolization is present

26.6.1
Papillary Fibroelastoma (Fig. 26.2)

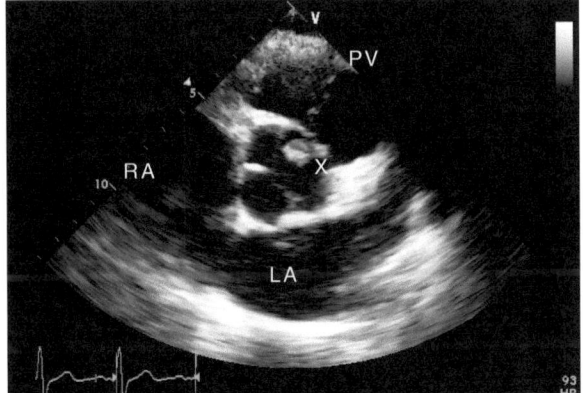

Fig. 26.2 Papillary fibroelastoma. Transthoracic short axis view of aortic valve. Round echodense fibroelastoma noted on the right coronary cusp (X)

26.6.2
Valvular Papillary Fibroelastoma (Fig. 26.3)

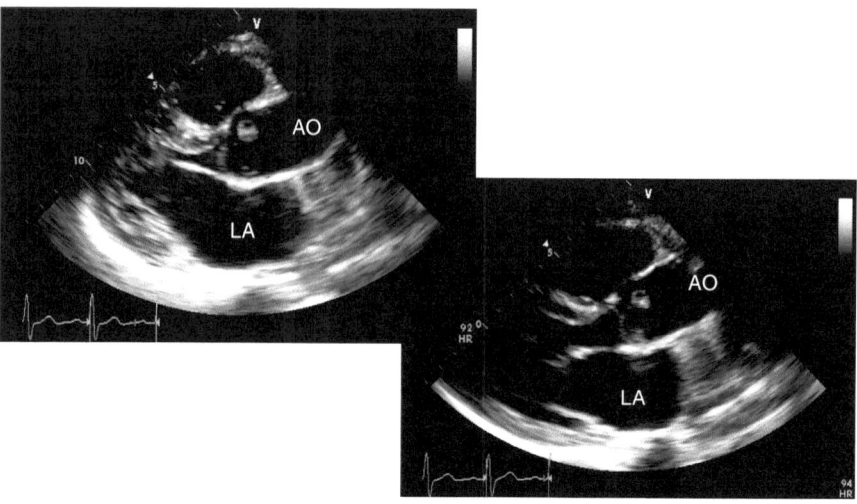

Fig. 26.3 Valvular papillary fibroelastoma. Transthoracic parasternal long axis view. Round tumor on a stalk on the aortic side of the aortic valve

26.7
Fibroma (Fig. 26.4)

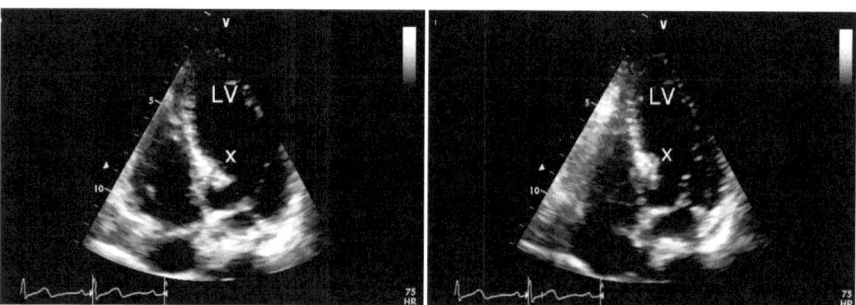

Fig. 26.4 Transthoracic four chamber view in diastole (*left image*) and mid systole (*right image*). Fleshy tumor mass on the proximal ventricular septum

26.8
Sarcoma

- Most common malignant cardiac tumor in adults, and second to myxomas in frequency though still rare.
- Derived from mesenchymal cells causing wide array of different histologic types: angiosarcoma, rhabdomyosarcoma, fibrosarcoma, leiomyosarcoma, osteosarcoma.
- These can be seen as bulky tumors in the chambers, and more so infiltrating the myocardium and pericardium.

26.9
Malignant Tumor: Burkitt B Cell Lymphoma (Fig. 26.5)

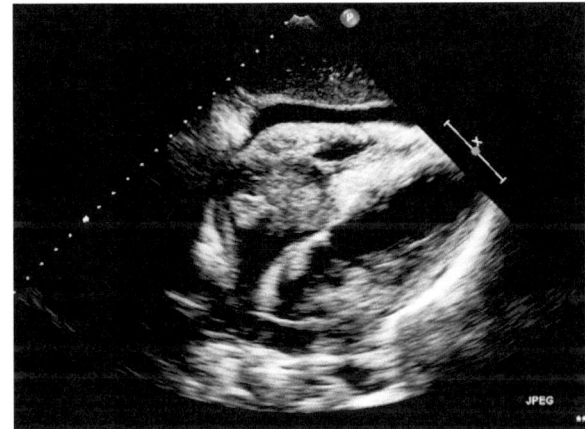

Fig. 26.5 Malignant tumor: Burkitt B cell lymphoma. Transthoracic subcostal view. Tumor mass in the right atrium, with infiltration of tumor in the myocardium. Pericardial effusion present

26.10
Mimickers of Cardiac Tumors (Figs. 26.6 and 26.7)

- Eustachian ridge and Chiari network: Normal variant of an embryologic remnant of the Eustachian valve from the IVC. This is a long mobile string like structure that can attach from the Eustachian ridge (IVC/RA junction) to the interatrial septum.

Fig. 26.6 Mimickers of cardiac tumors. Transthoracic parasternal short axis view. Chiari network – X

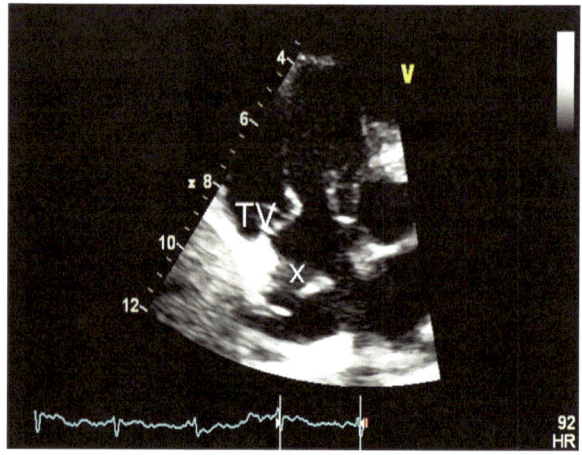

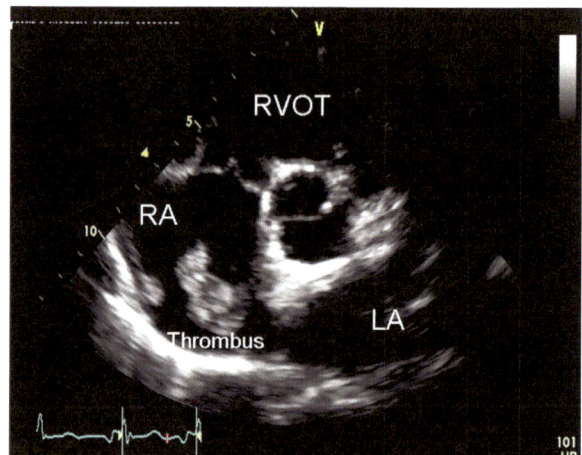

Fig. 26.7 Intracardiac thrombus in transit. Transthoracic parasternal short axis view

26.11
Lipomatous Hypertrophy TEE Bicaval View (Fig. 26.8)

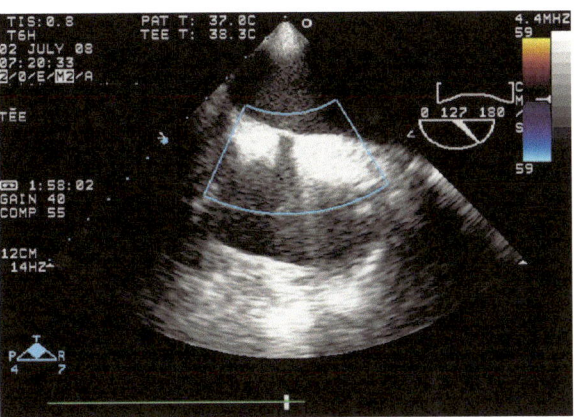

Fig. 26.8 Echogenic fatty tissue along the interatrial septum and sparing the fossa ovalis of the interatrial septum. Dumb-bell shape appearance and echogenicity of the tissue is characteristic of this anatomic variant

Cardiac Transplantation

27

James Mudd

27.1
Ventricular Assist Device

- Ventricular assist devices (VADs) are placed in the right, and most commonly, the left ventricle to support patients with end stage heart failure.
- Echocardiography is used to evaluate the following issues with VADs:
  - Apical cannula position
  - Assessment of ventricular unloading
    - Frequency of aortic valve opening
    - Position of the septum:
      - Leftward shift may indicate an under filled left ventricle from excessive unloading or abnormalities with preload.
      - Rightward shift may indicate poor LV unloading due to low pump speed or problems with pump filling.
  - Right ventricular size and function with left sided VAD

J. Mudd

T.P. Abraham (ed.), *Case Based Echocardiography*,
DOI: 10.1007/978-1-84996-151-6_27, © Springer-Verlag London Limited 2011

27.2
VAD: Parasternal Long Axis

- This view should attempt to show the VAD cannula protruding through the apex (arrow). The purpose of this view is to determine the orientation of the cannula and identify obstruction to blood inflow (clot or tissue).

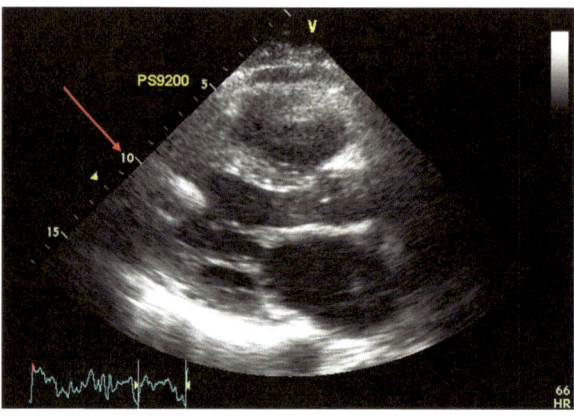

27.3
VAD: Apical Short Axis

- Much like the parasternal view, this view helps to determine if there is an abnormally aligned cannula or clot, or other debris preventing blood inflow through the cannula.

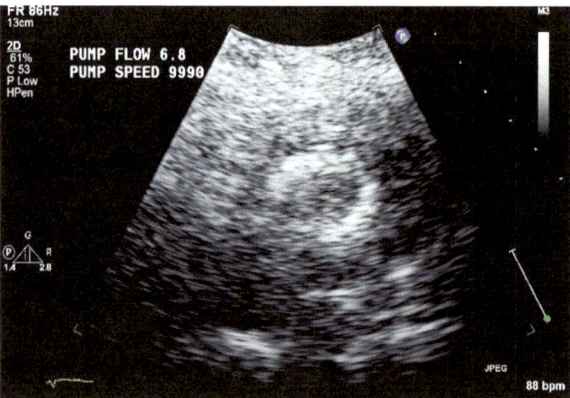

27.4
VAD: Aortic Valve Function

- Careful examination of the aortic valve with and without color flow Doppler should be performed capturing at least 10 beat in all views.
- Frequent opening of the aortic valve signals potential insufficient ventricular unloading either from low pump speeds or problems with pump filling.
- Significant aortic regurgitation may also develop.
- Continuous aortic regurgitation throughout the cardiac cycle is sometimes seen with an LVAD.

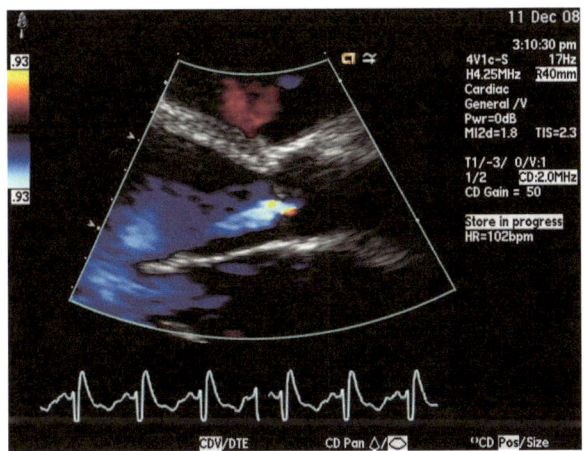

27.5
Heart Transplantation

- Important differences include larger atria and abnormal septal motion as seen after other cardiac surgeries.
- Most transplanted hearts are anastamosed with a bicaval technique resulting in a slightly larger left atrium and normal sized right atrium.
- Previous techniques resulted in biatrial enlargment as seen in this image.

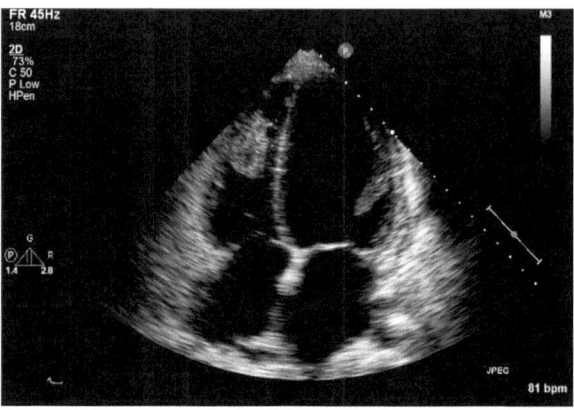

27.6
Echocardiography in Heart Transplantation

- Routine echocardiography is used to evaluate for changes in ejection fraction and/or regional wall motion abnormalities caused by:
  - Cellular or humoral immunologic rejection
  - Transplant associated coronary artery disease
- Transplant patients may also develop right ventricular dysfunction if there was preexisting pulmonary hypertension.
- Echocardiography can also be used to guide endomyocardial biopsy to evaluate for rejection.

27.7
Heart Transplant Rejection

Evidence of new hypertrophy in a heart transplant patient may be a sign of cardiac rejection as seen in this patient with suspected humoral rejection. The ejection fraction may be preserved, demonstrate regional wall motion abnormalities or diffuse hypokinesis in rejection

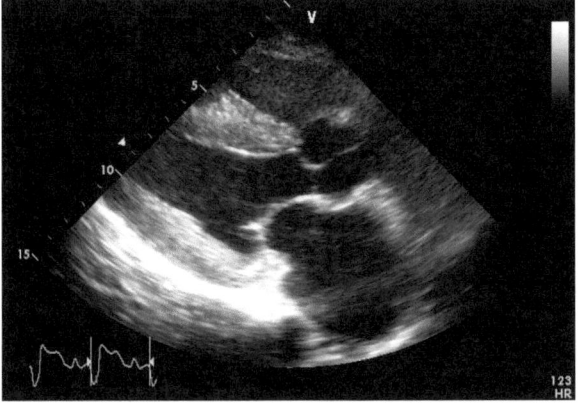

27.8
Dilated Cardiomyopathy

- Dilated cardiomyopathy refers to enlargement of the left ventricle and a depressed ejection fraction.
- Causes:
  — Coronary artery disease
  — Familial
  — Peripartum
  — Viral
  — Idiopathic
  — Sarcoidosis
  — Hemachromatosis
  — Primary valve disease
- Echocardiography is used to evaluate for:
  — Regional wall motion abnormalities
  — Severity of mitral regurgitation
    — Mitral regurgitation is common in dilated cardiomyopathy typically resulting from stretching of the valve annulus.
  — Presence of apical thrombus
  — Pulmonary hypertension
  — Aneurysm or pseudoaneurysm formation after myocardial infarction

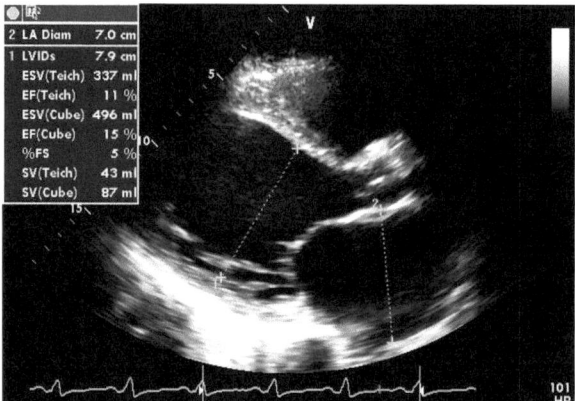

27.9 Dilated Cardiomyopathy Mitral Regurgitation

Apical four chamber view demonstrating eccentric mitral regurgitation.
Doppler signal demonstrates significant mitral regurgitant velocity

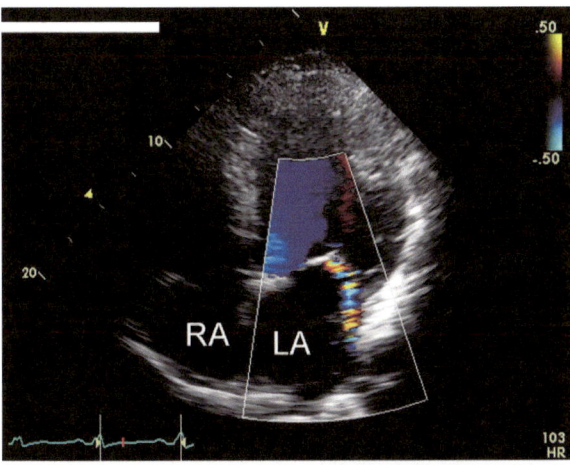

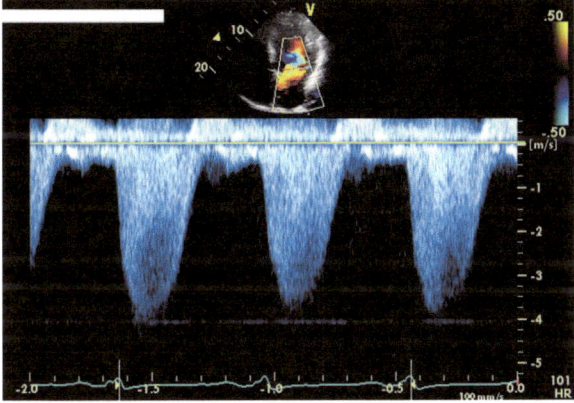

27.10
Dilated Cardiomyopathy

27.10.1
IVC Diameter

The IVC is often dilated in patients with heart failure and can be used as a metric for volume overload and/or right heart dysfunction. Lack of respiratory variation is also a sign of venous congestion.

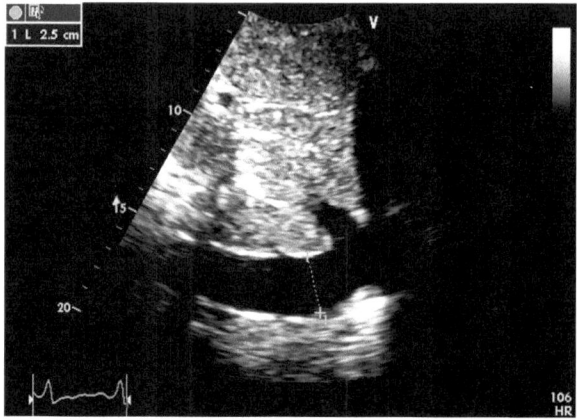

27.10.2
Ventricular Thrombus

RV thrombus.
Pedunculated LV trhombus

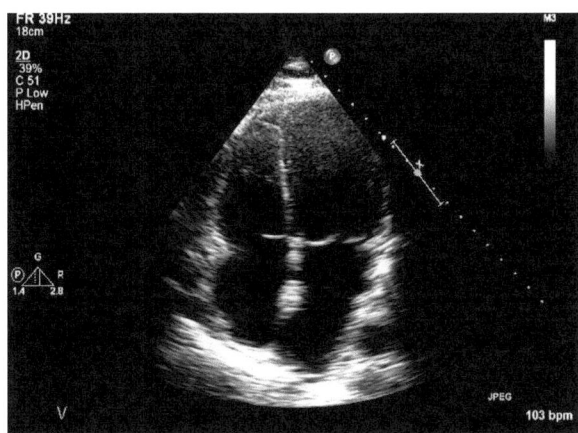

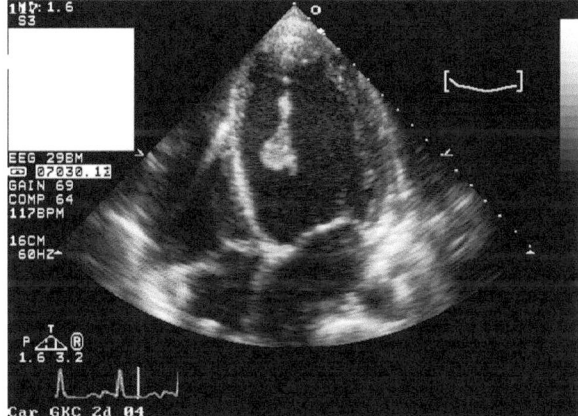

27.11
Amyloid Cardiomyopathy

Amyloid cardiomyopathy demonstrates significant hypertrophy, depressed left ventricular function. A distinguishing feature is a diminished mitral annular tissue Doppler signal.

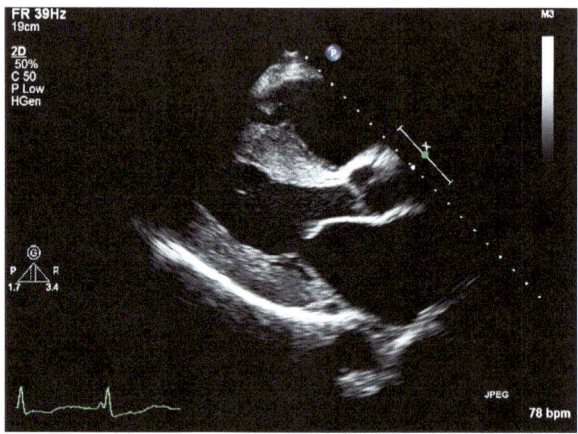

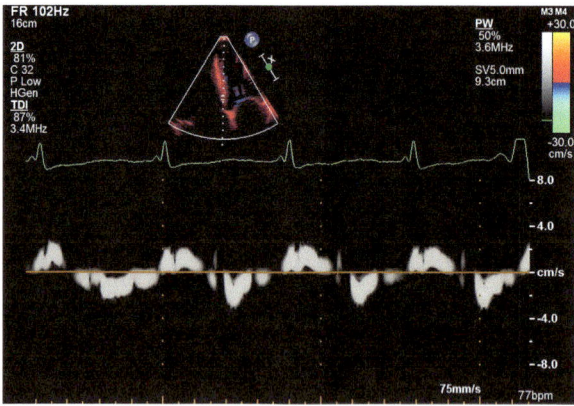

27.12
Bicaval Orthotopic Heart Transplant

- The recipient SVC and IVC are anastomosed to the donor heart without altering the size of the right atrium.
- The recipient pulmonary veins and some surrounding tissue are retained to anastomose to the donor left atrium.

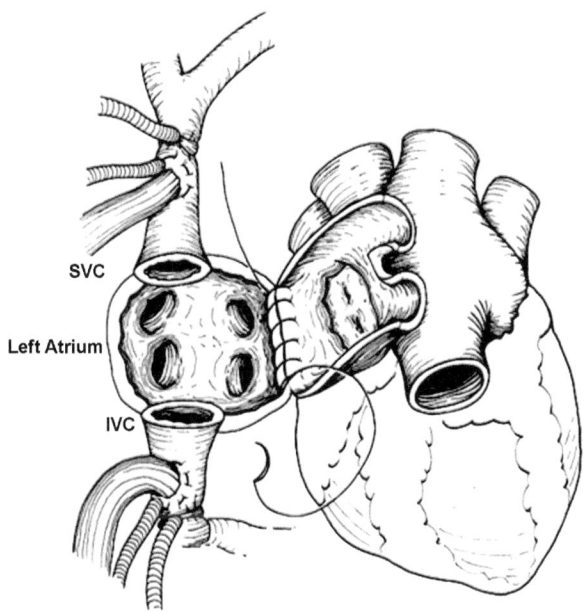

Vascular Imaging

28

Elizabeth V. Ratchford

28.1
Introduction

Vascular imaging has now become routine in many echocardiography laboratories. With increasing recognition of the systemic nature of atherosclerosis, cardiologists are becoming more involved in imaging outside the heart both for clinical and research purposes.

28.2
Outline

1. Vascular ultrasound principles
2. Carotid duplex
3. Abdominal aorta ultrasound
4. Research techniques in vascular imaging
   — Carotid intima-media thickness
   — Brachial reactivity
   — Augmentation index

E.V. Ratchford
Department of Medicine, Division of Cardiology, Johns Hopkins University School of Medicine, Baltimore, MD, USA
e-mail: eratchf1@jhmi.edu

T.P. Abraham (ed.), *Case Based Echocardiography*,
DOI: 10.1007/978-1-84996-151-6_28, © Springer-Verlag London Limited 2011

28.3
Vascular Ultrasound Principles

28.3.1
Vascular Ultrasound: Conventions

- Several principles and conventions are unique to vascular ultrasound:
  — The Doppler angle is set at 60°.
  — The head is on the left-hand side of the screen and the feet are to the right.
  — With color flow, red is for arteries and blue is for veins.
  — Flow *towards* the transducer is *positive*; flow away from the transducer is negative.

28.3.2
Vascular Ultrasound: Techniques

- All sampling should be done at an angle of 60° or less (between the beam and the flow direction or vessel wall).
- The sample volume should be at the center of the vessel and should be set as small as possible.
- The cursor should be parallel to the vessel wall.

28.3.3
Vascular Ultrasound: Diagnostic Criteria

- In any given artery, a doubling of the peak systolic velocity (PSV) on spectral Doppler generally indicates more than 50% stenosis.
- Percent stenosis refers to diameter reduction.
  — For example, 50% diameter reduction is equivalent to a 75% area reduction.
- The velocity in the area of stenosis (or just distal to the stenosis) is typically compared to a normal, more proximal portion of the artery.
- In general, diagnosis is based on velocity criteria and the presence or absence of plaque.
- While there are published criteria, each vascular laboratory is must establish and then internally validate its own velocity criteria.

28.4
Carotid Duplex

28.4.1
Indications for Carotid Duplex (Fig. 28.1)

- Carotid bruit
- Amaurosis fugax
- TIA/Stroke
- Follow-up of known stenosis or post-stent or post-CEA
- Syncope
- pre-CABG (controversial)

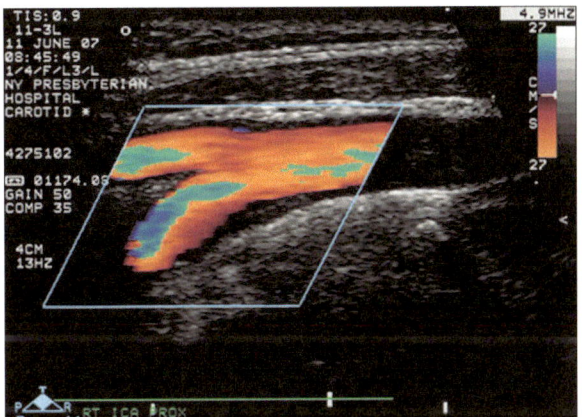

Fig. 28.1 Color Doppler image of the carotid bifurcation

28.4.2
Carotid Duplex Protocol

- Look for presence or absence of plaque
- Note morphology of the plaque
  - Calcified (echogenic) or echolucent or heterogeneous
- Degree of stenosis
  - Based on spectral Doppler (angle-corrected)
    A quantitative measurement of hemodynamic changes
  - Parameters include: peak systolic velocity (most important), end-diastolic velocity, and ICA/CCA ratio
    Spectral broadening – evidence of turbulence
    ICA/CCA ratio: peak systolic velocity in the ICA divided by the velocity in the distal CCA measured 2 cm proximal to the bifurcation.

28.4.3
Sample Carotid Diagnostic Criteria

Diameter reduction	Peak systolic velocity (cm/s)	ICA/CCA ratio	
Normal	<105	<1.8	No plaque
1–39%	<105	<1.8	Plaque imaged
40–59%	105–159	<1.8	
60–79%	≥160	1.8–3.7	
80–99%	≥240 (EDV ≥ 135)	>3.7	

EDV end-diastolic velocity, *ICA* internal carotid artery, *CCA* common carotid artery

28.4.4
B ("Brightness" Mode): Useful for Plaque Analysis (Fig. 28.2)

Fig. 28.2 An 8–11 MHz
linear transducer is typically
used to image the carotid
artery. This image illustrates
plaque in the bifurcation

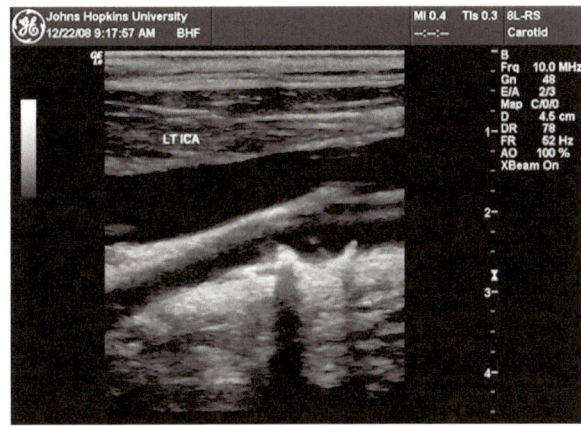

28.4.5
Color Doppler (Fig. 28.3)

Color Doppler is useful for detecting areas of turbulence to help localize stenosis.

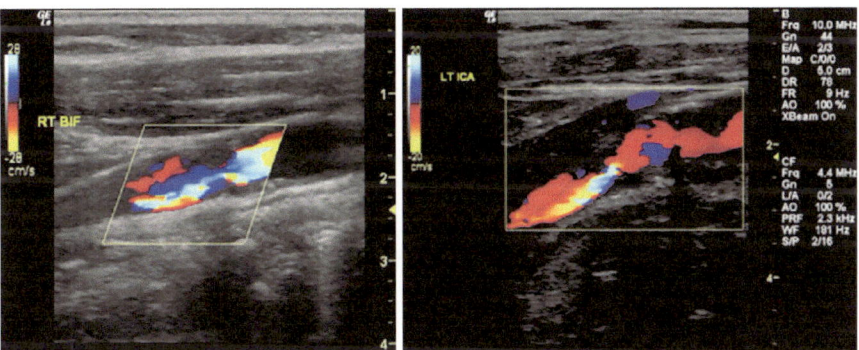

Fig. 28.3 *Left*; Color Doppler image of the stenosis at the bifurcation. *Right*; Color Doppler image
of the stenosis in the proximal ICA

28.4.6
Waveform Morphology (Figs. 28.4 and 28.5)

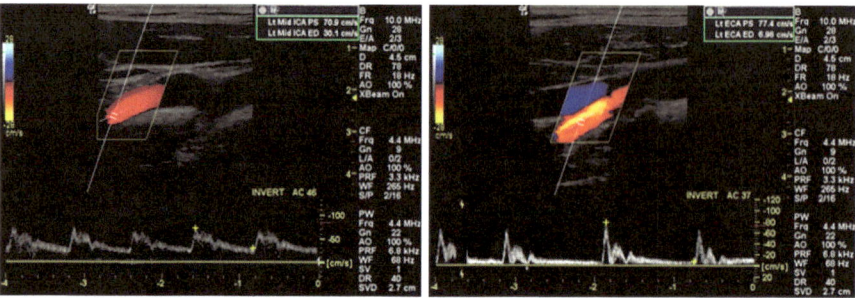

Fig. 28.4 The spectral Doppler waveform in the internal carotid artery (*left*) is typical of a "low resistance" vessel with more diastolic flow. The waveform in the external carotid artery (*right*) is "high resistance" with minimal diastolic flow

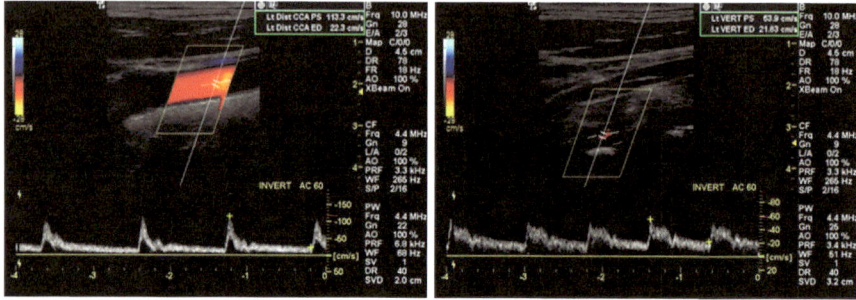

Fig. 28.5 The spectral Doppler waveform in the common carotid artery (*left*) shares features of both the internal and external carotid arteries which are downstream. The waveform in the vertebral artery (*right*) is "low resistance" with more diastolic flow similar to the internal carotid artery

28.4.7
ECA Versus ICA (Fig. 28.6)

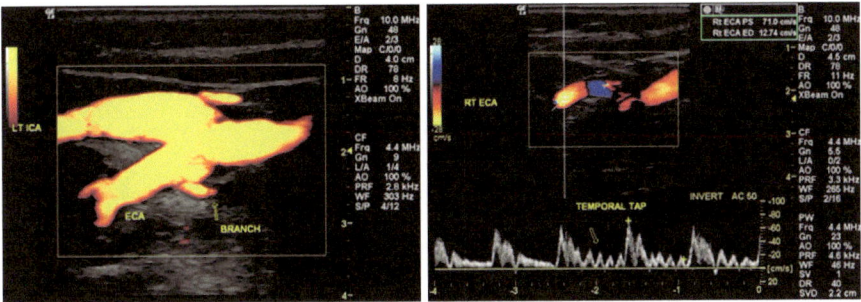

Fig. 28.6 In addition to the characteristic waveform morphology, several features help to distinguish the external carotid artery (ECA) from the internal carotid artery (ICA): (1) the ECA is typically smaller; (2) the ECA has branches (*left*); (3) oscillations can be seen in the ECA when the temporal artery is tapped, referred to as the "temporal tap" (*right*)

28.4.8
Vertebral Artery Waveform in Subclavian Steal (Fig. 28.7)

Fig. 28.7 Subclavian stenosis is suspected in a patient (most commonly asymptomatic) with a differential in brachial pressures of more than 12–15 mmHg. Retrograde flow may be seen in the vertebral artery (as shown here) in the presence of subclavian stenosis which is termed "subclavian steal." If accompanied by symptoms such as syncope or vertigo, it is referred to as "subclavian steal syndrome"

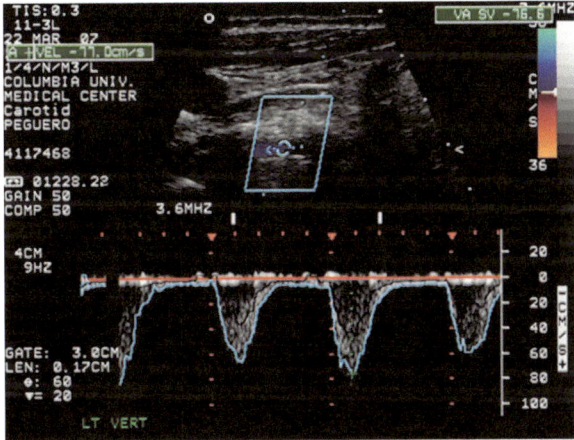

28.4.9
Carotid Stenosis (Fig. 28.8)

Fig. 28.8 This image illustrates 80–99% stenosis of the proximal internal carotid artery with a peak systolic velocity of 286.9 cm/s; the ICA/CCA ratio was 4.4. Turbulence is seen on color Doppler and spectral broadening is seen in the spectral Doppler waveform

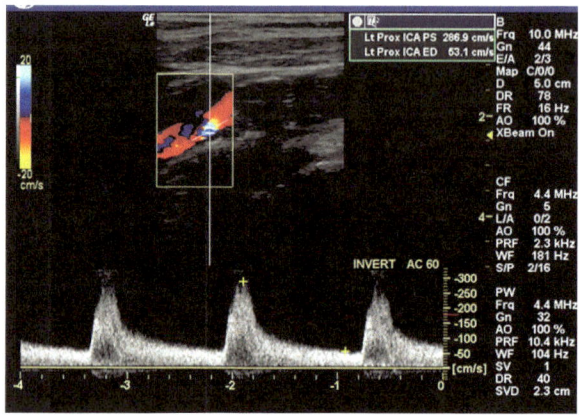

28.5
Abdominal Aorta Ultrasound

28.5.1
Abdominal Aortic Aneurysm (AAA)

- The abdominal aorta is easily imaged in the echo lab and can be seen with the cardiac transducer.
- A curvilinear convex (2–4 MHz) transducer is preferred.
- The patient must fast for 6–8 h prior to the exam to limit the interference of bowel gas.

28.5.2
AAA

- In general, an aneurysm is defined as an increase in the diameter of any artery that is 1.5 times normal.
- For example, the abdominal aorta is normally 2 cm in diameter, and AAA is defined as an aortic diameter greater than 3 cm.

28.5.3
Aortic Ultrasound (Fig. 28.9)

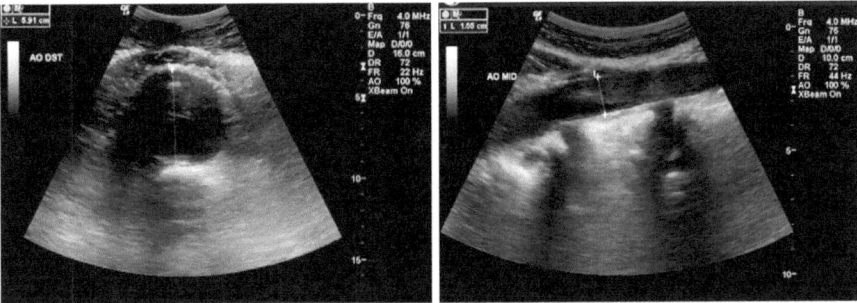

Fig. 28.9 Aortic measurements are obtained in both transverse (*left*; 5.9 cm aneurysm) and longitudinal (*right*; normal aorta) views. It is common to see plaque or thrombus within an aneurysm (*left*)

28.5.4
Aorta Protocol

- Transverse AP (anterior-posterior) and longitudinal AP measurements as well as spectral Doppler waveforms should be obtained:
  - In the proximal aorta near the superior mesenteric artery
  - In the mid aorta near the renal arteries
  - In the distal aorta near the bifurcation
  - In the bilateral common iliac arteries
- Normal aortic velocities are <100 cm/s

28.6
Research Techniques in Vascular Imaging

- Carotid intima-media thickness
- Brachial reactivity
- Augmentation index

28.6.1
Carotid Intima-Media Thickness

- Carotid Intima-Media Thickness (CIMT) measurement is a non-invasive ultrasound technique used most commonly in the assessment of subclinical atherosclerosis.
- Increased CIMT correlates well with cardiovascular risk.
- Sensitive and reproducible; protocols vary.

28.6.2
CIMT (Fig. 28.10)

- Once the CIMT measurement is obtained, it must be compared to an appropriate reference population depending on the protocol.
- Specialized "edge-detection" software and three-lead EKG monitoring for gated images are recommended.
- For further reference on CIMT, see the Consensus Statement of the American Society of Echocardiography (Stein et al., *J Am Soc Echocardiogr*. 2008).

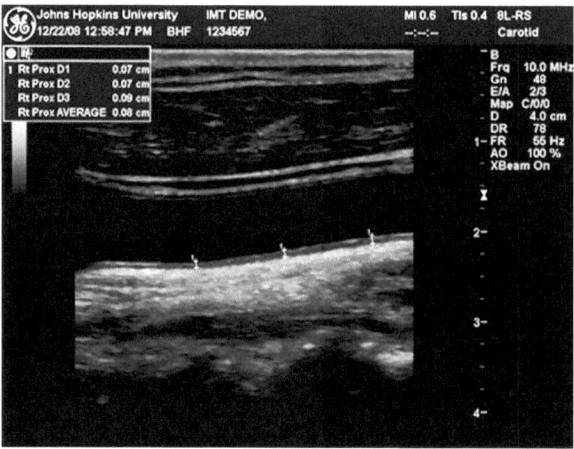

Fig. 28.10 The best method is to obtain R-wave gated images of the far wall of the distal common carotid artery. An example of CIMT measurement is shown here

28.6.3
Brachial Reactivity

- Brachial reactivity testing is used to measure endothelial function, a response referred to as "flow-mediated dilatation" (FMD).
- A blood pressure cuff is inflated to approximately 250 mmHg for 5 min and then rapidly released to induce reactive hyperemia; dilatation of the brachial artery occurs in response to shear stress.
- High-frequency ultrasound images of the brachial artery are gated to the R wave of the QRS complex.
- Reduced flow-mediated dilatation (FMD) is thought to be a sign of endothelial dysfunction and correlates with cardiovascular risk.

28.6.4
Augmentation Index

- Augmentation Index (AI) is a surrogate measure of systemic arterial stiffness.
- AI tends to be negative in young people, zero at approximately 35 years of age, and positive thereafter.
- Applanation tonometry may be employed at the radial artery to derive an ascending aortic pressure waveform.
- The AI is calculated as the difference between the first and second systolic peaks of the ascending aortic pressure waveform.
- The central pulse pressure is the systolic pressure minus the diastolic pressure.
- The AI is expressed as a percentage of the central pulse pressure.

Index

T.P. Abraham (ed.), *Case Based Echocardiography*,
DOI: 10.1007/978-1-84996-151-6, © Springer-Verlag London Limited 2011